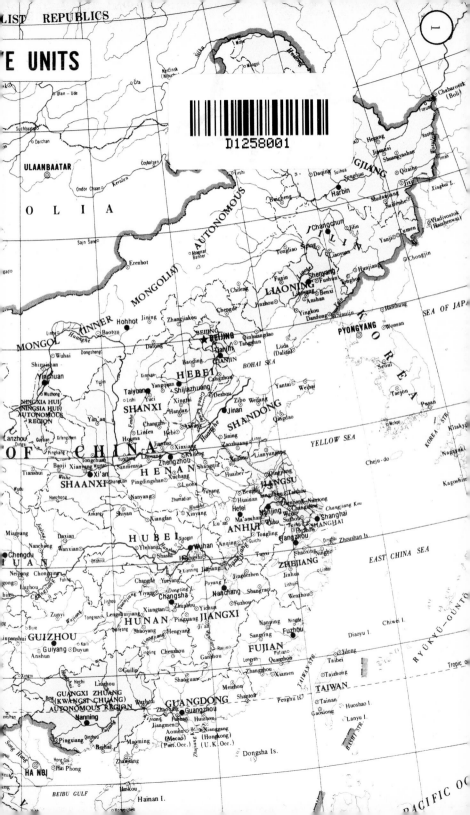

Health care and traditional medicine in China, 1800-1982

# HEALTH CARE AND TRADITIONAL MEDICINE IN CHINA, 1800–1982

S.M. HILLIER
and
J.A. JEWELL

Routledge & Kegan Paul
London, Boston, Melbourne and Henley

First published in 1983
by Routledge & Kegan Paul plc
39 Store Street, London WC1E 7DD,
9 Park Street, Boston, Mass. 02108, USA,
6th Floor, 464 St Kilda Road,
Melbourne, 3004, Australia and
Broadway House, Newtown Road,
Henley-on-Thames, Oxon RG9 1EN
Printed in Great Britain by
St Edmundsbury Press Ltd
Bury St Edmunds, Suffolk

Library of Congress Cataloging in Publication Data

Hillier, S.M. (Sheila M.), 1944-
Health care and traditional medicine in China,
1800-1982.
Includes index.
1. Medicine - China - History. 2. Medicine, Chinese -
History. 3. Medical care - China - History. I. Jewell,
J.A., 1950- . II. Title. [DNLM: 1. History of
Medicine, 19th century - China. 2. History of Medicine,
20th century - China. 3. Medicine, Chinese - History -
China. WZ 70 JC H4th]
R601.H5    1983    362.1'0951    83-3188

ISBN 0-7100-9425-6

# CONTENTS

# PLATES

# FIGURES

# TABLES

# INTRODUCTION AND
# ACKNOWLEDGMENTS

Our interest in China was derived from our experience of working in health care and health related disciplines in the United
Kingdom and promoted by an original visit to China in 1978.
Britain possesses the earliest system of large-scale socialised
health care, whose origins and development stem from a critical
fusion of socialist commitment, and pragmatic assessment of the
most efficient and economic means of bringing health care services to the British population.

To compare structures of health care in a relatively rich
Western country like Britain with those of poor populous China
may at first sight seem inappropriate. Yet we felt at the outset that both countries shared the necessity to distribute scarce
health care resources in an egalitarian fashion, and that China,
which had experienced a successful socialist revolution whereas
Britain had not, had tackled the problem with energy and commitment which was lacking in our own system, characterised,
despite its stated objectives, by inequalities of resource distribution between regions, medical specialities and sectors of
care with inequalities in sickness and life expectancy between
different social classes. We were not Sinologists but, along with
many other people, we found the Chinese model of health care
an exciting one, about which little detailed information (despite
many travellers' tales) was available. We decided to write this
book to explore parallels and contrasts between our own national
system of health care delivery and that of the Chinese, while
recognising that China's development may have some lessons
for other Third World countries both in its achievements and
mistakes. We would not be so presumptuous as to suggest what
the form of health care development in Third World countries
should generally be; many have begun to develop their own
initiatives, suited to their political, economic and social conditions; but the Chinese model, supported by strong political
commitment, still provides a useful experiment in confronting
for instance parasitic and infectious disease under conditions
of relative poverty and organising a thorough coverage of the
needs of a large population.

We have learnt much; we hope we can convey some of what we
learnt to our readers. Specifically, in tracing the origins of
China's health care system we saw important similarities between
the form of its development and that of our own: the need to
pacify professional interest groups, to control costs, to ensure
accessibility. We also noted differences particularly in relation

to China's turbulent history over the last century and the
marked cultural differences between our societies both of which
have an important influence on health care. In more recent
times the degree of direct political control of health services is
far greater in China than was ever true of the British system,
although political centralised control over health services is
now increasing here, paradoxically under the policies of a conservative administration.

We had many surprises too. On our first and subsequent visits
to China we began to recognise traditional medicine less as an
interesting curiosity, and more as a fundamental part of
Chinese culture. It is for this reason that we have attempted a
very full description and assessment of traditional medicine for
specialist and non-specialist readers.

The Chinese commitment to preventive medicine, which is as
ancient as Chinese medicine, was also seen by us to be fundamental to every aspect of medical care. This fact, which has
had to be rediscovered in the West, explains the prominence
which we, reflecting Chinese concerns, have given to the subject. But in our assessments of the objectives of the Chinese
health care system we have tried never to forget what econo-
mists call 'the real world', a confrontation with which is what
unites us with the Chinese as we too attempt to promote those
systems of health care which are efficient, effective, accessible,
appropriate, acceptable and advantageous.

A very real concern among Chinese health planners is the rate
of population growth, and our contributor Penny Kane, of the
International Planned Parenthood Federation, has attempted to
describe the political and economic pressures which have compelled the formulation of certain policies, and which may also
contribute to their failure.

The phrase 'health care' not only covers aspects of curative
and preventive medicine, but also those areas of life which promote good health. The nutritional status of the Chinese population is given appropriate attention in Dr Nancy Worcester's
chapter on nutrition in China, where she details dietary policies,
and contrasts Western and Chinese diets.

The care given to the mentally ill in any society is an indication of priority given to the recognition of non-physical states
which produce painful behavioural disorders. In China, inappropriate social behaviour has long been the subject of strong
normative controls, but there is also attention given to medical
treatment of the mentally ill, and recent approaches have utilised the latest psychiatric research, as well as more well
known methods of therapy. The emphasis given to community
care is indicative of the importance attached both to the re-
integration of individuals into society, and to the individual's
contribution to the prosperity of the whole society.

This book has therefore attempted a comprehensive survey of
major aspects of health care in China, and has also considered
the historical importance of non-Chinese influences in the

growth of the health care system. The introduction of Western medicine into China produced both benefits and drawbacks. The major disadvantage was that the style of Western medicine re-inforced an urban bias in health care which has subsequently been the focus of much political conflict.

Below we list our acknowledgments. Many people gave advice, encouragement and help. For the results, however, we bear sole responsibility.

## ACKNOWLEDGMENTS

Many library staff gave us their time and assistance. We should like particularly to thank the staffs of the Society for Anglo-Chinese Understanding (SACU) and the associated Anglo-Chinese Educational Institute, especially Alan Patterson. The unfailingly helpful librarians of the British Medical Association Library, the Wellcome Institute for the History of Medicine and the School of Oriental and African Studies, University of London, provided valuable material.

The London Hospital Medical College and the Medical College of St Bartholomew's Hospital were generous in their financial support for study visits to China for one of us (SMH), while the Department of Health and Social Security granted prolonged study leave to the other (JAJ) to go to Beijing for the International Acupuncture Training Course.

Many individuals, both in the fields of Chinese studies and in medicine and health care, helped us. Among them were members of the Socialist Health Association with whom we visited China in 1978; and Dr Robin Stott, consultant physician at Lewisham Hospital. Dr Joseph Needham and Dr Lu Gwei-djen gave us their valuable time for discussion on traditional medicine; Dr Howard Schubiner and Giovanni Maciocia for reading the traditional medicine section. Jessica Darling, Delia Davin, Stefan Feuchtwang, Giovanni Maciocia, Jonathan Mirsky, and Frances Wood were sources of intellectual stimulation, encouragement and practical help. We would also like to thank Professor Wu Chen-yi of the department of Medical Psychology, Beijing University, Dr Jiang Zuo-ning of the Anding Hospital, Beijing, and Dr Liu Xiehe of the Department of Psychiatry, Sichuan Medical College, for advice and information on Chinese Psychiatry. Others who gave us important help were Dr Chen of the Anti-tuberculosis Clinic, Luwan, Shanghai, Dr Liao Mei-ling of the Shanghai Chest Hospital, Dr Gao Li-sheng, Guananmen Hospital, Beijing, Dr Hsu, Xian Medical College, Dr Lin Yang, Nanjing College of Traditional Chinese Medicine, Dr Yuwen Yu, Institute of Materia Medica, Beijing, Dr Zhang Yuhuei, Cancer Institute, Beijing, Dr Ma Kan Wan, Academy of Traditional Chinese Medicine, Beijing, Dr Ma Haide, Ministry of Public Health, Beijing, and staff at the Institute of Acupuncture and Moxibustion, Beijing.

Several books have been quoted from extensively in the text, and require separate acknowledgment. The 'History of Chinese Medicine' (1932) by Wang Ji Min (Chimin Wong) and Wu Lian De (Wu Lien-teh) was a major source, as was the Science and Civilisation in China series of Joseph Needham, especially the more recent part of volume 6 with Lu Gwei-djen published separately under the title 'Celestial Lancets' (1980). Ralph Croizier's 'Traditional Medicine in Modern China' (1968) was an important work of reference which opened up the fascinating subject of the integration of Western and Chinese medicine. This was supplemented by the 'Chinese Medicine' of Pierre Huard and Ming Wong (1968). The well known 'Away with all Pests' (1971) of Dr Joshua Horn crystallised the optimism of the Cultural Revolution, and 'Serve the People' (1974) by Victor and Ruth Sidel was another book on health care in China which captured the imagination of Western readers. The more detailed publications of the John E. Fogarty International Center in Washington 'Medicine and Public Health in the People's Republic of China' (1972), 'China Medicine as we saw it' (1974), and the Josiah Macy Jr Foundation in New York, 'Public Health in the People's Republic of China' (1973), opened up the subject of health care in a thorough fashion. Finally, David Lampton's 'The Politics of Medicine in China' (1977) alerted us to the workings of the political process in China's health bureaucracy and is a scholarly, stimulating and altogether invaluable work on that subject.

We are grateful to the following for permission to reproduce paintings, drawings and photographs in their possession as indicated: the Wellcome Institute Library, London (Figure 1, Plates 1a, 1b, 3a, 3b, 4a, 4b, 4c, 6a, 6b); the British Library (Plates 2a, 2b, 5a, 5b); the President and Council of the Royal College of Surgeons of England (Plate 7a); Professor Preston Maxwell's collection (Plate 7b); Gordon Museum, Guy's Hospital Medical School, London (Plates 8a, 8b, 8c, 8d); Xinhua News Agency (Plates 9a, 9b, 10a, 10b, 13a, 13b, 14b, 15a, 15b, 16a, 16b); China Picture Service (Plates 11a, 11b, 12a, 12b, 14a).

The diagrams of the Chinese plants were taken from 'Chinese Herbs: Their Botany, Chemistry and Pharmacodynamics', John Keys, Tuttle, Tokyo, 1977 and 'Commonly used Chinese Medicinal Herbs: Illustrations and Text', Institute of Materia Medica, People's Health Publishing House, Beijing, 1970.

Our spouses, relatives and friends helped in several ways, by shouldering more than their fair share of domestic responsibilities, providing child care, or quiet places in which to work. We would like to thank Bill Hillier, Jane Rickell, Mary Thomas, Susan Dukes, Jean Daniel and John and Bridget Kelleher.

Finally, we wish to thank Dinah Mullineux. She typed the unwieldy manuscript several times and was unfailingly patient, methodical, sharp-eyed, skilful and good humoured. We could not have managed without her.

Sheila Hillier
Tony Jewell

# A NOTE ON ROMANISATION

Throughout the text we have used the pinyin System of Romanisation except in quotation and reference citations, where in the original the Wade-Giles System was used. In some instances, the sources quoted have used unorthodox romanisation. This is particularly true of nineteenth and early twentieth century historical material, and without access to the Chinese characters, accurate conversion to pinyin is impossible. Where this occurs, the original romanisations have been kept and sources cited.

Readers familiar with the Wade-Giles and other systems may find the thoroughgoing use of pinyin somewhat confusing, for example Guangzhou for the familiar Canton, Xianggang for Hongkong, Beijing for Peking, Mao Zedong for Mao Tse-tung, Taijiquan for Tai-chi Chuan. Although the pinyin for major political figures and place names is now becoming familiar some of the less well-known pinyin versions and their Wade-Giles equivalents are given below.

| W-G | Pinyin |
|---|---|
| Ch'ien Hsin-chung | Qian Xinzhong |
| Ho Ch'eng | He Cheng |
| Li Hsien-nien | Li Xiannian |
| Szechuan or Szechwan | Sichuan |
| Shensi | Shaanxi |
| Shansi | Shanxi |
| Hopei | Hebei |
| Honan | Henan |
| Hupeh | Hubeh |

We also decided to adopt the convention of using + and - instead of AD and BC as used by Joseph Needham in his major work 'Science and Civilisation in China'.

# A NOTE ON ROMANISATION

# MEDICAL FACILITIES IN THE
# PEOPLE'S REPUBLIC OF CHINA
# STUDIED BY THE AUTHORS

1978   Battery Factory Clinic, Anyang, Henan province
Linxian County Hospital, Henan
Yao Village Commune Hospital, Linxian county, Henan
Chiliying Commune Hospital, Henan province
Renho People's Commune Hospital, Guangzhou province
Henan Provincial People's Hospital, Zhengzhou, Henan
Zhongshan Hospital, Shanghai
Nanjing Road Neighbourhood Committee, Shanghai
Fengsheng Neighbourhood Committee and Resident's
   Committee Clinic, Beijing
Friendship Hospital, Beijing

1981   Institute of Acupuncture and Moxibustion, Beijing
   Cancer Institute, Beijing
Institute of Materia Medica, Beijing
Xian Medical College, Shaanxi province
Guananmen Hospital, Beijing
Bone and Joint Hospital, Dongzhimannei, Beijing
Chai Yuan Neighbourhood Committee Clinic, Beijing
Evergreen People's Commune Hospital and Production
   Brigade Clinics, Beijing
Jiangxi River Road School Health Service, Nanjing
Department of Neurology, Nanjing Medical College
International Peace Maternity Hospital, Shanghai
Anti-Tuberculosis Hospital, Luwan, Shanghai
Stonewell People's Commune Hospital and Production
   Brigade Clinics, Guangzhou province

# Part One

# HISTORICAL DEVELOPMENT OF HEALTH CARE

Part One

# HISTORICAL DEVELOPMENT OF HEALTH CARE

# 1 CHINESE AND WESTERN MEDICINE IN CHINA, 1800–1911

J.A. Jewell

For China, the ancient Celestial Empire and Middle Kingdom, the nineteenth century represents a period when she failed to adapt to the new aggressive forces represented by the rapidly industrialising Western countries. The political story of an Imperial state challenged by a new imperialism is reflected in developments in health care and changes were apparent by the turn of the century.

In 1805 Jennerian smallpox vaccination was introduced to China by the senior surgeon of the East India Company and others while the first Protestant missionary, Morrison, arrived in 1807. Peter Parker, the first medical missionary, started work in Guangzhou (Canton) in 1834. Following the Opium War of 1842 the Western nations gained Treaty Port concessions and after the Treaty of Tianjin (Tientsin) in 1858 these were extended. Thus 1860 is a turning-point and finds the Chinese Imperial State prostrated and open to widespread Western business, military and missionary penetration. By 1911 the old feudal bureaucratic order had collapsed and the Republic was formed.

As early as 1793 Lord Macartney, acting as ambassador for King George III, was politely received by Emperor Qian Long (1736-95) in Peking and his 'tributes' graciously accepted. However, the aim of the mission had been to seek more trade facilities than the East India Company had available in Guangzhou and Macao. It was explained to the delegation that the Middle Kingdom had no need to import goods from the barbarians and present arrangements should be sufficient for the foreigners' needs. The attitude of the Celestial Emperor infuriated and frustrated the industrialising Western nations keen to find sources of raw materials and markets for their products. The Manchu dynasty was unable and unwilling to change and during the nineteenth century the decline of the ancient feudal-bureaucratic state, both from internal rebellion and external imperialist invasions, was inevitable.

Despite frequent dynastic changes, the fundamental structure of the Chinese Imperial order had existed for two millennia. One of its major features was a well developed civil service. Access to the mandarinate, although largely from the gentry, was non-hereditary and achieved by passing the civil examinations.

The traditional Chinese medical system was in relative decline by the late Qing period, having blossomed in much earlier times.

An Imperial College which taught four main subjects - diet,
internal medicine, acupuncture and moxibustion, and exorcism
still existed in the Qing period although it had degenerated to
reciting the classics stored in the Imperial Library and only
supplied physicians for the Imperial household. The Court
Medical College consisted of thirty doctors, almost all of whom
had a degree in the mandarinate going generally from the copper
button (ninth and lowest grade) to the crystal button (fifth
grade).(1)

Medical care of the period consisted of a rather chaotic system
with numerous different practitioners involved and superstitious practices abounding. In the general population, however, medicine was the purview of the mainly urban-based
traditional practitioners. Hobson, an early medical missionary,
befriended such a doctor in Guangzhou and accompanied him
on his rounds. Apparently 'Ta wang seen-sang', or 'Dr Rhubarb' as he was nicknamed, because of his faith in the curative
properties of that plant drug, used first to consult at home
in the mornings before beginning his rounds in a sedan chair
carried by three or four men. Hobson describes a visit:

The doctor being ushered into the Hall or principal room is
met with bows and salutations by the father or the elder
brother of the family. Tea and pipes are offered in due form
and he is requested to feel his patient's pulse; if a male he
sits opposite to him, if a female a screen of bamboo inter-
venes, which is only removed in case it is requisite to see
the tongue ... [after pulse taking] ... perhaps a few questions are now asked of the father or mother concerning the
sick person but these are usually few as it is presumed the
pulse reveals everything needful to know. Ink and paper are
produced, and a prescription is written out, which consists
of numerous ingredients ... the prescription is taken to a
druggist to be dispensed; the prescriber seldom makes up
the medicine himself, and as large doses are popular so the
decoction made for the whole, amounts to pints or even
quarts which are swallowed in large portions with the greatest ease; powders, boluses, pills and electuaries are also
used. If the patient is an officer of the government or a
wealthy person, the nature of the disease, prognosis and
treatment are written out for the inspection of the family; for
this the Doctor's fee is a dollar (5s) but generally speaking
both the Doctor and the patient's friend are quite satisfied
with a verbal communication .... The fee is wrapped up in
red paper and called 'golden thanks' and varies from 6d to
2s 6d or more according to the means of the patient, the
chair bearers being paid extra. The Doctor returns to make
another visit if invited, but not otherwise. It is more common
if the patient is not at once benefited by the prescription
to call in another, then a third, then a fourth and even
more until tired of physicians, they have as a last resource

application made to one of the genii, or a god possessing wonderful healing powers.(2)

The mention of the prescription and the use of the druggist is a reminder of the important role the traditional pharmacy had in Chinese society. Many people used the pharmacy directly for advice and medicine and often doctors would be available in the larger stores for consultation. The remedies in the main were plant drugs, the herbs being stored in large jars and weighed out as per prescription. Pills, boluses and medical plasters were also sold and each shop had its own altar to one of the gods of medicine (see Figure 1).

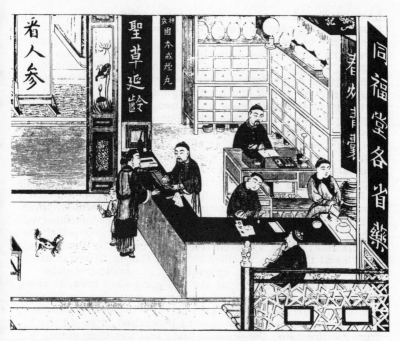

Figure 1   A print of a typical nineteenth-century Chinese pharmacy
Source:   Foundation Singer-Polignac, Paris, 1959.

The other category of 'wandering medical pedlars and pavement doctors' would offer a dazzling array of different types:

The practice of private medicine began at the street corner with soothsayers, geomancers, fortune tellers and other purveyors of para-medical advice. It continued with ocularists, aurists, dentists, herbalists, cuppers and the barber-masseurs. On a higher level there appeared the quack doctor who could be in one of several grades from the most humble setting out his remedies on the pavement, to the smartest who would have an expensively and carefully arranged stall either on a pavement pitch or as a moveable cart. In the suburbs, bonces and tao-shih practised in the shadow of the monasteries and distributed medical advice and amulets.(3)

Another author's list included in addition: 'bone setters, bruise curers, gland doctors, bullet and sword cut doctors, snakebite curers, corn-curers and the brass mule of Peking'. (4)
A colourful description of one such practitioner is given by Morse:

I was attracted by a large crowd in the market place surrounding a Chinese surgeon (?) who was executing the art
of surgery by means of needles in the operation of acupuncture. The dense crowd pressed in closely to watch and listen
to him. That man was no mean orator of the patent medicine
class and he had a forceful personality.... He was dressed
in a long gown which had been originally blue.... On his
feet were cloth-soled shoes which had incorporated in their
texture material of the general colour and consistency of
mud.... His shoes were an entomologist's paradise of un-
countable species. His finger nails were very long, thick and
stained with opium. On the ground before him were spread
four large charts. These charts explained something of his
supposed theory and were attractive because of their vintage
of four thousand years.... Suggestively placed on the charts
were coins, moxa and an assortment of twelve needles, three
to twenty-four centimetres in length. I saw needles inserted
deeply into the suprasternal notch and in the grooves above
the clavicle, which vibrated from their proximity to the great
arteries of the neck. Needles inserted five to fifteen centimetres into the liver and epigastrium.... Another needle
passed through the lacrimal sac and proceeded inwards along
the inner wall of the orbit apparently deeply enough to enter
the brain. One insertion was rather striking and gruesome.
The needle entered the nose until it reached, I would think
from its direction, the ethmoid plate and was then struck a
considerable blow, I presume piercing the ethmoid plate into
the brain!... He 'cleaned' the needle with his thumb nail
rubbed it through his hair and rubbed it off on his gown or
the sole of his shoe, he lubricated the needle with spittle
and drove it home. After a suitable time he removed the
needle, applied moxa, set it on fire and crushed the ashes
into the formed blister with his fingernail.(5)

Widespread magico-religious superstitious practices were found throughout the community. The feeling that diseases were caused by evil spirits was common and there were numerous deities worshipped and pleaded with in time of illness. There

were ten well-known physicians worshipped in the temples of
medicine and this deification of celebrated physicians is a tradition peculiar to China. It was said that if a patient was cured
by a doctor he usually said by way of praise that his doctor
is the eleventh celebrated physician.(6)

The twenty-eighth day of the fourth month in the lunar calen-
dar was observed as the birthday of the King of Medicine. On
this occasion the drug stores traditionally sold their medicines
at half price or set aside several drugs to be given away to
patients. Thousands of pilgrims went to the temples to burn
incense and to offer sacrifice of food to the Kings of Medicine.(7)
In Chengdu (Chengtu) there was the 'brass goat temple' (Jin
Yang Gong) and the people used to rub that part of the goat
that corresponded to the diseased portion of their body. In a
form of sympathetic magic, the eyes were frequently rubbed to
cure trachoma.(8) Prescriptions in temples were sometimes
selected by tossing numbered bamboo sticks while praying to
the God of Medicine. As one author put it, 'this holy medicine
was natural in composition but supernatural in prescription'.(9)

Whole communities could be involved in these practices and
there are examples of symbolically using an animal:

In the Lifan district the sins of a certain community are, by
the aid of a magical formula, transferred to a yak which is
then driven to the solitary wastes... masses of cliffs and
sombre forests behind the Monastery of White Negation.(10)

At a more mundane level it is reported that when the plague
struck his town in 1896 the Taotai of Mengzi assembled the
soldiers of his guard each evening in front of his Yamen and
made them fire salvoes in all directions to frighten the demon
of the plague.(11)

More commonly, messages were written to the gods on inflam-
mable material and burned - the smoke going to the heavens
carried the message. If a child was in coma, the mother and
relatives would light candles and paper money and pass the
child's jacket over the fire pleading for the return of his soul.
A missionary doctor records another example:

I was called to a woman suffering from post partum fever and
I found two women at the bedside one flourishing a sword
over the patient, the other beating a large brass pan; the
idea was to cause the devils of the disease to depart. The
bad spirits fear noise and swords.(12)

Over the centuries there had been many contacts with other
cultures and medical systems. The Arabic, Persian and Indian
traditions had all influenced Chinese medicine as well as the
particular Tibetan and Mongolian traditions. The post-Renais-
sance European influence may have begun when the Portuguese
established themselves at Aomen from +1557 but this achieved

only local influence. The Jesuits, and in particular Matteo Ricci
(+1552-1610), had developed an important influence in the
Imperial Court. Ricci brought watches, clocks and scientific
instruments over from Europe and established himself in the
Imperial bureau of astrology. Parrenin (+1669-1741) translated
an anatomical treatise and another Jesuit, Bernard Rhodes,
opened a dispensary in 1699. Brother Jean Joseph da Costa
followed this in +1715 and practised some minor surgery.(13)
Western anatomical knowledge interested Emperor Kang Xi
who characteristically restricted its distribution to the Court
for fear of its impact in the country, as it appeared to contra-
dict traditional anatomy. The Jesuit influence, although important, was limited to the insular Imperial household. When
Western doctors came to China during the nineteenth century
they confronted an ancient indigenous essentially rational
medical system with a strong superstitious medical subculture
that was in stark contrast to their own by then rapidly advanc-
ing, modern scientific medicine.

SMALLPOX INOCULATION

The East India Company had been trading at Aomen (Macao) and
Guangzhou since the early eighteenth century and their company
doctors had serviced employees, and occasionally outsiders.
In 1803 the Governor General of the East India Company was so
impressed by the new Jennerian smallpox vaccine that he dispatched some to China. This batch was unsuccessful but it was
was Dr Pearson, then senior surgeon to the Company, who
helped to introduce vaccination in 1805. There is some conten-
tion as to who first introduced the vaccine but Pearson in 1816
wrote:

> In the Spring of 1805 the vaccine was brought by Mr Hewit,
> a Portugese subject and a merchant of Macao, in his vessel
> upon live subjects from Manila - His Catholic Majesty having
> had it conveyed by suitable means and under the care of
> professional men across the South American continent to his
> settlement in the Philipine Islands. I observe that one of
> them (Don Francesco Xavier de Balmis) states himself to
> have introduced the practice in this country; but before his
> arrival in China it had been quite extensively conducted by
> the Portugese practitioners at Macao as well as by myself
> among the inhabitants there and the Chinese. The accompany-
> ing tract drawn up by me had been translated by Sir George
> Staunton into Chinese and published several months previous
> to his arrival.(14)

Smallpox 'variolation' as opposed to the new cowpox derived
'vaccination' had been practised in China since at least the
eleventh century. It was this practice which was transmitted to

Turkey and noticed by the British Ambassador's wife Lady Mary
Wortley Montagu who allowed the technique to be used on her
own family in +1718.(15) The work of Jenner on cowpox did not
take place until 1796 and in 1801 he prophesised the eradication
of smallpox which the World Health Organisation was able to
announce in 1979.(16) The traditional Chinese perspective on
smallpox was that it was transmitted 'in utero' and harboured
by everyone 'like fire concealed in the flint' until some external
influence precipitated its development. This is why the disease
occurred just once and why inoculation, referred to as 'cul-
tivating the heavenly flowers', was performed at an auspicious
time and was acceptable. Various methods were used such as
taking scabs of variolous lymph from pustules, drying and
powdering the material, and then introducing it into the nostrils
by blowing or on a damp cloth. Scarification techniques were
also used as were more crude forms like using the clothes of
smallpox victims. Inoculation was performed on healthy subjects,
particularly in spring when the weather was 'warm enough to
take off your coat but too cold to work in the fields'. Strict
rules were applied after inoculation and instructions given concerning diet, warmth and the avoidance of alarm and fright.
If the inoculation failed to cultivate a mild attack it was repeated
after fourteen days.(17)

Several Chinese were instructed by Dr Pearson in the art of
vaccination in 1806. One such was 'A Hequa' or You Hechuan
(Yan-Ho-Chün) who built up a reputation for it and at one time
was sent to Peking to introduce the technique there. He is
stated to have vaccinated upwards of a million people over thirty
years.(18) The practice spread through China from Guangzhou
and had important official recognition when Yuanyuan, the
Governor General of the two Guang Provinces (1817-26) and
later to become second minister of State in the Imperial cabinet, said:

> I grieve on account of the injury wrought by poisonous
> opium in China. I have done my utmost to put a stop to its
> use, but have not succeeded. As the practice of vaccination
> spreads throughout all the provinces, the lives of many
> children will be saved and thus the injury caused by opium
> will be in some measure compensated.(19)

The advantage of the Jennerian vaccination based on 'cowpox'
lymph was that it was a safer and more effective technique.
It was quickly taken up by the Chinese, and its Western origin
became blurred when the technique was absorbed into the
mainstream tradition. There was occasional resistance to the
'foreign flower' by priests with a vested interest in the
disease.(20) There were some other problems such as the difficulty in getting adolescent girls to expose their arms in public.
Unpockmarked girls of marriageable age were sometimes thought
still susceptible by the male's family, which damaged their
prospects. Also there was the problem of keeping the lymph

going on 'donor sites' until the following Spring season, but
with the large pool of poor and destitute people, many could be
found prepared to keep an active site on their arms for a small
fee.

## DISPENSARIES IN CHINA

Following Pearson other surgeons of the East India Company
made valuable pioneering contributions. In 1820 Dr Livingstone
opened a dispensary in Guangzhou for Chinese. He was interested in the Chinese Pharmacopoeia, for 'it might supply something in addition to the means now possessed of leavening human
suffering in the West'.(21) Dr Colledge opened a dispensary in
1827 and it was he who first suggested the sending of medical
missionaries to China. In a later pamphlet he said:

> Those societies that now send missionaries should also send
> physicians to this benighted race, who on their arrival in
> this land should make themselves acquainted with the lang-
> uage, and in place of attempting any regular system of teach-
> ing or preaching, let them heal the sick and administer to
> their wants, mingling with their medical practice such
> instructions either in religion, philosophy, medicine, chemi-
> stry etc. as the minds of the individual have been gradually
> prepared to receive.(22)

## MEDICAL MISSIONARIES ARRIVE

In 1834 Dr Peter Parker, recently qualified from Yale Medical
School, arrived in Guangzhou. By the next year he had opened
the Canton Missionary Hospital and thus started a long
line of predominantly Protestant medical missionaries. Four
years later he helped start the Guangzhou based Medical Missionary Society. His clinical burden consisted mainly of ophthalmic cases which indicates the prevalence of eye disease in
China at the time. His work had wonderful propaganda appeal -
that of restoring sight to the blind. He also records many
surgical cases with which, although performed in pre-anaesthetic and pre-antiseptic days, he had remarkable success.(23) In
1836 an initially reluctant patient agreed to undergo a successful limb amputation having been given fifty dollars by Dr Jardine, of the mercantile family, who was assistant.(24)
Surgery was relatively underdeveloped in China because of
reluctance among Confucianists to disfigure the body. So strong
was this feeling that relatives of condemned criminals would
plead for strangulation rather than decapitation of the prisoner.
The surgical tradition consisted mainly of tooth extraction,
puncturing of abscesses, closed reduction of fractures and
castration of the Imperial eunuchs. Parker records many cases

of large benign tumours with relatively narrow pedicles that he was able to excise in seconds. Some of the tumours showed scars where moxa cautery had been used as well as attempts to tourniquet. Clearly if a patient could walk in with a thirty-five kilogram tumour and be able to come out alive and with only a small scar to show, word would soon spread of the miraculous skill of the foreigner! He soon recognised the need to train an assistant and was successful with one of his apprentices Guan Yadu (Kwan Ato) who showed great aptitude and became the first Chinese to acquire a knowledge of Western medicine and surgery. In political terms Parker's success was seen to have been more productive than earlier efforts to 'open China' and he was said to have 'opened the gates of China with a lancet when Western canon could not heave a single bar'.(25)

Other medical missionaries were quick to follow Parker's example and when Xianggang (Hong Kong) was ceded to Britain after the 1842 Opium Wars it joined Aomen and Guangzhou as one of the early bases. By 1887 it was estimated that one hundred and fifty medical missionaries had come to China, the majority from America.(26) Their work took on three aspects: evangelism for the Christian faith; medical work for the sick; and medical education.

## WESTERN MEDICINE

It should be remembered, however, that the state of medical knowledge was still rudimentary at that time and the strength of Western medicine lay in its anatomical knowledge and related surgical skill. Although physiological knowledge was more scientifically advanced than traditional Chinese medicine, therapeutics was probably at about a similar level.

One early problem the medical missionaries encountered was that of language and terminology. This was crucial in medical education and one of the early pioneers, Hobson, made a major contribution. He wrote the following titles:

1851 Quan Ti Xin Lun   - Outline of Anatomy and Physiology.
1851 Tian Wen Lue Lun  - An outline of Natural Philosophy
                         and History.
1857 Xi Yi Lue Lun     - An outline of Western Medicine.
1858 Fu Ying Xin Shuo  - Modern Views of the Diseases of
                         Women and Children.
1858 Nei Xin Shuo      - Modern Views of Internal Medicine.
1858 Medical Vocabulary in English and Chinese.

His work was followed by Dr J.G. Kerr's 'Tract on Vaccination' and 'Tract on Hernia and Intermittent Fever' in 1859. Osgood and Whitney made a translation of 'Gray's Anatomy' in 1880.(27)

The content of these books helps us to gauge the state of

knowledge at that time. Hobson's first volume had a foreword by
his Excellency Yeh, Viceroy of Guangzhou, despite 'the indifference of the official class'.(28) The books were well illustrated
and attractively presented with detailed anatomical diagrams.
Writing prior to the development of the germ theory of disease,
Hobson considered gonorrhoea to be a symptom of bladder stone
and recommended venesection for the treatment of meningitis.
In his 'Modern Views of Internal Medicine' he enumerated the
causes of disease among which were:

> general weakness due to poor food, irregular eating habits,
> overwork, sexual excess and poor hygiene, exposure to cold,
> the eastern wind, cold wind, moisture, escape of bodily
> electricity in response to heat traumatic injuries and poison-
> ing.(29)

Henderson, writing in 1864, also demonstrates that 'modern'
Western medicine was still highly descriptive and, in China,
given to racial generalisation. The temperament classification,
notions of inflammation and plethora are all reminiscent of
Chinese traditional concepts:

> The type of disease among the Chinese is very different from
> what is seen in England or in Europe generally.
>    Among the Chinese there is no nervous or sanguine or
> nervo-sanguine temperament, indeed with the exception of
> perhaps one in ten thousand all Chinamen have the phleg-
> matic or lymphatic temperament. The bilious is met with
> among the upper and literary classes but is comparatively
> rare. The lymphatic temperament renders inflammatory
> diseases of an acute kind almost unknown.... The lympha-
> tic temperament of the people would partly account for this
> but the chief cause is their mode of living, the absence of
> all stimulating food and drink. Hence diseases produced by
> deficiency of blood are frequent while plethora is scarcely
> ever met with.(30)

THE OPIUM TRADE

Between 1842 and 1860 political developments took place that
were to affect the medical missionary movement and the whole
question of Western penetration into China: the growth of the
opium trade. Since the early days of trading by the East India
Company with China it had been apparent that a trade gap
existed. Quite simply, the West was interested in raw materials
such as soya beans, silk, tea, peanut oil, spices, bristles,
hides, tin and porcelain but the Middle Kingdom wanted little
in return, preferring payment in silver. The opportunity that
opium offered was irresistible. This could be grown, harvested
and processed in the Indian colony and exported to China,

being highly profitable in the process. Until 1733 the opium
traffic had been mainly in the hands of the Portuguese. In 1781
the East India Company took over and the trade expanded
rapidly, as the figures below show:(31)

| 1821 | 4,628 chests |
| 1825 | 9,621 |
| 1830 | 18,760 |
| 1832 | 23,670 |
| 1854 | 67,000 |

The trade was to continue long after the East India Company
lost its monopoly of trade in 1834 and in 1906 54,475 piculs were
imported, the equivalent to nearly 47,000 chests.(32) Between
1829 and 1839 China sent abroad as payment for opium some one
hundred million ounces of silver.(33) The profits to be made
were enormous, with margins of up to 2,000 per cent per chest
sold.(34) (Chest = 150lbs; picul = 125lbs.) The Chinese used to
refer to opium as 'Yangtu' meaning foreign dirt. This out-
rageous trade was opposed in a rather indecisive way by the
Chinese authorities but was enough to give Britain the chance
to exercise the 'gunboat diplomacy' for which it became famous
throughout the nineteenth century. The Jardine Matheson Company who had profited enormously from the opium trade had
been keen to find a base for their commercial activities outside
Chinese jurisdiction. A writer in Matheson's Guangzhou Register
noted in 1836: 'If the lion's paw is to be put down on any part
of the Southside of China let it be Hong Kong.'(35) After the
Opium War of 1842 the Treaty of Nanjing was signed and China
ceded Xianggang (Hong Kong) to Britain and opened five treaty
ports - Guangzhou, Xiamen, Fuzhou, Ningbo and Shanghai - for
trading. In the wake of the gunboats came commerce, consuls
and missionaries.
   Between 1853 and 1865 there was a major internal revolution
in China known as the Taiping Rebellion. The leader, Hong
Xinguan had received some instruction from the early missionary
Morrison and used Christian rhetoric in his propaganda against
idolatry and the Manchus. He called himself the 'Heavenly King'
(Tian Wang) and occupied the city of Nanjing for twelve years. The
rebellion was finally suppressed by Imperial troops, with the
assistance of the British General Gordon - later of Khartoum
fame. The death toll from this rebellion probably reached about
twenty million and was another factor in the weakening of the
Qing dynasty. Prior to the rebellion Britain and France had
been flexing their military might and in 1860 destroyed the
beautiful Summer Palace and 'sacked' Beijing (Peking). The
Treaty of Tianjin in 1858 helped to reduce China to a 'semi-
colonial' status and Beijing was opened to foreign residence,
opium importation was legalised and eleven new treaty ports
including Shantou (Swatow), Yantai (Chefoo), Ninzhuang
(Newchwang), Jiujiang (Kiukiang), Wuhan (Hankow), Tianjin,

Hangzhou and Tainan (on Taiwan) were 'opened up'. This paved the way for further missionary work and the opportunity for greater Western medical influence.


## PERIOD 1860-1911

*Social conditions*
Apart from the numerically small feudal elite and the developing 'compradore' class associated with foreign business the bulk of the Chinese people, most of whom were peasants, lived in squalid conditions that were overcrowded and unhygienic. As central government weakened and local corruption thrived the people's already difficult life became harder and throughout the nineteenth century the general standard of living deteriorated with the impact of frequent wars, local banditry, floods and famine.

Lockhart, who was one of the first missionaries to work in Shanghai, noted:

> The average of public health in the city of Shanghai has often been to foreigners, especially during the summer months, a matter of surprise.... The sewerage is moreover of the most imperfect kind. The drains are no better than a continuous cesspool, where filth of all varieties is allowed to accumulate and pollute the air. In truth were it not for the fact that the high market value of ordure of all kinds leads to the employment of a large number of men and boats in its deportation to the country for agricultural purposes the health of the city would be seriously deteriorated... the foreigner is almost prostrated by the offensive odours which assail him on every side in the Chinese city.(36)

As one astute observer put it, if bad smells were the cause of disease then the Shanghai population should be moribund! The same conditions pertained in the countryside:

> Even in the better houses one can find piles of rotted refuse, pools of stagnant water, uncovered buckets of nightsoil, geese covering the courts and walks with their excreta; other houses may shelter animals such as water buffalo used in ploughing or pigs.... Frequently the square floor of the court in the ancestral hall is full of filth - rotten straw and chaff, water and mud, ordure of poultry and animals.(37)

In addition to these impoverished social conditions natural disasters such as drought and floods occurred regularly.

The famine in Northern China of 1877-8 is relatively well documented thanks to the Customs Medical Service. Nine million people were recorded as destitute, there were reports of parents selling or destroying their children, others committing suicide and epidemics of dysentry and typhus followed:

> At first there was the hopeless sight of patchy drought and
> blighted crops; then the pinch of want and starvation, then
> the selling of clothes and furniture for a mere trifle; next
> the relinquishment of houses, lands and implements on the
> same terms; then parting with their wives and children, or
> leaving them utterly destitute.... Children were daily sold
> in the markets, the price paid for little girls of nine and
> eleven years old being nine hundred cash, equal to about
> 4s. 6d. sterling; in other instances young women were
> offered for nothing and even on such terms the difficulty
> was to get anybody willing to take them.... In several towns
> and villages the dead and dying lay unheeded in the streets,
> the dogs feeding upon corpses. Wolves rendered bold,
> prowled about in the immediate vicinity of human habitation,
> feeding upon the dead, carrying away famished children
> from the side of parents so weak as to be unable to defend
> against, far less pursue these animals.(38)

The human destruction was estimated between nine and a
half and thirteen million people. In Honan it was thought that
60 per cent of the population had died and 80 to 90 per cent
had disappeared. At Feu-shi-hsien out of the original population
of 120,000 inhabitants only 30,000 remained when the famine
had ceased. There were stories of people eating 'stone cakes'
made from soil and even of overt cannibalism.(39)

There are four other social indices which characterised society
at this time - self-mutilation, infanticide, foot-binding and
opium use.

*Self-mutilation*
Lockhart describes how he had a patient who had quite deliberately stuffed lime mortar into his eyes to blind himself for
the purpose of begging:

> His state was very lamentable; violent pain in his eyes, both
> cornea in a sloughy state, excessive suppuration flowing
> from the conjunctivae and the eyes totally destroyed. This
> plan is only one of several resorted to by the beggars to
> deaden the eyesight and make themselves objects of pity.
> They also blind their children in early life by means of lime
> and by puncturing their eyes with a coarse needle to destroy
> them.(40)

Lockhart tells of some beggars from Shandong who had their
lower limbs removed deliberately:

> The operation was performed by a beggar who made it his
> profession. He ties a piece of thin string as tightly as pos-
> sible around the middle of the calf... until mortification

ensues. When the soft parts are separated the bone is sawn through. The operation causes great suffering and many die in the process, but those who survive... are congratulated by their friends as having gained the loss of their limbs and an increase of fortune, from the contributions of the bene-volent.(41)

*Infanticide*
Infanticide is another phenomenon that reflects the nature of the society and was apparently a relatively common occurrence in some areas. Mainly baby girls were killed - an indication of the place of women in traditional Chinese society: 'In those districts where grinding poverty obliterates natural affection notices may occasionally be seen at the sides of pools to the effect that "Girls may not be drowned here". '(42) It is ironic that the 1980s should see a resurgence of this problem because of the desire for a son if only one child is permitted.

*Foot-binding*
Foot-binding of young girls was a common habit in Northern China, particularly among the richer class. The aim was to produce 'lotus flower' feet and the practice began between the ages of six and nine years. To produce the diminution of the foot the instep is bent on itself; the heel bone is thrown out of the horizontal position and what ought to be the posterior surface brought to the ground. Skilled binders existed but amateurs could cause even more damage. Parker in 1847 record-ed a case of a seven-year-old girl with bilateral gangrene of the feet following bandaging.(43) However, in the majority of cases it led only to a distortion of the normal anatomy and consequent difficulty in walking. The so-called 'tottering lilies' had an appearance not unlike the effect of stiletto heels and there was a well developed sexual culture and pornography surrounding tiny delicate white feet. In another sense of course

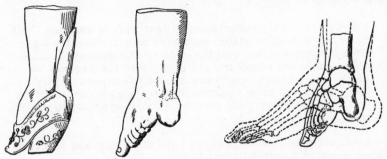

Figure 2    Illustration of decorative shoe, bound foot and outline of distorted anatomy
Source:    H.S. Levy, 'Chinese Footbinding - the history of a curious erotic custom', Walton Rawl, New York, 1966.

it demonstrated that the woman did not or could not work in the fields. Her mobility and hence her freedom were also restricted.

*Opium*
Opium use had a long history in China but there is no doubt that the extent of its use, especially by smoking, increased enormously with the importation of opium. The Dutch imported tobacco from Java in the seventeenth century and opium was mixed with it. As early as 1729 an Imperial edict forbade the sale of opium for smoking purposes.(44) The responsibility of the East India Company and the British State in fuelling the addiction throughout China and in distorting the economy by the massive levels of imports for silver exchange is clear. Although difficult to calculate the social effect of the opium habit, it ranged from the individual addict to the peasants obliged to grow the poppy by their landlords for cash crops and tax payments despite the near chronic state of famine. Even in the early twentieth century Dr Wu Lian De (Wu Lien Teh) tells of the 'mile upon mile of land covered with multi-coloured poppy plants in Manchuria, Shansi, Shensi, Jehol, Fukien, Yunnan and Szechwan from which the various warlords hoped to derive needed revenue for maintaining their troops'.(45)
   One estimate made in 1936 noted nearly four million registered addicts of whom about one third lived in Sichuan.(46) The use of agricultural land to cultivate the opium poppy in time of famine and the urban opium dens symbolise China's impoverishment at the time.


DEVELOPMENTS IN MEDICINE AND HEALTH CARE

From 1860 onwards there developed three main areas of medical practice: expansion of medical missionary effort; medical schools and training in Western medicine and the growth of the public health service.

*Preach, teach and heal - the medical missionary movement*
Following the early pioneering work by men such as Parker, which was mainly centred around Guangzhou and Aomen, the medical missionary effort spread to Xianggang and the five treaty ports after the 1842 Treaty of Nanjing. Xianggang, which had full colony status, became a centre for medical sciences. Shanghai, which in 1843 was referred to as 'an insignificant Chinese town of twenty-five thousand inhabitants'(47) became a prominent medical centre by the end of the century.
   In 1866 Dr J.G. Kerr opened a medical school at the Canton Missionary Hospital. His was to be both the earliest and most productive sector, having graduated seventy-nine doctors by 1897. Initially there were only twelve students under

instruction, including several traditional Chinese doctors or
their sons.(48) Kerr was superintendent of the Canton
Hospital for forty-three years and his other innovations included having two women students join his class in 1879; editing
the first Western medical journal in Chinese, the 'Western
Healing News', in 1881; writing several books on Western medicine in Chinese and founding the first mental hospital, the
'Refuge for the Insane', in 1897.(49) He also helped to start
the new China Medical Missionary Association in 1886 which
produced the 'China Medical Missionary Journal' in 1887 – 'The
first medical missionary journal published in heathen lands.'(50)
The first issue records that there were at least seventy-nine
medical missionaries belonging to twenty different missionary
societies. These are listed below:

| | | | |
|---|---|---|---|
| London Missionary Society | 1807 | American Board Commission Missionaries | 1830 |
| Church Missionary Society | 1844 | American Baptist Missionary Union | 1834 |
| English Baptist Missionary | 1845 | American Protestant Episcopal Missionary | 1835 |
| English Presbyterian Missionary | 1847 | American Presbyterian Missionary North | 1838 |
| Wesleyan Missionary | 1852 | Methodist Episcopal Missionary | 1842 |
| Methodist New Connection | 1860 | Seventh Day Baptist | 1883 |
| China Inland Mission | 1865 | American Baptist South | 1856 |
| United Presbyterian Church of Scotland | 1865 | Methodist Episcopal South | 1848 |
| Established Church of Scotland | | Woman's Union Mission | 1859 |
| | | American Bible Society | 1876 |
| | | Foreign Christian Missionary Society | 1886 |

The Xianggang (Hong Kong) Medical School was opened in
1887 with Dr Patrick Manson as Dean of Faculty. This medical
school was attended by Sun Yat-sen who later was to lead the
revolutionary anti-Manchu movement and become the new
Republic's first President. Sun Yat-sen's life was typical of
an increasing number of Chinese nationals who although numerically small had a decisive influence on the course of Chinese
politics. He was born and brought up in a small village in
Southern China and received a missionary education in Honolulu
where his elder brother emigrated. He became a Christian and
returned to China and later became one of the first group of
medical students in Xianggang. As a student he developed his
political interests. During his studies he befriended a Dr Cantlie, one of his teachers, who was later able to help free him
when in 1896 he was detained in the Chinese legation in London.
Sun Yat-sen referred to medicine as the kindly aunt that had

led him to the high road of politics(51) but in some senses he
was adhering to an ancient tradition:

> The superior doctor serves the nation
> The middle doctor the individual
> The inferior doctor treats physical ailments.(52)

In addition to the tasks of healing and teaching the medical
missionaries aimed to preach the Gospel and convert the Chinese
to Christianity. The question of the priority given to this side
of their work has always been difficult to gauge. In the first
edition of the Chinese Medical Missionary Journal the editorial
stated:

> Our calling as physicians is to relieve bodily suffering and
> to make this benevolent work auxiliary to the higher and
> more important object of making known the Gospel to those
> who are in ignorance of the message of salvation.
> We find prevailing in China not only false systems of
> religion but false theories of medicine and while we aim to
> give them a system of religion founded on external truth,
> we will also endeavour to introduce a knowledge of the
> sciences on which is founded a rational system of medical
> practice.(53)

The balance between service and evangelism was always difficult. Hobson for instance in the Report of the Shanghai
Hospital (1858) stated:

> Relieving suffering humanity is not the only object of a
> medical missionary, it is to place Christianity in an attrac-
> tive form and facilitate its diffusion among the people
> singularly suspicious of and averse to foreign influence.(54)

Other missionaries spoke of medical work not being a 'secular
attraction for a sacred purpose'.(55)
A Commission of Enquiry some forty years later stated:

> The use of medical or other professional service as a direct
> means of making converts, or public services in wards and
> dispensaries from which patients cannot escape is subtly
> coercive and improper.(56)

This report was published in 1932 and was countered by the
'Chinese Medical Journal's' Medical Mission Council who said:

> The Council desires to express its conviction that the pre-
> sentation of the full Gospel of the Love of God as revealed
> in Jesus Christ to every patient in a Mission Hospital is part
> of the work of the missionary physician.(57)

By 1877 there were 473 Protestant missionaries in China of whom over 90 per cent were from Britain or the USA.(58) The estimated number of Christian converts was 13,035 and by 1911 this figure had risen to 180,000. In 1889 the number of hospitals and clinics had risen to sixty-one(59) and by 1911 there were 4,628 missionaries and 170 mission hospitals.(60)

The expansion of the missionary effort paralleled the increasing Western domination of China and when anti-foreign feeling was growing among the people, especially in the 1890s and early twentieth century, the missionaries commonly sought help from their national consuls. This served to identify the missionaries with their countries' military and commercial interests in the minds of the Chinese. Even Western-educated Chinese noted the often patronising and racialist perspectives of some missionaries. As one, mindful of earlier missions in Chinese history, put it:

> It has often been assumed that missionary activities have been largely the work of fair skinned Europeans who having been blessed with an exalted faith and a high civilisation are determined to bring light and happiness to the rest of mankind.(61)

*Medical education*
With the growth of the missionary movement there was a corresponding increase in medical schools and in time Chinese graduates. By 1897 300 Chinese had been educated in Chinese medical schools, only five of which had more than ten students.(62) Many new schools including non-missionary ones were established. The first Chinese doctor to qualify abroad was Dr Huang Kuan (Wong Fun). He was from Guangdong province and attended the Morrison Education Society school. He took his first degree in America and then studied medicine in Edinburgh from 1848 to 1853. He returned to China in 1857 with the London Missionary Society.(63) In 1888 Miss Jin Yunmei (Yamei Kin) became the first Chinese woman physician to have graduated abroad. She lost her parents in an epidemic and was adopted by missionaries in Ningbo. She was sent to study medicine in the Woman's Medical College in New York and graduated in 1885.(64) An American graduate of the same College, Dr Trask, was sent to China as the second female missionary and arrived in Fuzhou in 1874. She was to start the first Women's Hospital in China in 1877.(65) The first foreign woman physician was Dr Combs who arrived in 1873 under the auspices of the Women's Foreign Missionary Society of the Methodist Episcopal Church. In 1901 Dr Mary Fulton opened the Guangdong Medical School for Women which later became the famous Hackett Medical College.(66)

In Tianjin there was a different but equally important movement under way. Viceroy Li Hong Zhang, who had made his reputation during the anti-Taiping campaign, was impressed by

Western superiority in medicine. This was partly due to its beneficial application to British troops. In 1861 the British occupied Tianjin and established a small hospital open to the general public in addition to its services for the 'Coolie Detachment'.(67) The Viceroy had a medical missionary, Dr Mackenzie, as his family physician. Li Hong Zhang was one of the so-called 'self-strengtheners' who sought to bring China up to Western levels of industrial development without destroying feudalism. In 1880 the 'Viceroy's Hospital' was opened under his patronage and a small medical school was started to train Western-style doctors for his Northern Army and Fleet. Yuan Shikai, who became increasingly important and powerful by the turn of the century, worked under Li Hong Zhang and was influenced by his pro-Western policy. He was later to become Viceroy himself and established a city Sanitary Service in 1901(68) and the Beiyang Military Medical School in Tianjin(69) in 1902.

There were some peculiarly Chinese cultural problems that confronted Li Hong Zhang's new graduates. Of the original class of eight students who had all been brought up in 'cultured American homes' and had received 'good English Education', six graduated from the three-year course. The Viceroy obtained for them 'civil rank' and the top student was enrolled in the ninth degree and was awarded a crystal button and honorary fifth rank (civil). This conferred the necessary status in the bureaucratic order. One of the students was placed with a General Chow who commanded 15,000 soldiers outside Tianjin. There was a Chinese traditional doctor there already, a well established middle-aged doctor who also professed to practise upon 'foreign principles'. The problem of where to place the new graduate was solved by calling together a panel of the senior officers who cross-examined the pair:

> Each candidate for the favour of the Court was expected to show all he knew but considering that one of the parties was an astute man of the world of fifty odd summers, equally conversant with Chinese etiquette and Chinese ideas of anatomy and disease, while the other not long entered upon man's estate, whose knowledge of human nature was drawn from the standpoint of the American youth of the nineteenth century while his anatomical and medical learning... differed in toto from the innate knowledge held by his examiners, the result may be readily imagined.(70)

The young doctor was posted away from headquarters and had little to do! Gradually a modus vivendi between traditional and Western medicine was worked out: Western medicine was regarded as good for external diseases, while Chinese medicine was superior in the treatment of internal diseases. As Dr Kerr put it:

In the field of internal medicine, there is so much room for
differences of opinion in regard to the effects of treatment,
that a Chinaman may very naturally doubt the superiority
of foreign methods to his own, but where he perceives the
evident good results following a skillful use of the knife, he
cannot but acknowledge that in this line at least foreigners
far surpass the natives in treatment of disease.(71)

Western medicine and surgery were not always so acceptable
to the often suspicious Chinese. It was thought that the 1868
riot in Yangzhou was precipitated by a physican who put a
dead human foetus in a bottle which was seen by the Chinese.
Similarly a report from Nanjing told of a doctor who enucleated
an eye from a boy and replaced it with a glass one. Threats
were made against him and he had to return the eye to the
family. Riots were threatened in 1891 in Shandong when the
Governor died in the presence of foreign physicians sent by
Li Hong Zhang. Rumours of foul play circulated and the
resident missionaries were threatened.(72)

*Public health*
With the development of China as a semi-colony a further crucial
development in health care occurred. This was the so-called
'Chinese Imperial Maritime Customs Service' which was established in 1863 and for many years run by an Englishman, Sir
Robert Hart. In many ways this was a typical colonial organisation. It carried statutory powers in the major ports, and was
an important source of revenues for the State through controlling the Customs taxes. As with other colonial developments
there was a progressive aspect to the organisation, namely the
development of the public health services.
    This was the era when the 'germ theory of disease' flourished.
Snow's work on cholera (1854) demonstrated how the disease
was spread by water supplies and poor sewage disposal. Lister
(1876) had demonstrated the benefit of antisepsis and its
application in surgery. Later work by Koch (1882) and Pasteur
(1895) showed that micro-organisms were involved in diseases
such as tuberculosis and rabies and that these agents were
infective.
    This new knowledge was applied in China through the Medical
Officers responsible to the Customs Service. In 1873 in Shanghai
the 'Sanitary Regulations for the Port' were promulgated by
the Taotai to prevent the spread of cholera in the city.(73)
From 1880 there were part-time medical officers under the name
of the Sanitary Department. A proper Municipal Health Authority
was started in 1898 with the appointment of Dr Stanley as
Medical Officer. In the early days, death notices of foreigners
had been kept and elementary control on house drainage and
food supply made. The staff consisted of a refuse removal over-
seer and one sanitary inspector. In 1898 they developed a
Chemical and Pathology Laboratory, Pasteur Institute and

Inspection service. In 1901 attempts were made to enforce by-laws concerning overcrowding, notification of infectious dis-eases, isolation of infectious cases and registration of medical practitioners. It is unclear whether these only applied to the foreign concessions which had 'extraterritorial status'. In 1903 free vaccinations for the Chinese were offered and by 1906 there were three health inspectors, an isolation hospital and disinfection station. Health education leaflets in Chinese were produced for distribution.(74)

The Customs Service had medical officers appointed who were asked to submit yearly reports of local health conditions and progress. One famous doctor associated with the service was Patrick Manson who worked at Xiamen (1871-1883). He demonstrated that the filarial worm that caused elephantiasis developed in and was transmitted by the mosquito although he thought that it was by contaminated water that man was then re-infected. This was the first evidence that a pathogen of man underwent obligatory development in an insect and pre-empted by some twenty years the discovery by Ross that mosquitoes were vectors of malaria. With this observation the science of modern tropical medicine was born, as it was subsequently proved that other diseases such as sleeping sickness and yellow fever also have an insect vector. Manson also made an important contribution to the understanding of the lung fluke (paragonimus Westermanii):

> On one occasion a petty Chinese mandarin came for consultation about an eruption on his hands which proved to be itch. During the examination he coughed and ejected the sputum on the floor of my consulting room. My disgust and anger at such an exhibition of bad manners evaporated on seeing that the sputum was tinged with blood. 'Here', I thought, 'is another opportunity', and taking a forceps I humbly picked up the sputum and transferred it to the microscope. To my astonishment I found not the expected filarial embryo but the operculated ovum of a different and to me quite new parasite.(75)

Later Manson, together with another Chinese missionary Dr Cantlie, founded the Society of Tropical Medicine and Hygiene. Manson was acclaimed at an International Medical Congress in 1913 as the father of modern tropical medicine.(76) The Society's motto 'Zonae Torridae Tutamen' was noted by 'The Times' of London (December 1929) to be 'the watchword of the new Imperialism which gives rather than gets'.(77)

The Customs medical officers had responsibility in checking incoming ships for infectious diseases and for vaccinating emigrants. These posts were much sought after and offered for sale in the 'British Medical Journal' and 'Lancet' because the charges for vaccination of emigrants made it a lucrative business.(78) If disease was suspected the new principles of isolation and quarantine were applied.

Other cities also had sanitary services. Some records of deaths and burials were kept in Guangzhou as far back as 1850.(79) In 1905 a Sanitary Department of Central Government at Beijing was established under the Ministry of Police (later the Ministry of Civil Affairs).(80) Public hospitals were developed, some of which offered both Western and Chinese medicine. In 1906 a semi-official water company was established in Guangzhou.(81) With increasing industrialisation the basis for a future industrial health service was being laid. In 1885 the Colliery Hospital at Tangshan was the first industrial hospital in China.(82) Later the railways were to provide company based services and even medical colleges.

Over a hundred years the character of medicine in China, linked inseparably with Western imperialism, changed from a variegated, patchy scheme, with little overall organisation and practitioners of varying levels of skill, to one where the latest developments in Western medicine were applied through the administrative structures of Western commerce and religion. Towards the end of the century Western medicine was welcomed by those nationalists who sought to modernise China. After the fall of the Manchu dynasty new possibilities of an organised system of health care under the Republic emerged.

## NOTES

1 Pierre Huard and Ming Wong, 'Chinese Medicine', London World University Library, London, Weidenfeld & Nicolson, 1968, p. 61.
2 J. Henderson, The Medicine and Medical Practice of the Chinese, 'Journal of the North China Branch of the Royal Asiatic Society', new series, no. 7, December 1864, pp. 54-5.
3 Huard and Wong, op. cit., pp. 61-2.
4 'Chinese Medical Missionary Journal', ('CMMJ'), vol. V, no. 3, September 1891, Book Notices, p. 176.
5 W. Morse, 'Chinese Medicine', New York, Hoeber, 1934, pp. 155-7.
6 Lee Tao, Ten Celebrated Physicians and their Temple, 'Chinese Medical Journal' (CMJ), vol. 58, September 1940, pp. 267-74.
7 Ibid.
8 Morse, op. cit., p. 48.
9 C.K. Wong and Wu Lien-teh, 'History of Chinese Medicine', Tientsin Press, 1932, pp. 91-2.
10 J.H. Edgar, The Sin Bearer, a Note on Comparative Religion, 'Journal of the West China Border Research Society', vol. 3, 1926-9, p. 151, quoted in E.H. Hume, 'The Chinese Way in Medicine', Baltimore, Johns Hopkins University Press, 1940, p. 2.

11 Huard and Wong, op. cit., p. 70.
12 Morse, op. cit., p. 113.
13 Wong and Wu, op. cit., pp. 130-6.
14 Thompson, Rev. J.C. 'CMMJ', China's First Foreign Medical Benefactor. Dr Alexander Pearson, vol. 1, no. 3, September 1887, p. 96.
15 Joseph Needham, 'Clerks and Craftsmen in China and the West', Cambridge University Press, 1970, p. 375.
16 Ibid., p. 376.
17 Lockhart, 'The Medical Missionary in China. A Narrative of Twenty Years Experience', London, London Missionary Society, 1861, pp. 239-42.
18 'CMMJ', vol. 1, no. 3, September 1887, op. cit., p. 93.
19 Ibid., p. 94.
20 Ibid., p. 99.
21 Wong and Wu, op. cit., p. 169.
22 Wu Lien-teh, 'Plague Fighter - The Autobiography of a Modern Chinese Physician', Cambridge, Heffer, 1959, p. 348.
23 E. Gulick, 'Peter Parker and the Opening of China', Cambridge, Mass., Harvard University Press, 1973.
24 Hospital News, ('CMJ'), vol. 49, no. 2, February 1935, p. 193.
25 Beadle quoted by Thompson In Memoriam - Dr Peter Parker, in 'Chinese Recorder', vol. xix, May 1888, p. 231, also in Wong and Wu, op. cit., p. 177.
26 Wong and Wu, op. cit., p. 313.
27 Thompson, Medical Publications in Chinese, 'CMMJ', vol. 1, no. 3, September 1887, p. 115.
28 Yang Chi-Shih, Some of Dr Hobson's Medical Works in the Chinese Language, 'CMJ', vol. 53, pp. 323-34, April 1938, p. 327.
29 Ibid., p. 332.
30 Henderson, op. cit., p. 58.
31 Figures from Wu Lien-teh, op. cit., p. 472; and Fitzgerald and Roper, 'China a World so changed', London, Heinemann, 1973, p. 40.
32 Wu Lien-teh, op. cit., p. 478.
33 Fitzgerald and Roper, op. cit., p. 40.
34 B. Inglis, 'The Opium War', London, Hodder & Stoughton, 1976, p. 47.
35 Ibid., p. 181.
36 Lockhart, op. cit., p. 36.
37 D.H. Kulp, 'Country Life in South China', vol. I, New York, Columbia University Press, 1925, p. 57.
38 Surgeon General C.A. Gordon, 'An Epitome of the Reports of the Medical Officers to the Chinese Imperial Maritime Customs Service from 1871 to 1882', London, Balliere, 1884, p. 385.
39 Ibid., pp. 386-8.
40 Lockhart, op. cit., p. 251.

41 Ibid., pp. 260-1.
42 R. Douglas, 'Society in China', London, Innes & Co., 1894, p. 354.
43 Lockhart, op. cit., p. 338.
44 Wu Lien-teh, op. cit., pp. 471-3.
45 Ibid., p. 471.
46 Kan Nai Kuang, The Treatment of Opium and Narcotic Addiction, 'CMJ', 51, June 1937, pp. 815-20.
47 M. Bernard, 'Strange Vigour', London, Heinemann, 1944, p. 88.
48 Wong and Wu, op. cit., p. 247.
49 C. Selden, The Life of John Kerr, 'CMJ', 49, no. 4, April 1936, p. 366.
50 Items and News, 'CMMJ', vol. 1, no. 1, March 1887, p. 38.
51 Sze, Four doctors and a famous kidnapping, 'CMJ', 61, no. )2, April-June 1943, pp. 172-83.
52 E.H. Hume, op. cit., p. 59.
53 Editorial, 'CMMJ', vol. 1, no. 1, March 1887, p. 29.
54 Lockhart, op. cit., p. 154.
55 Borst-Smith, 'Mandarin and Missionary in Cathay', London, Seeley Service, 1917, p. 80.
56 Report of Appraisal Commission of the Laymen's Foreign Mission Inquiry on the work of medical missions in the Far East (Sponsored by seven Protestant denominations), 'CMJ', vol. XLVI, no. 12, December 1932, pp. 1211-13.
57 Council on Medical Missions, 'CMJ', vol. 47, no. 2, February 1933, pp. 191-2.
58 Wu, op. cit., p. 512.
59 R. Croizier, 'Traditional Medicine in Modern China', Cambridge, Mass., Harvard University Press, 1968, p. 38.
60 'Christian Mission Year Book', 1911; also Wu, op. cit., pp. 513-14.
61 Wu, op. cit., p. 500.
62 Wong and Wu, op. cit., p. 368.
63 Ibid., p. 228.
64 Ibid., p. 333.
65 Ibid., p. 274.
66 Ibid., p. 380.
67 Ibid., p. 226.
68 Ibid., p. 382.
69 Ibid., p. 404.
70 Mackenzie, Viceroy's Hospital Medical School, 'CMMJ', vol. 1, no. 3, 1887, pp. 102-3.
71 'Book Notices', 'CMMJ', vol. V, no. 3, September 1891, p. 172.
72 Editorial, The Medical Missionary and the anti-foreign riots in China 1891, 'CMMJ', vol. VII, no. 2, June 1893, p. 114.
73 Wong and Wu, op. cit., p. 253.
74 Ibid., p. 403.
75 'CMJ', op. cit., 61, no. 2, April-June 1943, pp. 172-81.
76 'CMJ', xliv, no. 6, June 1930, pp. 572-4.

77 Ibid.
78 Wu, op. cit., p. 406. He mentions the posts being adver-
   tised for £5,000-£6,000.
79 Jordan, Municipal Health Administration in International
   Settlement in Shanghai, 'CMJ', vol. xliii, no. 4, April 1929,
   p. 338.
80 Wong and Wu, op. cit., p. 405.
81 Ibid.
82 Ibid., p. 299.

# 2 THE DEVELOPMENT OF CHINESE HEALTH CARE, 1911–49

J.A. Jewell

## POLITICAL BACKGROUND

In 1911 the Qing dynasty was finally overthrown by the Nationalist forces which were mainly southern-based. Dr Sun Yat-sen
was recalled from abroad and proclaimed First President of the
Chinese Republic. This new government was based on the
Western democratic model but because China was still a traditional peasant society there was a weak social basis for it and
the honeymoon was short-lived. There followed years of political struggle mainly between powerful war-lords asserting
political control in different regions. It was only in the 1926-8
period that the Nationalist Guomindang (GMD) under their new
Leader Jiang Jieshi (Chiang Kai-shek) managed to unite the
country. The Chinese Communist Party had been formed in
1921 and had grown rapidly. The communists formed a United
Front with the GMD to assist unification. The GMD-inspired
massacre of communists and trade unionists in Shanghai and
Guangzhou in 1926-7 destroyed this brief alliance and shifted
Communist attention to the peasantry. The Japanese invasion
and subsequent occupation in the early 1930s led to war in
1937, which had a devastating effect on China. After the
Japanese surrender, the Communist forces working from their
'guerilla base' areas were able to extend their influence over
the corrupt and demoralised GMD. They were victorious in
1949 and declared the formation of the Peoples Republic of
China while the rump of the GMD sought exile in Taiwan.

## CHANGES IN HEALTH CARE

With such a political background it is perhaps surprising that
any progress in health care was made at all. The frequent
political upheavals contributed to a worsening of the social
conditions in China. Sun Yat-sen always noted that China had
'the poor and very poor' and because it was essentially a rural
society this meant an impoverished peasantry. The four areas
of change in health care provision over this time were: improvement of public health; expansion of western type medical
schools; introduction of state medicine; application of guerilla-
base experience.

## RURAL AND URBAN HEALTH CONDITIONS

R.H. Tawney reported how:

> An eminent Chinese official stated that in Shensi at the
> beginning of 1931, three million persons had died of hunger
> in the last few years, and the misery had been such that
> four hundred thousand women and children had changed
> hands by sale.
>    There are districts in which the position of the rural popu-
> lation is that of a man standing permanently up to the neck
> in water, so that even a ripple is sufficient to drown him.
> The loss of life caused by the major disasters is less signi-
> ficant than the light which they throw on the conditions
> prevailing even in normal times over considerable regions.(1)

In the cities early industrialisation was creating new health
problems to add to the picture of increasing rural impoverishment. Dame Adelaide Anderson, a factory inspector, visited
China in 1923-4 and described her experience:

> A drooping little girl of seven or eight years of age in the
> steaming atmosphere of a semi-industrial silk filature, with
> a swollen body and mask like face of helpless suffering,
> whom I found standing during a long day, making the mono-
> tonous movements needed for stirring cocoons in nearly boil-
> ing water to moisten them for the reelers; a small boy of not
> more than eleven years discovered in a rambling old match
> factory boxing white phosphorus tipped matches, face swol-
> len with suppurating wounds at the cheekbone under the
> left eye and the expression of one who endures great suffer-
> ing; a large ill lighted cotton-spinning room, dusty and
> extremely hot, where numerous children, streaming with
> perspiration work strenuously (on the night and day shift
> system) under Chinese foremen amid inadequately guarded
> machinery; ill lit stuffy, dark rug making workshops (that
> are also sleeping and messrooms) where rows of closely
> packed boys, who work together seated on narrow planks
> slung up to the rising level of the hand made rugs, with
> bowed shoulders and inflamed eyes, infect each other with
> the trachoma that is so common in China.(2)

Another horrifying picture is of the Yunnan tin mines during
the 1930s:

> About 50 per cent of the fifty thousand workers in the Yun-
> nan tin mines are under the age of fifteen years of age....
> This unhealthy occupation gives them a green complexion
> and swollen legs. Their clothing is scanty and filthy, many
> of them are racked with coughing or suffer from inflammation
> of the eyes. Facilities for bathing, washing or changing

clothes do not exist even though at the bottom of the pits
the temperature frequently reaches 120°F. The living quarters match these conditions; twenty workers were found
sleeping in a room of less than thirteen feet by ten feet.
Horses and buffaloes are housed in the same building with
the workers. No means of sanitation are provided.

The mortality is estimated at 30 per cent of the roll
annually. Survivors are not considered likely to live long,
for the tin ore at Kochin contains from 8 to 12 per cent of
arsenic oxide.... Private mines give no medical aid to their
workers believing neither in Chinese nor in foreign medicine,
the sick buy medical herbs from women priests.... The
chief causes of sickness among the workers are diseases of
the respiratory system and digestive tract. Skin and eye
diseases are also common. Trachoma is common; 70 per cent
of the workers are affected by it and the resultant blindness creates a serious social problem.(3)

EPIDEMIOLOGICAL STUDIES

Epidemiological data were becoming available by the 1930s. Estimates of crude birth rates, death and infant mortality rates
were for the country as a whole (Table 2.1).

Table 2.1  Vital rates for China, 1934

|  |  |
|---|---|
| Crude birth rate | 35/1000 |
| Crude death rate | 25-35/1000 |
| Infant mortality rate | 200-300/1000 |

Source: Birth Control in Peiping, First Report of the Peiping
Committee on Maternal Health, Marion Yang, 'CMJ' 48,
1934, pp. 786-9.

In human terms the cost was enormous. Given a population of
approximately 450 million people this meant 11,250,000 to
15,750,000 deaths annually. Compared to the death rates in
the West at this time there was an excess death rate in China
of some 4 to 8 million people. The total loss of life in Europe
for the four years of the First World War was estimated at 10
to 11 million. The excess deaths for four years in China, exclud-
ing infant mortality, are 50 to 200 per cent higher than the
total death toll of the First World War.(4)

There were a large number of studies of infant mortality in
different parts of the country (Table 2.2). Of course these
surveys are not all strictly comparable methodologically. One
obvious bias was that usually urban populations were studied,
although the Dingxian experiment was rural. They do confirm
the extremely high infant mortality rates, particularly in the
southern areas, and it was estimated that approximately 80

Table 2.2 Infant mortality rates in selected areas

| | Year | IMR/1000 live births |
|---|---|---|
| Guangzhou (5) | 1925 | 350.8 |
| Beijing (6) | 1930 | 110.7 |
| Jinan (7) | 1933 | 121.3 |
| Nanjing (8) | 1933 | 122.6 |
| Shanghai (9) | 1936 | 199.4 |
| Dingxian (10) | 1937 | 185.2 |
| Beijing (11) | 1939 | 141.0 |
| Xianggang (Hong Kong)(12) | 1939 | 345.0 |
| Qujing (Kutsing) (Yunnan)(13) | 1939 | 165.3 |
| Chengdu (14) | 1944 | 126.5 |

per cent of these deaths were from infectious diseases and could be prevented by scientific methods, e.g. hygienic midwifery.

MIDWIFERY

Childbirth was mainly supervised by the family or by 'old style midwives' who paid scant attention to antisepsis. One eyewitness reported:

The single large room where she lay in a poster bed, was crowded with thirty or more people... a week the young woman had been lying there while from between her thighs protruded the cord, now dried and shrivelled, and attached to the cord the skeletal baby between her feet.... All that week, the after birth had not come down, the local untrained midwife had tried to bring it down by massaging the stomach and later by introducting her hands within the girl's body. Meanwhile the cord had not been cut to release the baby for according to the old way in Szechwan, the cord was only cut after the placenta was expelled.

That the girl was dying was obvious, she was quite green, could not speak, could not swallow, lockjaw (tetanus) was very common in Szechwan and many babies died of it after the cord had been cut with dirty knives or scissors, and it was customary to plaster the umbilicus with rice straw and with mud.(15)

Midwifery training was recognised to be important both to produce a new brand of modern midwife but also to train the 'old style' midwives in basic hygiene. The First National Midwifery school was opened in Beijing in 1929 with Dr Yang Zhong Rui (Marion Yang) as Director. They offered a range of courses from the full two-year training of senior high-school graduates to six-month training for graduate nurses and basic rural mid-

wives. They also provided 'improvement courses' for old style
midwives, teaching them principally aseptic techniques of
delivery. A second national midwifery school was formed in
Nanjing in 1933 and in addition to these two urban centres there
were three rural 'maternity and infant welfare projects'.(16)

One series illustrated the impact of modern midwifery supervision (Table 2.3).

Table 2.3 Modern midwifery and infant mortality rates

|  | Live births | Infant deaths | IMR / 1000 |
|---|---|---|---|
| Old style midwife + others | 3,257 | 504 | 154.7 |
| Modern physician + midwife | 1,716 | 125 | 72.9 |

Source: Cheng Mei Yu, An Investigation of Infant mortality and
its causes in Chengtu, 'CMJ', 62, 1944, pp. 47-54.

The same series showed the effect of social class with the
inequality being fivefold - a familiar story even today in Western societies (Table 2.4).

Table 2.4  Vital rates by economic background

|  | Live births | Deaths | IMR / 1000 |
|---|---|---|---|
| Very poor | 1176 | 243 | 206 |
| Poor | 2005 | 246 | 122 |
| Middle | 1457 | 126 | 86 |
| Rich | 335 | 14 | 42 |

Source: as for Table 2.3.

The investigators also noted that:

of the 235 total deaths under one month, only 16 occurred
after scientific obstetrical care with no cases of tetanus;
219 occurred when no scientific methods had been used with
193 cases of tetanus, i.e. 80 per cent of neo-natal deaths.


MAJOR CAUSES OF DEATH

Although it is difficult to get a precise record of general causes
of death for the population and actual death rates, Table 2.5
shows the six most important categories in two different
series:

Table 2.5  Major causes of death in urban and rural series

| | Death rate/100,000 | |
| --- | --- | --- |
| | Beijing (Peiping) series | Dingxian (Tinghsien) series |
| Respiratory TB | 303 | 397.5 |
| Other respiratory diseases | 260 | 225.0 |
| Digestive tract } Diarrhoea and enteritis | 244 | 137.0 |
| Cardio-renal | 166 | 123.8 |
| Convulsions | 125 | 150.0 |
| Senility and apoplexy | 120 | 123.8 |

Source: Peiping series: Grant and Yuan, A note on the causes
        of mortality and their classification in Peiping, 'CMJ',
        46, 1932, p. 1187. Ting Hsien series: Ch'en, Public
        health - rural reconstruction at Tinghsien, Annual
        Report 26, 1933.

These categories are rather broad and ill defined but it is clear
that TB was the major killer with other respiratory diseases
and enteritis next. 'Convulsions' included the large number of
infant deaths from tetanus neonatorum.


MORBIDITY

For an assessment of morbidity in the 1930s the 'First General
Epidemiological and Morbidity Survey of China' by Gear for
the period 1933-4 is helpful. Out of necessity the survey was
hospital based and therefore rather urban biased. He achieved
the return of all new cases in the wards and outpatients from
seventeen hospitals in 1933 and twenty-five hospitals the
following year.
    These patients were largely adolescent and young middle-
aged, with a sex ratio of two males to one female. This is an
indication of the place of women in society rather than their
state of health, for they were less likely to be admitted to
hospital! The top eight diseases were as follows:

Table 2.6  Morbidity in China

| Disease title | No. cases | % of total |
| --- | --- | --- |
| Diseases of the skin and cel- lular tissue, bones and organs of locomotion | 45,186 | 21.7 |
| Conditions of violence (excl. suicide) | 22,426 | 10.8 |

| Disease title | No. cases | % of total |
|---|---|---|
| Diseases of digestive system (excl. diarrhoea, appendicitis, hernia, anal fissure and liver disease) | 15,935 | 7.7 |
| Venereal disease | 12,943 | 6.2 |
| Tuberculosis | 10,263 | 4.9 |
| Eye disease (excl. trachoma) | 8,967 | 4.3 |
| Genito-urinary (excl. nephritis) | 7,742 | 3.7 |
| Trachoma | 6,905 | 3.3 |

Source: Gear, CMA Special Report Series no. 11, June 1940, p. 31.

The 'diseases of the skin' were mainly chronic ulcerative conditions that occur commonly in malnutrition and with some parasitic diseases. The three major infections were tuberculosis, venereal diseases, and eye disease. A survey of 2,700 railway workers showed 48 per cent of the defects noted were related to the eyes, of which trachoma was the cause in 31 per cent.[17] Of the thousand-strong workforce of the Yanjing rug factory in Beijing examined in 1926, 90 per cent had trachoma.[18] A later survey of 2,000 blind people found that 90 per cent had been caused by infection of the conjunctiva and cornea of which 39 per cent was due to trachoma.[19]

*Social diseases*
Tuberculosis is a 'social disease' which is an index disease pointing to the conditions of life and work prevailing in society. It was recognised that the high incidence reflected 'extreme poverty, malnutrition and undernourishment, congestion in the urban areas, unhygienic dwellings, sharing of common feeding bowls and chopsticks and the universal habit of expectoration',[20] and that profound social changes were required to stamp out the disease. In 1948 an estimated 6.8 per cent of the population suffered from active TB and over 90 per cent had been primarily infected before puberty.[21]

Venereal diseases also reflect social conditions. Social disorder, particularly under war conditions with occupying armies, leads to high rates. Gear noted the highest incidence in the Menzies Memorial Hospital, Hwaitang, where 15 per cent of all patients were reported as attending hospital for treatment of venereal disease.[22] Syphilis (3.3 per cent) and gonorrhoea (2.6 per cent) were the two major infections and as usual the males presented in the ratio of five to one in the case of gonorrhoea.[23] Gonorrhoea (GC) was another cause of eye disease and blindness and Gear received an interesting letter:

Our cards this time show a heavy lot of GC eyes. This is due to some forty odd cases coming down to us from the

41st Army over in Shansi. The first lot of twenty-six men
came over a very rough mountain pass with one man who
could see. They each clung onto the overcoat tail of the man
in front and came through very, very dangerous mountain
paths. On the plain they walked three abreast, the outside
ones touching the shoulders of the man in the centre, who
held in turn to the shoulders of the man in front. The front
centre man could see and the rest were blinded. Of twenty-
six there were ten odd who were hopelessly blind and the
rest all lost one eye.(24)

Prostitution was obviously an important factor and local taxes
on brothels were often a major source of income for police forces.(25)

In 1928 Feng Dja-chien reported that there were in Shanghai
more than 5,100 public prostitutes in 805 brothels in the International Settlement and the French concession.(26) One unse-
lected survey on 137 prostitutes in Jiangsu found 48.9 per cent
had positive serological tests for syphilis.(27) Later surveys
suggested that gonorrhoea was more common than syphilis and
a study on 876 prostitutes in Peiping found 89.2 per cent
infected on repeat testing.(28)

*Faecal diseases*
Another major group of infectious diseases was the so-called
'faecal-borne diseases'. Broadly these could be divided into:

| 1 Bacterial: e.g. | Bacillary dysentery |
| | Typhoid |
| | Cholera |
| 2 Protozoan: e.g. | Amoebic dysentery |
| | Giardia |
| 3 Helminthic: e.g. | Schistosomiasis |
| | Ankylostoma (hookworm) |
| | Ascariasis |
| | Trichuriasis |
| | Clonorchiasis |

These are an extremely important group of diseases in the Third
World and offer the possibility of control by sanitary hygiene.
They occur both as endemic and epidemic disease. In 1932 an
epidemic of cholera broke out spreading to twenty-three provinces and claimed over 100,000 victims with nearly 34,000
deaths.(29) The extent of faecal-borne infection can be gauged
by Winfield's estimate of sixty million people infected with amoe-
bic dysentery.(30) The economic and social effects can be extra-
polated to a frightening extent. For instance, ascariasis does
not cause severe disease but it is parasitic and surveys showed
that approximately 80 per cent of people examined in different
parts of the country were infected. On the basis of a four hundred million population Winfield calculated the cost as follows:

We therefore arrive at an estimate that there are 335,600,000 people in China that are parasitised by a total of 6,080 million adult ascarids. This huge population of ascarids is maintained because this number of worms is capable of producing 220,000,000,000,000,000 eggs per year. This mass of adult worms would weigh about 48,640,000 catties or 24,300 metric tons, which is equivalent to the weight of about 442,000 men. If it is assumed that it costs as much to nourish a cattie of worm tissue as it does to nourish a cattie of human tissue and that a man can be fed for $4.00 per month or $48.00 per year, then it costs $21,000,000 Chinese currency annually just to feed China's ascarids.(31)

In addition to the faecal-borne disease there were other important endemic and epidemic diseases. In 1935 a survey of Notifiable Diseases was made by the Central Field Station in Nanjing from replies from 204 hospitals. The total number of cases reported was 29,468 (Table 2.7).

Table 2.7  Communicable diseases in China, 1935

| Total cases 29,468 | In-patients 12,639 | Out-patients 16,829 | Male:Female 280 : 100 |
|---|---|---|---|
| Most common diseases: | Malaria | | 50.2% |
| | Ankylostomiasis | | 13.1% |
| | Typhoid and para- | | |
| | typhoid | | 11.1% |
| | Kala-azar | | 7.8% |
| | Diphtheria | | 5.0% |

Source: Hsu and Ke, An Investigation of 19 communicable diseases in China, 'CMJ', 51, June 1937, pp. 833-50.

The importance of malaria is confirmed in a later survey of the number of cases of communicable diseases reported throughout the country in 1941, from eighteen different provinces (Table 2.8).

Table 2.8  Major communicable diseases in China, 1941

| | |
|---|---|
| Malaria | 351,431 cases |
| Dysentery | 101,686 |
| Typhoid | 15,218 |
| Relapsing fever | 12,800 |
| Smallpox | 11,966 |
| Typhus fever | 5,320 |
| Diphtheria | 2,382 |
| Plague | 1,146 |
| Cerebro-spinal fever | 1,040 |
| Scarlet fever | 880 |

| Cholera | 349 cases |
|---------|-----------|

Source: K'ing, Epidemic prevention and control in China,
'CMJ', 61, January-March 1943, p. 2.

Malaria was more common in South China in climates suitable
for the anopheline mosquito. However war conditions facilitated
its spread and caused epidemics in new areas.

In the hyperendemic regions the disease had devastating
effects with underpopulation and impoverishment. The so-
called 'lazy native' was probably suffering from at least three
major diseases.

Winfield's report was in agreement with Gear's conclusions,
that:

'prevention is better than cure' is not the unanswerable
dictum it should be in all medical circles in China and the
great lesson of the survey is surely the call for simple
education in personal hygiene and in sanitary measures
throughout the country.(32)

*Malnutrition*
One last important factor is malnutrition. Even in Third World
countries today this is the basis for a great deal of ill health
and particularly susceptibility to infections. This explains why
some childhood diseases such as measles which are considered
to be relatively minor in the West are frequently fatal in developing countries. In China in the early part of the twentieth
century deficiency diseases were of enormous importance and
included beriberi, vitamin A deficiency, pellagra, scurvy and
rickets. A Chinese delegation to a UN Conference on Food and
Agriculture in 1943 said:

The large majority of the population, even under pre-war
conditions, have suffered from insufficient food.... The
most important reason for this is the low purchasing power
of the average person or family. With the average income
per person per year before the war (1937) as low as forty
to fifty Chinese dollars [= US$13-16] the purchase of an
adequate amount of food becomes indeed impossible. The
inevitable consequences are general undernourishment,
prevalence of deficiency diseases, lowered resistance against
infection and very much lowered expectation of life.(33)

Beriberi (vitamin $B_1$ deficiency) was the most common deficiency disease and one study in Shanghai showed that 15 per
cent of patients admitted to St Luke's Hospital, Shanghai, were
suffering from it.(34) The British colony of Xianggang (Hong
Kong) was a particularly high risk area for the disease which
partly explains their high infant mortality and general death
rate (Table 2.9):

Table 2.9   Vital rates in 1939 in Beijing and Xianggang

| | | |
|---|---|---|
| General death rate/1000 | 16.3 | 46 |
| Infant mortality rate/1000 | 141 | 345 |

Source: L. Fehily, Prevention of Beri-beri, 'CMJ', 60, July
    1941, pp. 53-65

In a Xianggang Infant Welfare clinic it was found that 18 per
cent of infants showed symptoms of beriberi while 26 per cent
were suffering from bronchitis and 20 per cent from pyodermias
(infected skin ulcers). Further, 25 per cent of mothers on their
first visit to an Infant Welfare centre were observed to have
either numbness, weakness of the extremities or oedema of the
feet, all symptoms associated with beriberi. In fact due to the
frequent occurrence of paresis or paralysis during pregnancy
and the puerperium, these symptoms were regarded by Chinese
in Xianggang as the physiological effects of childbearing.(35)
The key to this particular problem lay in the use of partly
milled rice rather than the white highly milled rice which was
the exclusive food staple in Xianggang.


PUBLIC HEALTH MEASURES 1911-24

*Vaccination and measures against infection*
It is perhaps no surprise that 'prevention' and public health
measures had not become universally accepted and applied in
China. One of the first preventive techniques in modern times
had been the use of Jennerian vaccine for smallpox prophylaxis
in the early nineteenth century. Over a century later its
introduction had not been applied in any systematic form, for
'Vaccination was apt to be looked upon as a hobby of the practising physician, a benevolent deed of a philanthropic organisation, or a means of earning a living by a "self styled physician
quack".'(36)
    Because of the neglect in ensuring community immunity by
systematic vaccination epidemics would break out from time to
time. Not until proper state organisation of public health
measures took place was the social potential of the vaccination
technique realised. Following the 1911 Revolution the Imperial
Maritime Customs service, which had enforced health measures
in the treaty ports, was reorganised as a department of the
Ministry of the Interior. Although this body had statutory
responsibility for public health its scope and jurisdiction were
very limited. However, sanitary bureaus were opened in the
principal cities and were under the control of a modern scientific doctor.

*Manchurian Plague*
A major milestone was achieved in 1911 following the epidemic of

pneumonic plague in Manchuria (similar to the 'black death' in Europe) which claimed approximately 60,000 lives.(37) Dr Wu Lian De (Wu Lien-teh), who had recently arrived from Malaya to take up a post in Beiyang Medical College, was asked to direct the Chinese part of the operation. He had trained in Britain (Cambridge and St Mary's Hospital) and studied bacteriology in Germany and Paris.

When he arrived people were dying at a rate of 3,413 per month.(38) The epidemic was brought under control within a month by isolating cases, disinfection, bacteriological testing, inoculation and cremation.

There were a number of unprecedented proposals that were carried out with Imperial permission. For instance the legitimation of post mortems and mass cremation of bodies ran counter to Confucian ideals. Similarly the legal detention of contacts, house to house searches and the use of disinfection were new in China.

The reputation of traditional Chinese doctors suffered badly in this epidemic. Dr Wu Lian De (Wu Lien-teh) noted that as they had no conception of the 'germ theory' of disease they were at a disadvantage.

The native practitioners as a rule entertained wrong ideas of the cause of pneumonic plague and when called in for consultation, normally sat facing the coughing patient without wearing any protective masks though the need for taking the utmost precaution had been continuously impressed on them. At Changchun among a population of one hundred thousand with only a limited number of Western trained doctors around, the services of native practitioners were more sought after; here the number of their dead was seventeen out of a registered total of thirty-one.(39)

The satisfactory results achieved by modern trained anti-plague staff gave a 'great fillip to scientific medical practice throughout China'.(40) A Plague Conference that was held in Shenyang in April 1911 was the first international scientific gathering ever held in the 'Old Empire' to deliberate upon the hygienic aspects of mankind! At his opening address Viceroy Xi Liang said:

We Chinese have believed in an ancient system of medical practice, which the experience of centuries has found to be serviceable for many ailments but the lessons taught by this epidemic, which until practically three or four months ago had been unknown in China, have been great, and have compelled several of us to revise our former ideas of this valuable branch of knowledge.(41)

The North Manchurian Plague Prevention Service was formed to continue research into plague and search out the plague focus. In 1913 a Presidential mandate was issued legalising and regulating the dissection of dead bodies.(42) In 1915 an isolation hospital was built in Beijing and in 1917 when a new attack of plague broke out in Shanxi province a Central Epidemic Prevention Bureau was established.(43)

The public health movement continued when Guangzhou became the first city to begin to organise a Municipal Department of Health in 1913.(44)

In 1925 the Beijing Health Demonstration Station was set up in conjunction with the National Epidemic Prevention Bureau but it required the formation of the National Health Administration in 1928 before these pioneering efforts were co-ordinated and developed.

*Mass campaigns in Fuzhou and Jiangxi*

A well documented example of Public Health work done by voluntary missionary organisations was in the anti-cholera campaign in Fuzhou in 1920. This was co-ordinated by the Council on Health Education, was highly successful and had many features that the Chinese Communists were later to use. The major limitation was that it was an isolated campaign, a fact implicit in a congratulatory telegram on behalf of the citizens of Fuzhou: 'Fuzhou was an island of safety in a sea of danger.'(45)

The impetus behind the campaign was the 1919 cholera epidemic that left an estimated 19,000 dead. There was no Health Department and the people responded by flocking to the temples or joining 'idol processions'. It was even reported that the Governor had donated money to the priests to enlist their aid. A group of medical missionaries and Western trained Chinese doctors opened a cholera hospital and used saline infusion therapy with some success. This group was asked to suggest precautions before the expected outbreak the following year and to organise a mass health education campaign in Fuzhou.

This campaign was held in June 1920. In one week 247 meetings were conducted in fourteen districts of the city. By count 110,000 people attended. A cholera parade visualising the wrong and right ways of using water, food and human excreta was seen by approximately 220,000 people.

Three hundred thousand pieces of illustrated cholera literature were distributed free. To do all this work, there were 2,480 volunteers, mostly students, but including also some of the most prominent people of the city. The cost of the campaign was provided by a few businessmen and others of Fuzhou.(46)

The public shows were extremely striking:

China's load of disease was visualised on stage by a Chinese man carrying a heavy bag. He was asked to do various kinds

of work but he failed because so much of his time and strength
had to be given to this load on his back. The bag was
opened to examine the contents. It revealed blocks of wood
on which were printed the names of various diseases such
as smallpox, cholera, plague, typhus, all of which came out
quite readily, and other blocks such as hookworm and TB
which were brought to the mouth of the bag with difficulty.
The lecturer explained the relationship between poverty,
ignorance and disease. Once this load was lightened, the
man was able to do more work, make more money to support
his family, send his children to school and thus be a better
citizen.(47)

The result of this health propaganda was that Fuzhou, a city
of about half a million people, was spared during the next
cholera epidemic.

The Council on Health Education was also active in other parts
of the country initiating school medical examinations, vaccination
campaigns, conferences and health education courses. Organisations such as the Rockefeller Foundation, Rotary Clubs and
Missionary Societies figured prominently in financing activities.
Later there were examples of municipal and provincial health
authorities promoting mass preventive campaigns. For instance
in 1935 the Jiangxi Provincial Bureau reported:

An intensive health campaign was started on Saturday June
15th attended by over twenty thousand people in which the
whole staff in the city participated. In the Sun Yat Sen
Memorial Hall there was a large health exhibit, and in various
public gardens there were health plays, health lectures and
attractive showings of lantern slides. Health talks were broadcast over the radio. In the clean up campaign which was
one feature of the activities citizens co-operated in giving
a thorough cleaning to houses, streets and schools and
other public buildings. Travelling clinics gave free preventive inoculation against cholera and typhoid.(48)

The success of the Fuzhou experiments and the Jiangxi
campaign were evident. They illustrated the need for public
health and preventive medicine to be properly organised and
planned which is impossible under an individualised private
practice model. This realisation formed part of the pressures
toward the socialisation of medicine.

It is worth mentioning that these pioneering activities often
met with problems. For instance we are told of a woman heard
to say in front of an enlarged picture of a housefly: 'If we had
flies as big as this in China, we would certainly have to be
careful also.'(49) One missionary, referring to Peter Parker,
the first medical missionary to China, replied to a preventive
medicine circular that 'China was opened with a lancet and not
a fly swatter'.(50)

*Health care organisation under the Guomindang*
The Moral Welfare movement was the title given to a group of
representatives from about a dozen religious charitable associations formed in 1918.(51) Their aim was to abolish commercial-
ised vice in the community. In 1919 the ratepayers of the
International Settlement decided to appoint a Special Vice Committee. They later produced a report recommending the registration and gradual elimination of brothels of all nationalities.
In 1930 an association to look after the interests and welfare
of Chinese prostitutes was organised at Hangzhou by the 'leading
gentry'.(52) A 'purity campaign' was started in 1921 by the
Canton Christian Council against sexual evils. In 1920 Shanghai
was visited by a Commission appointed by the British National
Council for combating VD.(53) The YMCA and the YWCA were
active in promoting the cult of 'mens sana in corpore sano'.

A similar development promoted by the Guomindang was the
New Life Movement, a set of precepts based on the Confucian
mode of teaching. Developing original republican ideas of
'social welfare of the people', it nevertheless degenerated into
a barren list of rules, which attacked ignorance and bad health
rather than the fundamental social difficulties which caused
them. This is an example of 'victim blaming'. The New Life
campaigns were referred to bitterly as 'toothbrushes for starv-
ing people'.

The other scourge that attracted attention from the Christian
moral welfare movement and the government was the opium and
narcotic problem. During the nineteenth century the opium
market had rapidly expanded and even in 1906 more than seven
million pounds weight of opium were imported. In 1908 the
Chinese and British government signed a Ten Years' Agreement to decrease the Indian export of opium with the aim of
ceasing in a decade.(54) The gap in the market was filled however by an increase in domestic cultivation.

The Nationalist Government of 1928 appointed a National
Opium Suppression Commission and attempted to deal with the
problem. By 1936 there were a total of 970 anti-opium hospitals
and stations. The number of registered opium smokers, which
is always an underestimate of total users, was 3,786,368 in
1936.(55) The criminal fraternity that supported the network
of opium dens and brothels were going to be a formidable problem for a new reforming government.

*The role of the Red Cross*
The International Red Cross organisation also worked in China
and is still active today. The first involvement was in the 1894-5
Japanese War and the Newchwang Red Cross Hospital was
opened in 1894.(56) It is interesting to note that, unlike in
predominantly Christian or Muslim countries:

The meaning of the cross to most of the people in China
was unclear to them, the not very illuminating name of

the Society in many places was a literal translation of the
'Red Ten Character Society' - the cross being taken as the
arithmetical sign for the Chinese numerical ten.(57)

The Red Cross made an important contribution in emergency
relief work and during the anti-Japanese War had some five
hundred chapters with 380,000 members, forty-five hospitals
and 200 clinics and welfare centres.(58) Sun Yat-sen's widow,
the late Soong Chingling, continued to play an important role
in this organisation until her death in 1981.


MEDICAL EDUCATION

*The development of medical schools by foreigners*
Medical education was gradually being transformed over the
first three decades of the twentieth century. The pioneering
efforts of the missionary movement were being supplanted by
foreign philanthropic organisations such as the Rockefeller
Foundation, foreign universities such as Yale. in the USA, and
foreign organisations and government investments with German,
Japanese and French universities. Indigenous developments
were also moving forward with the Army Medical Colleges
followed by national and provincial level medical schools. There
were also the extremely important if small group of students
who were trained abroad and those who graduated from the
small private medical schools of variable quality.
   The Peking (Beijing) Union Medical College (PUMC) was
founded in 1906. It was formed by the combined efforts of
several missionary groups, both Anglican and non-denomi-
national. They all helped to develop and maintain the College
until 1915.
   The Rockefeller Foundation decided to undertake a programme
of medical philanthropy in China. John D. Rockefeller's financial
advisor Frederick Gates was a crucial person in this decision,
which started with the Oriental Education Commission which
spent six months in China, India and Japan in 1909.(59) It
recommended that when conditions were more favourable,
medical schools should be developed in China.
   The Rockefeller Foundation sponsored the China Medical
Board which assumed full responsibility for the Union Medical
College which was governed by a board of trustees. In 1937 it
was reported that the Foundation had given over fourteen
million dollars to the China Medical Board and to PUMC in
particular roughly eighteen million dollars.(60) PUMC was the
elite medical school providing an extended course of eight
years, taught largely in English. It had few students and by
1932 had only graduated sixty-four doctors. Not surprisingly,
of their 208 postgraduate years, 58 per cent was spent in their
Alma Mater, 14 per cent abroad, 10 per cent in private or
contract practice, 7 per cent in mission hospitals and none in

public service.(61) American plans for PUMC intended that it should finally be taken over by the Chinese. John Rockefeller Jr, in a speech at the 1921 dedication ceremony, said:

> Clearly whatever Western medical science may have to offer to China, it will be of little avail to the Chinese people until it is taken over by them and becomes a part of the national life.(62)

The College was the focus of massive investment by American philanthropy and reflected the aspirations for the new institutionalised scientific medicine of its corporate benefactors. The investment was successful as the graduate output later formed a high proportion of influential Chinese doctors who made major contributions before and after 1949.

St John's College, Shanghai, incorporating St Luke's Hospital, came to an agreement in 1914 with the trustees of the Pennsylvania Medical School to link up. A similar story was that of the Xiangya Medical College, Changsha, Hunan, which was founded in 1913 as a joint venture between the Hunan Provincial Government and the Yale-in-China Association. It was commonly referred to as the Hunan-Yale College.(63) Other countries were also involved. The German Paulun founded Donaji Medical College in Shanghai in 1907. The faculty was German with Chinese students. A smaller project was also developed in Qingdao. The French Doumer Hospital was opened in 1900 in Guangzhou and the Franco-Chinese Medical School was founded by the French government in association with this hospital in 1914. The Jesuits opened the Aurora University in 1903 and the Sisters of Charity founded St Mary's Hospital in 1907.(64)

The Japanese founded the South Manchuria Medical College of the South Manchuria Railway in Shenyang in 1911. Unlike other colleges where at least the students were Chinese, here the majority of teachers and students were Japanese and most returned to Japan on qualifying. The first Chinese was admitted in 1913 but even in 1929 there were 216 Japanese students and only 23 Chinese.(65)

The British in addition to their widespread influence through the Protestant medical missions had acquired the colony of Xianggang (Hong Kong), and the Hong Kong College of Medicine for Chinese was founded in 1887.(66)

Professor Eugene Vincent from Lyons in France, when he visited China, articulated the competition between foreign powers. He urged that a medical faculty be established at Aurora in Shanghai not only for humanitarian reasons but to extend French influence:

> The Germans work with a tenacity, large sums of money and soldiers to conquer a very important place in China, they follow us step by step to profit from our long work in all branches of the civilisation.(67)

Similarly a contributor to the 'British Medical Journal', referring to the threat of a 'Russian nightmare' in China, urged companies such as the Asiatic Petroleum Company, the Anglo-American Tobacco Company and the cotton industry to invest in a 'first rate hospital' in Hankow.(68)

Another means of influence was in the training of medical students abroad. On their return they were known as Western-style doctors of the 'German-Japanese school' or the 'Anglo-American school'. Returned students used to form their own Association and clubs. The numbers were small but influential (Table 2.10):

Table 2.10    The number of Chinese students studying medicine abroad

|         | 1932 | 1933 |
|---------|------|------|
| Japan   | 29   | 44   |
| Germany | 9    | 15   |
| USA     | 7    | 6    |
| France  | 3    | 6    |
| GB      | 2    | 7    |
| Austria | 2    | 1    |

Source: Lee Tao, Some statistics on medical schools in China for the year 1933-34, 'CMJ', 49, 1935, pp. 894-902.

One Chinese doctor drew attention to the consequence of foreign training:

graduates are better qualified to handle the social problems of Germany and America than those of China. The most prevalent epidemic diseases of China are trachoma, smallpox, dysentery, typhoid, cholera, etc. yet there are fourth-year medical students who do not know how to make a diagnosis of trachoma or to vaccinate a person against smallpox, much less to improve the sanitation of any locality.(69)

An editorial of the 'Chinese Medical Journal' also noted that:

It is very natural for a man trained in Germany to equip a hospital with an 'X' ray machine from Siemens, hemocyto-meter from Leitz, microscope from Zeiss, surgical instruments from Jetter-Scheerer and to prescribe drugs such as Omnadin, Prontosil etc.(70)

In 1930 Dr Rajchman, representing the League of Nations, commented:

Hospitals in China are, as a rule, in foreign hands... the majority of the subordinate staff is frequently Chinese...

there are only a handful of Chinese doctors in China today
who have had experience as the administrative head of
hospitals.(71)

## State medical schools
Apart from the relatively small number of private hospitals
owned by Chinese businessmen and doctors that also provided
some medical education, there was an increasing number of
State-funded schools. This was in line with the move forward
on State medical services that became formalised in 1928 with
the Ministry of Health which later was called the National Health
Administration. Medical schools were formed at national,
provincial and army levels. The total number of students at
this time was 3,616 of whom 638 were women. The number of
medical graduates in 1934 was 532, but this number excluded
those produced by the smaller medical institutions.(72)

## Medical education for women
There are early historical records of women practitioners. The
Han Annals mention that a woman doctor was called to the
palace to treat the queen. In the Song dynasty women versed
in medicine were selected and examined by the court physi-
cians.(73) With the Western medical missionary movement early
Chinese women recruits were either daughters of Chinese pas-
tors or adopted children. For example one of the first Chinese
women to qualify in Western medicine was Miss Jin Yunmei
(Yamei Kin), who graduated in 1885 from the Women's Medical
College in New York. Later the opportunity for women's medical
education in China became available at the Guangdong Medical
College in 1899. This was followed in 1902 by the Hackett
Medical College for Women. By 1909 over thirty students had
graduated from Hackett and in 1933 it affiliated to Lingnan
University.(74)

The Methodist Episcopal Church South established a Women's
Medical School in Suzhou in 1891. This moved in 1919 to Shanghai and amalgamated with the Margaret Williamson Hospital. In
1924 it became the Women's Christian Medical College under
charter from the District of Columbia (USA).(75)

The Peking Union Medical College for Women was started in
1908 with two students. This was later transferred to Jinan to
merge with the Medical Faculty of Shandong Christian University. With the Republican Educational Laws of 1912 co-education
became permissible and by 1932-3 out of twenty-eight medical
schools there were only two male- and two female-only schools.
By 1934 16.9 per cent of graduates were female and there were
approximately 550 qualified women physicians.(76) Medicine was
the only profession in which women had established themselves
and credit for this must go to the early missionary pioneers.

## The quality and quantity debate in medical education
An important issue in medical education was the length of train-

ing required to produce an adequate doctor. There was by that stage a distinction between the university course of six years and the 'Zhuan Ke' (second grade) medical course of four years. The Faber Report (1930) had suggested one of the 'Zhuan Ke' for each province. Attached to the medical schools would be schools for nurses, midwives, pharmacists, technicians and health officers. By the early 1930s the Ministry of Education was attempting to draw up a model curriculum for each course. There was also a keen debate on the enormous need for rural health workers. The basis for a quality/quantity conflict lay in the demands of the rural areas against the high quality college graduate symbolised by the eight-year graduate of PUMC. The Chinese Medical Association (CMA), formed in 1932, was an amalgamation of two earlier professional associations, the older missionary organisation and the predominantly Chinese National Medical Association. It was keen to maintain standards in medical education and practice and introduce professional registration. This would exclude traditional practitioners and thus legitimise Western medicine only. The CMA stood for high-quality college graduates of Western medicine. Dr Arthur Wu stated in his presidential address

> The creation of a special grade of medical practitioner by lowering the standard of entrance into the profession will not, I fear, minister to the crying need of the rural districts. Rather it will help to flood the commercial cities and large towns with another army of men ready always for a consideration to attempt more than their knowledge warrants. This can only bring discredit to the profession and drive the public back into the arms of the old style herbalists and pulse feelers.(77)

Others were not so sanguine:

> The position of our Association [CMA] at its conferences a little recalls the story of Nero fiddling while Rome burns. Nearly all the time at such meetings is taken up with abstruse scientific discussions while the people are perishing not from rare diseases requiring minute scientific investigations but from common ailments of which we largely know the causes, prevention and treatment.(78)

The League of Nations expert Knud Faber had recommended that medical schools should be brought up to minimal standards and private schools of insufficient standard should only be registered provisionally.(79)

A National Commission on Medical Education was set up soon after the National Health Administration was formed with its terms of reference to include 'the fundamental measures to be adopted for the reformation of medical education before the laissez faire policy has cast it into indestructible moulds unadaptable to this country'.(80)

## DISTRIBUTION OF RESOURCES

The maldistribution of resources was easily demonstrated. To begin with, there were too few doctors. In the 1930s approximately five thousand qualified doctors produced a ratio of one in 80,000 of the population. This was compared to figures such as one in 800 in the USA and one in fifteen hundred in England.(81) In other words if each Chinese physician had looked after as many patients as a doctor in Europe, less than 2 per cent of the population of China would have been able to receive modern medical care!

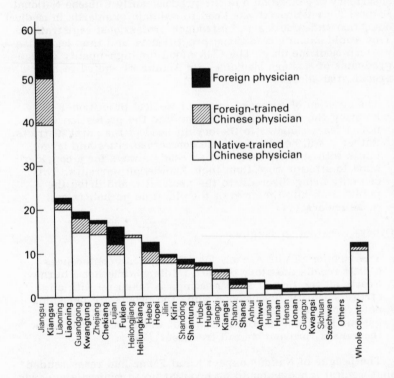

Figure 3    Comparative number of physicians per one million
            population in provinces of China, 1936
Source:    Hsi-Ju Chu and Daniel G. Lai, 'CMJ', 1936, p. 545.

Apart from the gross numbers there was also a maldistribution, with the bulk of doctors practising in the major coastal cities. One study in 1933-5 found a total of 5,390 qualified doctors of whom 87 per cent were Chinese. Of the Chinese, 83 per cent were graduates from Chinese medical schools. Nearly half the physicians were concentrated in the two coastal provinces of Jiangsu and Guangdong.(82) (See Figures 3 and 4.)

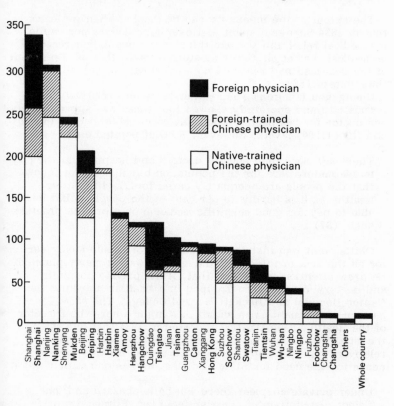

Figure 4   Comparative number of physicians per one million
           population in cities of China, 1936
Source:   Hsi-Ju Chu and Daniel G. Lai, 'CMJ', 50, 1936, p. 547.

The market forces of private practice resulted in a massive urban bias, especially towards the more wealthy cities. It was estimated that Shanghai had about one quarter of the nation's wealth, and 22 per cent of the physicians concentrated there. The 'inverse care law',(83) which states that where need is greatest the least resources are found, was clearly at work.

Under the present system of private practice, one does not wonder that out of 5,390 physicians on our record, 22 per cent are located in this city, particularly in the International settlement and the French concession.

Outside these, there are very few physicians residing in the districts of Greater Shanghai, which has altogether more than two million inhabitants, and has very little medical care as compared with the prosperous sections.(84)

The extent of the inequality can be gauged when we learn that in 1934 Shanghai spent just over four dollars per capita for medical relief and yet one third of the population received no medical care at all.(85) One study showed that 36.2 per cent of the deceased had received no medical care of any sort during their illness.(86)

Guangzhou (Canton) was another large and relatively prosperous city and one study showed that there was approximately one doctor for 905 people which was comparable to USA (1:800) and GB (1:900) levels. However, F. Oldt pointed out:

There are more than enough doctors and hospitals in the city to adequately care for the population but it does not follow that the people are adequately cared for.... In Canton wealthy as it is hardly 10 per cent of the people would be able to pay for good scientific medicine on a private practice basis.(87)

Oldt's point was that Guangzhou's doctors could easily care for all the sick in the city if the service was properly planned. He drew attention to the fact that all the private hospitals and doctors' offices were grouped in a small area around the Canton Hospital and Hackett Medical College. The same pattern of inequality was shown in Nanjing where the Director of the Health Administration reported in 1934 that one third of the municipal population received no medical care despite a relatively high per capita expenditure.(88) All this was evidence for the need for State Medicine, and as one author put it:

Under private auspices there will be haphazard and inefficient distribution of curative facilities. Rural territories would be insufficiently served and in cities there would be areas of unjustified proximity of hospitals each maintaining unnecessary duplication of expensive equipment to the disadvantage of inadequately served districts.... The eventual cost of State medicine would be no more than the present haphazard distribution of private facilities and the former would give the bulk of the people much more efficient protection.(89)

While there were about one third of urban dwellers without medical aid it was recognised that the rural population who make up about 90 per cent of the population had no medical care to speak of:

In Li Ch'eng County, which surrounds Tsinan the capital of
Shantung, there are over five hundred thousand people, 90
per cent of whom are farmers. Apart from two rural clinics
maintained by Cheeloo, no provision has yet been made to
carry the benefits of scientific medicine to the people of this
county, though worthless and expensive patent medicines
are sold everywhere. This condition is typical of 139 out of
141 counties of this province and so over thirty million
people are involved.(90)

Cultural problems were acute in the countryside with illiteracy,
poor educational levels and superstitions hindering health work
and causing waste. For instance:

Smallpox is not only a vital health problem in rural Kiangsi
but a source of much wasted wealth. One unit reported that
in its districts within a radius of ten Li, fifty altars were
built to the smallpox goddess the previous spring and that
the superstitious and ignorant farmers must have spent, it
was estimated, at least $500 for each altar.(91)

In the same district a 'young and unmarried' modern trained
midwife who was viewed with suspicion had a successful case.
A congratulatory poster was nailed to her clinic door which
eulogised her as the 'living Buddha'. The other pattern of
behaviour would be to use worthless patent medicines until
the disease had progressed and then for the family to mortgage
itself to pay a 'witch doctor' or local traditional practitioner in
a last desperate attempt to save the patient. This serves as an
example of wholly inappropriate use of limited resources.

The perennial problem which prevails still today in China and
other Third World countries is to persuade doctors and other
health workers to go to the countryside. At the graduation of
Cheeloo students in 1934 President K'ing Chu stressed that
while the countryside was characterised by ignorance, illiteracy,
poverty, disease, unhygienic practices, disorder and banditry,
he urged new graduates:

who are altruistically minded there is a great scope for helping these rural districts, and to those who have the mind
that was in Jesus Christ there is a great life work of sacrifice and service open in these areas.(92)

The reasons for the reluctance to go to the countryside were
familiar:

The doctors cannot come to the country places because the
common people are too poor to pay for their services. The
doctor cannot enjoy the social conditions he had been taught
to require, nor can he get an education for his children.(93)

## THE DINGXIAN (TINGHSIEN) MODEL

Dr Chen Zhi Qian (C.C. Chen) of the Dingxian rural health
centre, one hundred miles west of Beijing, calculated that the
average family consisting of not less than five members paid
at most one dollar fifty per year for buying medicines for the
whole family. This amount should be compared to the cost of
two or three dollars per day per person for hospital treatment.
It was calculated that ten cents per person per year was the
amount the average Chinese rural community could afford for
medical services.

Scientific medicine had to be introduced within the financial
reach of the population and in essence this meant an emphasis
on prevention and simple treatment of common ailments. It was
estimated that over 70 per cent of the deaths were due to easily
preventable disease. By efficient grassroots organisation using
village health workers with well organised expert back-up,
basic preventive work was done. Mass health education stressing
personal hygiene, registration of births and deaths and public
co-operation with public health measures were all undertaken.
The village cadre was trained to give vaccinations, render first
aid, treat common skin conditions and simple surgical wounds,
and keep a register. Only elementary education was required
and training was by apprenticeship. Health workers received a
fixed salary and were recruited locally. They were the predecessors of the famous barefoot doctors of a later era.

In other areas the 'mobile medical team' existed too:

Our clinics have been held in the country districts 30 to
140 *li* from the hospital. They have usually been held in a
chapel in market towns, although a wayside inn once served
and two operations were performed on the outside food table
made of stone.... In a clinic held 90 *li* to our West in the
mountains early this year, two nurses and one doctor treated
523 patients in six days.(94)

## THE FORMATION OF THE MINISTRY OF HEALTH

The political unification of the country with an initially reforming government, the recognition that China had too few medical
personnel for a population with enormous health needs and that
these meagre resources were maldistributed helped create the
conditions for state medical organisation. The historic inaugura-
tion of a Ministry of Health in October 1928 was a major step
forward. Prior to this public health matters had been handled
by the Central Sanitary Bureau of the Ministry of the Interior.
The 1928 government mandate read:

Up to the present, public health has in a large measure been
carelessly neglected in this country; during this period it is

particularly important to develop healthy bodies, to train
sound minds and to control and prevent epidemic diseases.
Therefore by this order, a Ministry of Health shall be
established.(95)

The Ministry was divided into four main departments, which
dealt with administration and control of hospitals and sanatoria;
supervision of matters relating to the sale of drugs; matters
concerning doctors, pharmacists, midwives and nurses; and
supervision and support of local health affairs.

*'Chinese Pharmacopoeia'*
Another important step was the production of the 'Chinese
Pharmacopoeia' in 1930. This book contained both Western drugs
and some Chinese herbal drugs and drew heavily from the US,
British, Japanese and German Pharmacopoeias for the Western
drugs. The drugs were named in Chinese with Latin titles and
official American Pharmacopoeia abbreviations. Where German
and Japanese names differed these also were added. Metric
weights and measures were used but obviously there were
problems with the crude drug standards for some of the Chinese
herbs.(96)
Although Chinese Pharmacopoeia was an important first step,
it is questionable how much it affected everyday life. The
secretary of the Shanghai Pharmaceutical Association noted in
1933 that

those regulations governing trade in drugs, and governing
importation, manufacture and sale of pharmaceutical preparations exist only on paper: there are no authorities en-
forcing the regulations in question. For it is known to the
Health Authorities of the Foreign Settlements that 90 per
cent of the dispensaries in Shanghai are run by unqualified
people and the importation and sale of pharmaceutical products is in the hands of laymen.(97)

This kind of situation was ideal for pharmaceutical companies
to pursue profit 'unethically':

China is regarded by smaller as well as bigger manufacturing
enterprises abroad as the only country in the world that can
be flooded with all kinds of worthless medicines... which
the makers would not dare to sell in the country of origin.(98)

Ethical considerations apart, the advertisement of tranquillisers
and hormone extracts for menopausal symptoms hardly seems
appropriate for the needs of the country.

*Preventive work*
There were other important responsibilities assumed by the new
National Health Administration which included setting up com-

missions to look into midwifery training and medical education,
industrial and school health services. It assumed responsibility
for epidemic control, vital statistics and quarantine regulations
as well as promoting public health work in the provinces. One
mechanism used was to establish model or demonstration centres
for experimental education and publicity purposes. The first
Midwifery School in Beijing and the Dingxian rural health
centre referred to above are examples of such models.

By 1934 the Director of the Administration was able to report
on progress. A five-year programme on maternal and child
health had begun, and a national midwifery school established
in 1929. They ran short courses for rural midwives, as well as
longer professional courses, refresher and 'improvement' courses for traditional midwives. Two city-based and two rural
child health projects were begun.

A school health programme in seventeen schools of the major
cities was started. A communicable disease programme offered
free inoculations and there were mass campaigns of smallpox
vaccination. Health education campaigns were initiated, and
health teachers for schools were trained in Nanjing. Most
importantly, in 1932 a fledgling rural health service began in
three experimental centres: Dingxian, Gaoqiao and Tangshan.(99)

While this is an impressive record in many ways at grassroots
level it probably had little impact. Although it illustrates a well
planned structure, presumably encouraged by progressive
League of Nations experts, the real test would be the degree
of consistent influence such changes would have on the health
of the people.


## ORGANISATION OF HEALTH SERVICES FOR RURAL AREAS

Private medicine had failed to provide for the mass of the people
and State medicine was the only policy able to offer basic medical protection for the population in an efficient manner. The
difficulty was both in finding adequately qualified health
workers and in providing a service at a level the community
could afford. Medical services in themselves were only a partial
solution and the undernourished and impoverished peasantry
required political reform and rural economic reconstruction.
However, the structure that the NHA suggested for rural areas
was:

> For a unit of five to ten thousand population there should
> be a rural health sub-station to take care of simple medical
> and health work and for every five or ten such substations
> there should be a district health station to render more
> fundamental health and medical services to the people. In
> a *hsien* (xian), there should be a health centre which
> includes a hospital, a simple laboratory and an administrative

organ for the supervision of medical and public health works
under its jurisdiction. Similarly a provincial health centre
should be built on a larger scale to supervise and assist the
different *hsien* centres and to take care of certain types of
health work beyond the scope of a *hsien* administration.
Above all there should be a national health organization to
supervise the medical and health work throughout the
country.(100)

At the basic rural sub-station it was recognised that some
form of 'medical assistant' or 'village aid worker' would be
necessary:

Firstly the supply of doctors is so limited that it is estimated that the provision of one doctor per two thousand of
population will be difficult to realise within two decades.
With so few a number and relatively large territories to
cover it is essential that they be provided with assistants to
undertake that part of their work which does not require the
degree of technical skill and knowledge of the doctor. Further, personnel may even be required at times to work in
villages more or less remote from a doctor, they must on
occasions be able to function independently of him.(101)

Another problem was that public health and prevention would
be ignored because of the curative demand:

The danger that the urgency of medical relief may dominate
preventive measures, which are even more productive of
results, is very great unless the minimum preventive measures to be undertaken are from the beginning clearly defined and subsequently held to by a system of competent
supervision reaching down to the smallest peripheral unit
and personnel.

The preventive measures emphasised health education, epidemiology and a sanitary environment together with 'the development of social machinery adequate for the maintenance of
health'.(102)
With increasing experience in attempting to introduce rural
health schemes it became obvious that effective medical and
social organisation was a prerequisite:

Far too often, one comes across a health officer hardwork-
ing and extremely anxious to show results, but who fails to
realise the limitations of a single person or institution. What
he should do is to build a basic organisation, however humble
it may be at the outset, whereby his efforts can be multiplied
... only in localities where the local government, the economic organisation and other phases of social life are undergoing
reform are there signs of the medical service taking root.(103)

It was recognised that the village aid workers should not be paid per item of service and that this and other safeguards were needed to remove incentives for going beyond the prescribed scope of activities. Services should be free and supervised both by a more qualified person and by the local community.

By 1937 only 74 'xian' health centres and 144 rural health stations were in operation. This number is infinitesimal when compared to the total of about 2,000 xian and 100,000 villages and between one and two million hamlets!(104)

The level of financial investment was at a very low level absolutely and relatively. In 1937 the NHA budget was only about 1.2 per cent of the total national budget. The most well endowed 'xian' was Jiangning, but even there the health service only got nine cents per capita out of a total per capita expenditure of three dollars.(105)


## WARTIME HEALTH SERVICES AND POST-WAR DEVELOPMENTS

The Japanese invasion had an immediate effect on the health services. Many casualties were added to the disease burden. In addition, of the thirty medical schools only a couple avoided being moved once or twice during the war. The total enrolment dropped to not more than 3,000 students with about 500 graduates per year.(106) There were so few graduates that of the Guomindang's 30,000 Army medical officers only 2,000 were medical college graduates.(107) No plans for rapid production occurred however. Indeed Surgeon-General Lin Ke Sheng (Robert Lim), speaking at the conference of the CMA, confirmed the inadequate number of doctors and said that the present number must be augmented twelve times, and this could only be achieved through careful planning over a period of thirty to forty years.(108) Even at this time three-quarters of the hospitals were non government and the majority of these were still missionary.

There were some more humorous inconveniences of war such as the CMA members left in Shanghai after the Japanese takeover:

It seems that the Chinese doctors in Shanghai are carrying on with their practices successfully in spite of the numerous emergency obstacles. All motor cars have been taken over by the Japanese military authorities, so transportation difficulties are particularly great. However we hear that Dr A.S. Wong has been fortunate in securing a motor-cycle which he uses on his daily visits, while Dr W.S. Fu has borrowed a tandem bicycle for two persons, himself sitting at the back while his former chauffeur pedals and steers in front.(109)

The United Nations Relief and Rehabilitation Administration was formally established in 1943 and called into China in the

1945-47 period. Their report set the scene:

Even before the war the Chinese people, with severe population pressure, an extremely low standard of living and a
minimum of surplus production available as reserve against
disaster, were constantly beset by recurrent droughts,
floods, epidemics, famines and civil unrest. The new Nationalist Government had just begun the gigantic task of encouraging modernization and new economic development.
During the war, havoc was widespread and economic
deterioration deepened steadily. Civilian casualties were
innumerable. Millions of people were forced to flee as refu-
gees from their homes. Huge tracts of fertile farmland were
flooded. Agricultural production declined. Starvation increased;
nutritional and contagious diseases spread. The nation's
meagre transportation system was largely disrupted or
destroyed. Industrial centres were bombed, shelled and
looted. Thousands of cities, towns and villages were laid
waste.(110)

The resulting disease pattern was overwhelming

Between 1937 and 1949 outbreaks of cholera occurred every
year. There were 34,519 cases of cholera in the epidemic of
1939.... Plague broke out in North East China every year
during the Japanese occupation. Infant mortality during the
war markedly increased. For instance the statistics of one
district of Beijing showed the IMR rising to 190 per thousand
during the war years.(111)

The causes of death were mainly related to malnutrition,
prematurity, tetanus neonatorum and pneumonia. A comparative
study on Shanghai schoolchildren of the same age-group for
the years 1938 and 1946 showed that 60 to 80 per cent of the
children in 1946 had marked retardation of development in
weight and height.... In 1948, 18.2 per cent of the students
of Peking University suffered from tuberculosis.(112)
Some eighteen years after the grandiose plans for the new
NHA had been laid little change for the mass of the people had
been achieved. Inadequacy and maldistribution of health care
resources and the underdevelopment of public health remained
major problems. As a 'CMJ' editorial said in 1944:

China has never had a competent health service... in Nanking in 1929 the foundations of a modern public health
service were laid. But a very small percentage of the population could be reached and vast problems in the public
health field, e.g. sanitation, control of epidemics, infant
and maternal welfare, general medical care and social diseases
were barely touched upon. However a model programme was
worked out for health organization in the provinces, cities

and rural districts so that a minimal service could be given to the people.(113)

The reason for this failure was partly due to the devastation of war but also to the incompetence and corruption of the ruling Guomindang.

## HEALTH CARE ORGANISATION IN THE COMMUNIST-BASE AREAS

In the communist-base areas under very primitive conditions a different kind of development was taking place. The Chinese Communist Party moved their base to the countryside in the 1926-7 period. They had managed to form 'soviets' in some country areas but were kept on the move by Jiang Jieshi's 'extermination' campaigns. The legendary Long March was undertaken to evade encirclement and eventually more secure 'guerilla-base areas' were founded in Northern China with head-quarters in Yanan. In these areas the Communists were able to support fundamental social change with land reform and the overthrow of feudal social relations. Co-operative ventures were encouraged including rural medical co-operatives, which brought basic medical care within reach of the peasants.

The immediate and continuing problem, however, was how to cope with war casualties. In Yanan caves were dug in the loess hillside and converted into wards. One witness reports:

The hospital is an unusual place. Rows of caves in a steep, yellow hillside are its wards, with over 200 beds. The doctors' and nurses' caves at the bottom of the hill are surrounded by vegetable gardens where all the staff and even patients who are well enough do their production work. The 'corridors' and 'elevators' of the hospital are steep, narrow paths, slippery with mud when it rains. The hospital has no electricity, no running water and no pressure sterilizers. The only X-ray set is practically unserviceable for lack of spare parts and films....

On my way through the various departments I saw instrument sterilizers made of old gasoline cans, catgut containers used as test tubes, cuticle scissors serving the ophthalmologists for eye operations, and strange contraptions of old dye cans and cardboard for eye testing. I heard of doctors who for days carried test tubes with bacterial cultures on their bodies to secure the even temperature which is needed for their growth.(114)

The blockade by the Japanese and Guomindang meant very few modern drugs were available, and those were kept firmly under lock and key. Permission for use was only granted after joint consultation between the doctors. Traditional herbal

medicines were widely used, and traditional prescriptions tested.
This experience was crucial in moulding the Communist Party's
view on the role of traditional medicine. Home production of
smallpox vaccine and injections such as 'sheep liver extract'
were carried out. The sheep guts were used to make 'catgut'
thread and the bones turned into medical charcoal. Calcium was
obtained from ground-up eggshells, while willow twigs boiled
in vinegar substituted for aspirin. Toasted wheat husks wrapped
in cloth took the place of hot water bottles and silk worms
were cultivated for silk thread. Glass ampoules for injection
were manufactured and surgical instruments were made out of
bomb fragments and other scrap.(115)

One hospital in Yanan was called the Bethune Memorial International Peace Hospital after the Canadian surgeon who worked
in the guerilla-base area. He died of septicaemia from an infected
cut caused whilst performing emergency surgery. One of his
major contributions was to encourage mobile medical units to
keep near the fighting. He emphasised mobility and the benefit
of early treatment for the war wounded. Medical assistants
were trained in the principles of first aid and surgical dressing
with little formal education. Temporary hospitals were made
from old temples, inns or peasant houses wherever necessary.

There were other International Peace Hospitals (IPH) and
they came into being following the International Peace Campaign
Conference in 1938, and the efforts of the China Defence League.
Dr Norman Bethune was sent by the American and Canadian
League for Peace and Democracy and became the first Director.(116) By the end of the struggle there were eight central
hospitals and forty-two branches accommodating 11,800 beds.
There was not a single IPH that did not have to move once and
many were continually mobile. Following Bethune's death in
1939 eight Bethune medical schools were established in connection with the IPH. In addition to this, numerous short-term
training courses for first-aid workers, sanitation workers,
nurses and midwives were set up. The China Medical College
in Yanan had a teaching staff of fifteen and trained 210 students
in medicine and surgery. They had shorter courses of three
years.(117)

Perhaps of equal significance was the basic public health and
hygiene work that was carried out in the army and villages.
The fact that this was taken seriously by the Communist
leadership was shown both by constitutional statements and
the level of leadership involvement. For instance the 'People's
right to freedom from ill health' was affirmed in item 3 of the
'Rights of the People' in the constitutional principles of the
Shaanxi-Gansu-Ningxia border region. In the Shanxi-Qahar
Hebei border region article 11 of the Administrative Programme
pledged 'to promote the hygiene and sanitation movement and
to improve public health in order to prevent disaster caused by
disease'.(118)

An independent outsider supported the view that public

health work was treated seriously:

> The importance attached to anti-epidemic work for example
> can be judged from the fact that the Chairman of the central
> anti-plague committee of the newly established administrative
> council is a vice-Premier of the central government. This
> committee has recently dealt with an outbreak of plague in
> Chahar province and as part of the rigorous measures of
> control used only 144 cases occurred whereas during the
> epidemic of 1947 there were over 30,000 cases. Insecticides
> were not used but a *cordon sanitaire* was created by the use
> of inoculation and the destruction of fifteen million rats. In
> Manchuria during the summer and autumn of 1949 nearly
> eight million people, a fifth of the total population, were
> inoculated against cholera, typhoid and plague.(119)

The same report tells of the *xian*-based mobile teams who
could respond to emergencies or epidemics. They worked in
co-operation with the village health workers and involved the
peasants themselves in the task of securing and maintaining
hygienic conditions. Villages challenged each other for the
title of 'cleanest village in the district'. The locally formed
medical co-operatives had elected representatives and co-
ordinated local activity. One task was to fight against the 'witch
doctors'.

> The witch doctors are banned, they are dangerous. We got
> rid of them by introducing them in 'yangko' plays so that
> the people laughed at them and we got them better jobs –
> gave them farms – anything as long as they would stop harm-
> ing the people. The herb doctors, the acupuncturists and
> the midwives we kept but we gave them training in the
> essentials of Western Medicine. Chinese herb-doctors have
> done an enormous lot of good.(120)

The encouragement of local initiative was part of the so-
called 'mass line' which was to be so crucial in the post-1949
period.

> The mass movements are of central importance to us; all
> our policies are carried out through them. To carry on a
> prolonged war and to achieve progress in every field, we
> have to rely on the masses of the people. We could not rely
> on bureaucratic methods or a dictatorship if we did not want
> to fail as the KMT did. We had to mobilise the masses, to
> awaken, educate and guide them to the goal of self help.(121)

It was this kind of attitude and example that the communist-
controlled areas shared. The experience in public health work,
preventive medicine, mass movements and integration with
traditional Chinese medicine was to be crucial in determining

future policies. The civil war that followed the Japanese capitulation in 1945 culminated in the Communist victory in 1949. The victory had widespread popular support and it offered a new hope for China after years of war.

NOTES

1 R.H. Tawney, 'Land and Labour in China', George Allen & Unwin, London, 1932, pp. 76-7.
2 Hodgkin, 'Living Issues in China', London, Allen & Unwin, 1932, p. 101.
3 News and Notes, Labour Conditions in Yunnan Tin Mines, 'Chinese Medical Journal', 52, 1937, pp. 294-6.
4 Marion Yang, Birth Control in Peiping, 'CMJ', 48, 1934, pp. 786-9.
5 P.L. Fan, Chinese Infants and Children. A Study of the Infant and Child Mortality, size of the family and sex ratio on 2,500 cases, 'CMJ', 47, 1933, p. 657, quoted from Canton series of Chan and Wright, 'CMJ', 39, 1925, p. 687.
6 Hsu and Chu, Statistics concerning births and deaths in the children of 2168 Chinese families, 'National Medical Journal of China', XVI, 1930, pp. 744-55.
7 P.L. Fan (Cheeloo University Hospital, Tsinan), Chinese infants and children. A study of the infant and child deaths, size of the family and sex ratio on 2,500 cases, 'CMJ', 49, op. cit., 1933, pp. 652-61.
8 Hsu and Wang, A study of infant mortality in Nanking, 'CMJ', 50, 1936, pp. 573-80.
9 Chang, Lai, Chu, A note on the IMR in Kao-chiao, Shanghai, 'CMJ', 50, 1936, pp. 581-2.
10 Vital statistics of Ting Hsien, 'CMJ'. 51, 1937, pp. 1021-2.
11 Lydia Fehily, The prevention of beri-beri, 'CMJ', 60, July 1941, pp. 55-6.
12 Ibid.
13 Lai and Chu, The Kutsing (Yunnan) Health Demonstration Centre. A review for 1939-40, 'CMJ', 59, 1941, pp. 468-75.
14 Cheng Mei Yu, An investigation of infant mortality and its causes in Chengtu, 'CMJ', 62, 1944, pp. 47-54.
15 Han Suyin, 'Birdless Summer', London, Jonathan Cape, 1968, p. 162.
16 J. Heng Liu (Director of the NHA and of the Central Field Station), Hygiene and public health - some phases of public health work in China, 'CMJ', 48, 1934, pp. 70-3.
17 Huang, Developing a railway health service, 'CMJ', 49, 1935, pp. 973-89.
18 Yao Hsun-yuan, Industrial health work in Peiping special health area, 'CMJ', 43, 1929, pp. 379-84.
19 Chang, Blindness among the Chinese, 'CMJ', 67, March 1949, pp. 169-70.
20 E. Burnett, General principles governing the prevention

of TB, 'Quarterly Bulletin of Health Organisation', Geneva
1: 489, 1932.

21 Chiao, Project on BCG vaccination for China, 'CMJ', 66,
October 1948, pp. 568-75.

22 Gear, CMA 'Special Report Series', no. 11, June 1940,
p. 75.

23 Ibid., p. 87.

24 Ibid., p. 83.

25 S. Gamble, 'Peking - A Social Survey', New York, Doran,
1921, p. 249.

26 Lai and Chang, Syphilis and prostitution in Kiangsu, 'CMJ',
42, 1928, pp. 558-63. From Feng Dja-chien, 'Prostitution
in Shanghai', MA thesis, Shanghai College Library, 1929,
pp. 195-202.

27 Ibid.

28 Chu and Huang, Gonorrhoea among prostitutes, 'CMJ',
66, June 1948, pp. 312-18.

29 Wu Lien-teh, Chun, Pollitzer, Wu, C.Y., Cholera - A
manual for the medical profession in China, 'National
Quarantine Service', Shanghai Station, 1934, p. 197.

30 G.F. Winfield, Studies on the control of fecal-borne diseases in North China, 'CMJ', 51, February 1937, p. 221.

31 Ibid., p. 223.

32 Gear, op. cit., p. 159.

33 Heng Liu and Chu, Problems of nutrition and dietary
requirements in China, 'CMJ', 61, April-June 1943, no. 2,
p. 107.

34 P.T. Kuo, Cardio-vascular manifestation of beri-beri,
'CMJ', 55, 1939, p. 427.

35 Lydia Fehily, The prevention of beri-beri, 'CMJ', 60,
July 1941, pp. 53-65.

36 Chen, Yu, Li, Seven years of Jennerian vaccination in
Tinghsien, 'CMJ', 51, June 1937, no. 6, pp. 953-62.

37 Wu Lien-teh, 'Plague Fighter - The Autobiography of a
Modern Chinese Physician', Cambridge, Heffer & Sons,
1959, p. 33.

38 Ibid., p. 25.

39 Ibid., p. 37.

40 Ibid., p. 38.

41 Ibid., p. 41.

42 Ibid., p. 351.

43 C.K. Wong and Wu Lien-teh, 'History of Chinese Medicine',
Tientsin Press, 1932, p. 439.

44 Ibid., p. 434.

45 W.W. Peter, Director of Council on Health Education, The
field and methods of public health work in the missionary
enterprise, 'CMJ', vol. XL, no. 3, March 1926.

46 Ibid., pp. 185-6.

47 Ibid., p. 210.

48 Public Health Notes: Nanchang Health Campaign, 'CMJ',
49, no. 7, July 1935, p. 705.

49 Peter, op. cit., p. 206.
50 Lennox, A self survey of Mission Hospitals in China, 'CMJ', vol. XLVI, 1932, p. 530.
51 Wong and Wu, op. cit., p. 455.
52 Ibid., p. 455.
53 Ibid., p. 496.
54 Wu, op. cit., p. 478.
55 Kuang, The treatment of opium and narcotic addiction, 'CMJ', 51, 1937, pp. 815-20.
56 Wong and Wu, op. cit., p. 361.
57 Ibid., p. 429, 'as in other parts of the world it is called the Red Crescent Society in Muslim areas'.
58 Tung Fang-ming, The National Red Cross Society of China, 'People's China', 16 August 1952.
59 J.E. Bowers, American private aid at its peak: PUMC, in Bowers and Purcell, 'Medicine and Society in China', New York, Josiah Macy Jr Foundation, 1974, p. 85.
60 News and Notes, 'CMJ', 52, July 1937, p. 119.
61 Lennox, The distribution of medical school graduates in China, 'CMJ', vol. XLVI, 1932, pp. 404-11.
62 J.E. Bowers, 'Western Medicine in a Chinese Palace - PUMC 1917-1951', New York, Josiah Macy Jr Foundation, 1972.
63 Prospectus of Medical Schools, 'CMJ', 49, 1935, pp. 998-1034.
64 J.E. Bowers, American private aid at its peak, op. cit., p. 85.
65 Wong and Wu, op. cit., p. 456.
66 Ibid., p. 319.
67 Bowers, op. cit., p. 85.
68 Wills, The Chinese doctor, 'British Medical Journal', 33, 22 September 1928, pp. 536-7.
69 Ch'en, State medicine and medical education, 'CMJ', 49, 1935, pp. 951-4.
70 Editorial, 'CMJ', 62, October-December 1944, no. 4, p. 389.
71 Rajchman, 'CMJ', vol. XLIV, no. 7, June 1930, China Medical Association, League of Nations Health Organisation. Proposals of the National Govt. of the Republic of China for collaboration with the League of Nations on Health Matters.
72 Lee Tao, Some statistics on medical schools in China for the year 1933-4, 'CMJ', 49, 1935, pp. 894-902.
73 S.M. Tao, Medical education of Chinese women, 'CMJ', 47, 1933, pp. 1010-28.
74 Wong and Wu, op. cit., p. 333.
75 S.M. Tao, ibid.
76 Ibid.
77 Arthur Woo, Presidential Address, 'CMJ', vol. XLIII, no. 2, February 1929, pp. 152-63.
78 The hospitals, 'CMJ', 48, no. 10, October 1934, pp. 1080-2.
79 Knud Faber, Editorial and Report on medical schools in China, 'CMJ', vol. XLVI, no. 1, January 1932.
80 Medical Education, 'CMJ', 49, 12 December 1935, pp. 1062-5.

81 W.G. Lennox, The distribution of medical graduates in China, 'CMJ', vol. XLVI, 4 April 1932, pp. 404-11.

82 Hsi-Ju Chu and Daniel G. Lai, Distribution of modern trained physicians in China, 'CMJ', 49, 1934, pp. 542-52.

83 J.T. Hart, The Inverse Care Law, 'Lancet', I, 1971, p. 405.

84 Chu and Lai, op. cit., p. 547.

85 Ibid., p. 549.

86 T. Huang, Development of Health Centres, 'CMJ', 55, June 1939, pp. 546-60.

87 F. Oldt, Scientific medicine in Kwangtung, 'CMJ', 48, 1934, pp. 663-71.

88 Wang and Wang, The potential field of medical and public health work in Nanking, 'CMJ', 49, 1934, p. 549.

89 Grant, State Medicine - a logical policy for China, 'National Medical Journal of China', 14: 119, 1928.

90 Struthers, The relations of medical school to the rural health program, 'CMJ', 52, September 1937, pp. 447-9.

91 Public Health Notes, Health work in Kiangsi, 'CMJ', 52, January 1937, p. 102.

92 Universities and Colleges, (Cheeloo University, Tsinan), 'CMJ', 48, no. 1, p. 81.

93 Correspondence (George Pearson, Paoking, Hunan), 'CMJ', vol. XLVI, no. 6, June 1932, pp. 643-4.

94 Henke, Equipment for a country clinic, 'CMJ', vol. XLVI, 1932, pp. 908-10.

95 Min Ch'ien and Tyau, 'Two years of Nationalist China', Kelly & Walsh, Shanghai, 1930, p. 263.

96 Bernard Read, Chinese Pharmacopoeia, 'CMJ', vol. XLIV, no. 6, June 1930.

97 Barat, The pharmaceutical situation in China, 'CMJ', 47, no. 4, April 1933, p. 405.

98 Ibid.

99 Heng-liu, Hygiene and public health - some phases of public health work, 'CMJ', 48, no. 1, January 1934.

100 Yen, Medicine of future China, 'CMJ', 50, 1936, p. 156.

101 Wu Lien-teh, Fundamentals of state medicine, 'CMJ', 51, no. 6, June 1937, p. 789.

102 Ibid., p. 790.

103 Ch'en, Some problems of medical organisation in rural China, 'CMJ', 51, June 1937, pp. 803-14.

104 Ibid.

105 Ibid., p. 813.

106 Difficulties of a Chinese army surgeon, editorial, 'CMJ', 61, no. 2, April-June 1943, p. 182.

107 Ibid.

108 Proceedings of the 7th General Conference of CMA, 5-10 May 1949, 'CMJ', 65, July-August 1947, p. 297.

109 News and Notes, 'CMJ', vol. 61, no. 1, January-March 1943, p. 89.

110 Operational Analysis Papers no. 53, UNRRA in China

1945-1947, April 1948, United Nations Relief and Rehabilitation Administration Washington DC, p. 3.

111 Fang Shih-shan, Effects of war on the health of the people, 'CMJ', 71, no. 5, September-October 1953, p. 322.

112 Ibid., p. 323.

113 Editorial, 'CMJ', 62, no. 1, January-March 1944, p. 83.

114 Gunther Stein, 'The Challenge of Red China', London, Pilot Press, 1945, pp. 216-17.

115 Accounts of Gunther Stein and Ma Hai-teh, The International Peace Hospitals in The twenty years of the China Welfare Institute, 'CWI', 1958, pp. 77-80.

116 See Ted Allan and Sydney Gordon, 'The Scalpel and the Sword: The Story of Doctor Norman Bethune', New York, Monthly Review Press, 1952.

117 Ma Hai-teh, op. cit., p. 71.

118 Hsia Tao-tai, Laws on public health (p. 113), in J. Quinn (ed.), 'Medicine and Public Health in the Peoples Republic of China', Washington, John Fogarty Center, 1972.

119 W. Tuckman (Friends Service Unit), Rural health problems in China, 'Lancet', 8 March 1950, p. 509.

120 R. Payne, 'China Awake', London, Heinemann, 1947, pp. 358-61 (interview with Ma Hai-teh in Yenan).

121 G. Stein, 'The Challenge of Red China', op. cit., p. 175.

# 3 HEALTH CARE AND WELFARE IN CHINA – THE 'TEN GREAT YEARS', 1949–59

## J.A. Jewell and S.M. Hillier

The Chinese Communist armies moved swiftly through the country from their Northern bases in 1948 and 1949. Mao Zedong was able to declare the formation of the People's Republic of China on 1 October 1949.

In health care terms what faced the new government was daunting. The United Nations Relief Organisation had reported in 1948 that:

China presents perhaps the greatest and most intractable public health problem of any nation in the world. Underlying this problem is the excessive pressure exerted by a vast and still growing population against limited economic resources and production.(1)

The task that faced the new leaders was enormous. Their experience over twenty years had been in a state of siege in very isolated rural and mountainous areas. These guerilla bases were quite different from the cosmopolitan centres, such as Shanghai, Guangzhou and Beijing, over which they would now assume control. Despite this the leadership adhered to the principles developed during their guerilla experience and were thus able to swiftly formulate their national policy.

On 29 September 1949 'The Common Programme of the Chinese People's Political Consultative Conference' was adopted and Article 40 stated: 'National physical culture shall be promoted. Public health and medical work shall be expanded and attention shall be paid to the protection of the health of mothers, infants and children.'(2)

Within a year the new Ministry of Health had called the First National Health Conference which declared three fundamental principles for the Administration: to serve the workers, peasants and soldiers; to emphasise preventive medicine; and to unite 'old-style doctors' and those trained in modern methods.(3)

These objectives were to remain the cornerstone for health policies over the following thirty years with political changes reflecting degrees of emphasis rather than complete redirection. Baseline data for the period is inevitably imprecise but some estimates for a health profile of China at this time are shown in Table 3.1.

These figures showed a poor, growing, largely rural population, suffering from malnutrition, infectious diseases, and

Table 3.1 Vital rates and health care resources in China, 1949

| | |
|---|---|
| Estimated population | c. 450-550 million[a] (85% rural) |
| Crude death rate | c. 30/1000[b] |
| Crude birth rate | c. 40/1000[b] |
| Infant mortality rate | c. 200/1000[b] |
| No. of Western trained doctors | c. 10-40,000[c] |
| No. of traditional practitioners | c. 276,000[d]-500,000[b] |
| No. of hospital beds | c. 70-90,000[e] |
| No. of hospitals | c. 600[f] |

(a) L.A. Orleans, Population dynamics in J. Quinn (ed.), 'Medicine and Public Health in the PRC', Washington, John Fogarty Center, 1972, estimated 540 million. The UNRRA estimate in 1948 was 450 million ('Operational Analysis Papers', no. 53, April 1948, p. 119).

(b) H. Chabot, The Chinese system of health care, 'Trop. geogr. Med.', 28, 1976, p. S98-S102.

(c) Ibid. Low estimates start at 10-12,000 (Chen, 1961) with the highest being 40,000 (Orleans). The CMJ recorded 13,000 registered practitioners in 1947, (65, 1947, p. 265, 7th General Conference of the CMA). Ma Wen Kan from Ministry of Public Health Sources (1981) gives 38,000.

   T.H. Chen, Science, scientist and politics, 'Sciences in Communist China', 68, Washington, American Association for the Advancement of Science, 1961.

   L.A. Orleans, Medical education and manpower in Communist China, in C.T. Hu (ed.), 'Aspects of Chinese Education', New York, Columbia University Teachers' College Press, 1969.

(d) Ma Wen-kan, Ministry of Public Health, Beijing, personal communication August 1981.

(e) Li Teh-Chuan (Li Dequan), Health work in New China, 'People's China', vol. II, no. 7, October 1950, p. 11.

(f) H. Chabot, op. cit., estimated 600.

poor housing. The ill health this generated had to be dealt with by a limited urban-based medical service, and biased towards curative acute style medicine rather than public health or preventive work. China in 1949 was the 'sick man of Asia'. Today it is not. This makes the story of the transformation relevant for political leaders and people of the developing world.

EARLY PUBLIC HEALTH WORK, INOCULATION AND EDUCATION

An adequate public health policy was regarded as the key to success. In 1950 an American journalist noted the following reaction to the new public health campaign:

'Sure its been overdue for centuries' was a familiar refrain at the French Club Bar 'but only the Communists are crazy

enough to undertake it!' My amah, Fu Ma, a rugged indi-
vidualist in all things, dismissed it with a contemptuous
'Nobody is going to stick us with needles!' Sze Shing, the
office boy at the Review, chuckled, 'Suddenly all sickness
will stop and everyone will live ten thousand years'.(4)

Despite those attitudes the Minister of Health was able to
report that in the first six months of 1950 health workers gave
fifty million vaccinations and inoculations against smallpox,
TB, cholera, plague and typhoid.(5) She also reported on the
work of special anti-epidemic teams, and an anti-plague campaign in north-east China which had mobilised the people to
kill 14,590,000 rats in 1949. Basic refuse clearance and clean-
up campaigns were organised such as that which involved
73,537 volunteers in Beijing, who shifted 201,638 tons of
garbage.(6)

After just two years the Ministry of Health reported that over
200 million people had been vaccinated against smallpox and
that no new cases had been reported for the major cities and
only sporadic cases in the countryside. Over 30 million people
in potential cholera areas had been inoculated and quarantine
stations and water purification schemes had been established.
No new cases of cholera had been reported by then.(7)

Environmental measures were crucially important in public
health work, and city clean-ups were undertaken:

Outside the East Gate of Yenching lay Ch'eng-fu village
....Rubbish lay in its streets, odd corners and waste
patches became public conveniences. Mangy dogs scrounged
round the garbage dumps. A stream which ran between
Ch'eng-fu and the university wall was a stinking open
sewer, with broken-down banks. Whenever it rained the
mud roads became ankle deep in sludge. In our thirty years
of proximity and sporadic good intentions Yenching had
been unable to get the village cleaned up.

But as soon as the People's Army came to be quartered on
the village soldiers began to sweep the streets and build
proper latrines. Then with the new administration came more
basic changes.

A system of refuse collection was started and the people
became proud of the new appearance of the village. Our cook,
who lived there, told us proudly that the village had won a
red silk banner for civic responsibility.(8)

A summary of the main urban public health policies was outlined by the Director of Beijing's Health Department in 1952.
They included refuse control, clearing of dumps and street
cleaning, latrines to be closed and some septic tanks provided.
A supply of clean piped water was made available. Measures to
control dogs were also instituted. Mass health campaigns particularly against flies and mosquitoes were carried out, using the

mass organisations, with one person responsible for organising ten households. Posters, meetings, plays and contests were used with the slogan 'Everybody needs health' and 'To protect the health of the People is the People's duty'.(9)

Health consciousness amongst the public was increasing and the authorities achieved this through propaganda and by example. An interesting aspect was the changed attitude to sports and fitness:

> During 1951 and 1952 we observed a profound change in the attitudes of our students to exercise. For thirty years the university administration had struggled against the old scholars' attitude - that manual labour was undignified, exercise was a waste of time and defeat in sports a loss of face. Students being urged to play football are said to have retorted: 'If you need to have that ball kicked about you can pay coolies to do it'.(10)

The new government, recognising the poor state of health of the students, proposed after consultation that a '50-1-8 system' should be adopted. This recommended no more than fifty hours' of work each week, one hour's exercise each day and eight hours' sleep at night. Students themselves began to organise their games and it was during this period that the early morning radio exercises were introduced. Newspapers published diagrams with instructions and later there was even a complete set of forty postage stamps intended to popularise the exercises. Each morning at 7.15 a.m. university staff, students and workers turned out to do their physical jerks during the 12-minute musical sequence.(11) These examples perhaps give some idea of the new optimism that had spread through the country in the early 1950s and revolutionised people's attitudes and values.

## BACTERIOLOGICAL WARFARE

Hopes of a complete unification of the country and peaceful reconstruction were dashed by the blockade of the Taiwan straits by the US Navy, protecting Jiang Jieshi, and the outbreak of the Korean War. The new government sent volunteer military units up to the Korean border area. The most important consequence of this development for the new health services was the problem of bacteriological warfare.

There had been reports of the Japanese using such tactics in 1940. The Director General of National Health Service Administration under the Guomindang in a lengthy report said that:

> Japanese planes again visited Kinghwa in Chekiang and there scattered small yellowish granules of shrimp egg size which contained numerous gram negative bipolar stained

micro-organisms that resembled morphologically the plague
bacilli. . . . On the strength of this evidence, it was believed
that the plague in Ningpo and Chuhsien was the result of
Japanese attempts at bacterial warfare.(12)

The Communist government now alleged that the Americans
were using bacterial warfare against the Koreans and Chinese.
To investigate this an International Scientific Commission was
set up by the World Peace Council in 1952.(13) This Commission,
which included Joseph Needham, toured North China and
reported on the evidence that the Chinese authorities had
amassed. Disease vectors such as insects, voles, seafood, rags,
feathers and grain were dropped from aircraft carrying strains
of plague, cholera and anthrax. Suspicion was aroused by
epidemic outbreaks which did not correlate with climatic conditions or occupational risk factors.
The Chinese response to this challenge was thorough and
efficiently organised. For example, when 717 plague infected
voles were dropped in Gannan 'xian' in Heilongjiang province
the authorities responded immediately:

Traffic cordons were thrown around infected areas, and the
public advised to patch up holes in the walls and use DDT
sprays. Rats and mice were killed, and their holes sprayed.
Cats and dogs were killed, the population inoculated and
houses and wells thoroughly cleaned.(14)

The co-ordination and discipline of the large numbers of
people mobilised impressed the Commission who noted:

As one listened to all these people one began to see something previously unknown - a terrible, strange and touching
epic unfolding itself in front of one's eyes. One could see
hundreds, indeed thousands of people with improvised
masks, hand protection and chopstick-tweezers made of
cornstalks in their hands, move slowly day after day over
their own countryside stopping to collect small insects and
feathers one by one.(15)


MASS CAMPAIGNS

The Central Government launched a mass patriotic health and
sanitation campaign in the spring of 1952 and, as they noted,
'one of the important factors for the success of this patriotic
movement has been the indignation and hatred aroused in the
people towards the US imperialists who are waging bacteriological warfare against Korea and China'.(16) This became more
formalised when a special Patriotic Public Health Campaign
Committee was set up in December 1952 on instructions from
the Government Administrative Council.(17) Their task was to

plan for a massive spring campaign in 1953.

Public health campaigns became a regular feature in Chinese life under the Communist government. Particular dates would be chosen for 'shock attacks', e.g. Spring Festival or May Day. Particular targets would be chosen such as flies or mosquitoes, the spitting habit, house and street cleaning. Thousands would be mobilised - workers, students and schoolchildren with loud-speakers, banging drums, marched with banners, charts and diagrams. Street theatres would also be used to spread the message. Sanitation committee members would even tour the area doing random household inspections.(18) Of course not all the campaigns were well organised and criticisms arose about the unnecessary disruption of production; some questioned the need for them while some cadres and intellectuals felt it was 'beneath them'.(19)

One writer describes a campaign to kill grain-eating sparrows.

I was one of the warriors in the Peking battle against the birds, which demonstrated the ingenuity and organizational skill of the Chinese. One Spring day was set as the time for the final crushing assault. On every building, in every street in front yards, in backyards, people stood or sat and waved white cloths and shouted, whistled or beat on pans, wherever sparrows appeared. I was perched on a high garden wall with a pillowcase and I flapped and whooshed for hours.

Confused and hungry the birds plunged into net snares, alighted on limed branches, ate poisoned food laid out in areas purposely left open. Thousands upon thousands were eliminated that day.(20)

Later the authorities realised that the sparrows were an inappropriate target and bedbugs were substituted instead!

The results of this unprecedented public health movement showed up in the rapidly improving health statistics. The infant mortality in Beijing had fallen from the 1949 level of 117.6/1,000 live births to 59.3 in 1953.(21) Maternal mortality was almost halved and there have been no epidemics of cholera or smallpox between 1950 and 1956.(22) In the rural areas the changes were less dramatic but were beginning. Apart from the mobile anti-epidemic units that operated throughout the country there were some specific campaigns, for example sandfly control to prevent the spread of kala-azar, and campaigns against malaria, schistosomiasis and hookworm.(23) The county health centres were seen as the basic organisational unit for the rural areas and by 1952 they were in operation in 85 per cent of all counties.(24) There were also 1,498 'zhu' sub-district centres. They formed the framework for a rural health network in which, because of the scale involved, transportation and communication difficulties were to prove to be the greatest challenge. Sending trained medical personnel to China's vast rural areas has been likened to 'tossing grains of sand into the ocean'.


## THE CHINESE MEDICAL PROFESSION AND THE COMMUNIST PARTY, 1950-7

The impact the new Communist government had on the medical profession of Guomindang China was dramatic. Many of the well established doctors had fled the country of course in the 1948-9 period and thus contributed to the already severe shortage of trained personnel. Those that remained waited anxiously for the People's Government to act. Their worst fantasies, developed under the Guomindang regime, did not come about and soon the 'Chinese Medical Journal' was able to report 'An Appreciation'.

> Since the liberation of Shanghai on 25th May 1949 the Journal has not met the fate predicted by many. On the contrary our Journal was registered with the proper authority and was among the few in the first batch of journals approved by the Military Control Commission.(25)

*Traditional medicine*
One of the first contentious issues between the profession and the Communist Party was that of traditional Chinese medicine. The Chinese Medical Association, representing doctors qualified in modern scientific medicine, had always wanted proper registration of doctors and ultimately the exclusion of traditional practitioners from recognition as bona fide medical practitioners. A group of CMA members had met in June 1949 to discuss plans for the future under the new government. These plans included the eradication of traditional medicine.(26) This attitude of Western trained practitioners was to be a source of recurring conflict between the Party and the profession, throughout the 1950s.

These discontents were to surface again during the Hundred Flowers Movement in 1957. Criticism was made of the poor research record of the Institute of Traditional Medicine and it was suggested that its task should be merely to write the history of traditional medicine. The feeling among Western trained doctors was that much of traditional medicine was quackery which deceived the patients and ultimately delayed more appropriate treatment.


*Specialisation*
Apart from this question there was also the obvious political differences a Communist government would expect from a conservative profession. One of these differences was about the role of expert knowledge; the health care needs of the country were huge, but relatively little attention was paid by Western-trained doctors whose aspirations were for a medicine with the

same worldwide scientific status as found in major Western countries. The president of the CMA felt obliged to comment on this attitude:

The *Chinese Medical Journal* is of course a specialised and learned publication, and we do not expect it to be a periodical for the masses. But we should insist on having more articles which answer the needs of the people. In our Journal there are very few articles on health work in the country-side, in factories and mines and with the armed forces. There are also very few articles on Chinese medicine and popular cures.(27)

The first eight presidents of the CMA had been European or American trained.(28) The group was very influential and well represented in the Ministry of Health. Mao recognised this early, and in 1953 on two separate occasions he criticised the Ministry for not exercising leadership and for deferring to doctors.(29) Traditional Chinese doctors were only permitted to join the CMA in 1954 and by 1956 they only numbered 1,037, some 6 per cent of the 15,059 membership.(30)

*Relations with the Soviet Union*
Further problems were posed to the profession by the role of medicine, for the Soviet Union was the principal ally of the new government. In 1953 the CMA president exhorted the members:

We should oppose the blind worship of America and Britain and set ourselves against narrow conservatism. We should fully realise that vigorous growth and development of medical science in China is possible only through learning from the Soviet Union.(31)

There is no doubt that Soviet aid was extremely important to the new People's Republic in the early post-liberation period. Doctors and medical equipment were sent and hospitals built with Soviet assistance. Special advisers had influential positions, and medical education was modelled on the Soviet experience. Medical schools were separate from other university faculties, had early specialisation and there were three basic divisions:

higher medical college training - 4-5 years;
intermediate medical school training - 2 years;
basic level training - 3-6 months.

The creation of a group of 'intermediate' doctors ran counter to the CMA's long-held position of maintaining 'quality over quantity' but the Ministry of Health accepted the three-tier system which promoted the Soviet 'feldsher' health worker with limited two-year training. Higher level medical education was retained, however. There were ninety-four two-year 'feldsher' type middle-grade schools. A total enrolment of 55,592 students were studying in 228 nursing and 101 midwifery and doctor's assistant schools. There were also the basic-level schools which 'hundreds of thousands' had been through.(32)

Chinese students were also sent to study in the Soviet Union and in the Five-Year Plan for 1953-7, of the 2,000 students to be sent abroad to study, 1,400 were to go to the Soviet Union and 700 to the People's Democracies and other countries.(33)

Other Soviet influences made themselves felt, too. The design of new hospitals tended to follow the Soviet pattern. Pavlovian theory dominated much psychiatry and tissue therapy was in vogue. In the control of venereal disease in China, the Soviet doctors espoused legalistic methods, like fines and imprisonment, which were inappropriate in the Chinese context. Rather than penicillin, they preferred to prescribe long-term bismuth and mercury injections which were difficult to use, especially in the infected national minority peoples.(34)

In their opposition to Soviet orthodoxy, the doctors had an unusual ally - Mao Zedong. The relationship between the Communist Parties of Russia and China had traditionally been uneasy. The former had experienced an urban, proletarian revolution - the latter a peasant-based guerilla struggle. The intense Chinese nationalism that had developed in the CCP was important in resisting Soviet influence. Mao Zedong referred to the early dogmatism:

> I couldn't have eggs or chicken soup for three years be-
> cause an article appeared in the Soviet Union which said
> that one shouldn't eat them. Later they said one could eat
> them. It didn't matter whether the article was correct or
> not, the Chinese listened all the same and respectfully
> obeyed. In short the Soviet Union was tops.(35)

*Private practice*
The Guomindang government had partly developed a State medical service, but had generally failed to distribute limited resources equitably. The Communist Party was opposed in principle to private practice, but as in other areas of policy their strategy was not to ban outright but to gradually create the conditions which would replace outmoded structures. The aim therefore was to gain some control over private medicine and to encourage its gradual absorption into the State system. A directive on the subject was issued in April 1950 which indicated that private practitioners should be encouraged to join semi-co-operative, united or joint hospitals and clinics. It was hoped to introduce a standardised fee schedule and private practitioners were warned that private hospitals must shoulder part of the responsibility for public health work. The April directive also condemned the view the medical work was simply another form of commercial activity and urged that

private practitioners should concern themselves with service and not just money.(36) In January 1951 provisional regulations governing the management of all private hospitals and clinics were promulgated. An exception was made for clinics operated by Chinese herb doctors. The local government was empowered to issue essential licences and to assess the schedule of fees used. Advertising was to be scrutinised and 'false claims' prohibited.

The directive emphasised the responsibilities of private hospitals in the event of an epidemic, and to preventive work, as well as stating that they could not without proper reason refuse treatment to any person.(37) The main development was that the larger hospitals became public-private joint ventures while the individual private practitioners were encouraged to join together in groups and use a fees-pool system. Individual payment for consultation and treatment persisted for most people in China, but in urban areas at least the medical service became more hospital based. This semi-nationalisation of private facilities meant that in the cities, facilities remained far superior to what was available in rural areas, or small county towns.

## NEW WELFARE PROVISION - LABOUR INSURANCE

*Welfare schemes*
One of the most ambitious schemes that the new Government introduced early on was the Labour Insurance Regulations which came into effect on 1 March 1951.

Under this scheme workers in the larger factories were protected 'from the insecurity that once came from old age, disease, death, disabilities and permanent injuries'.(38) The main benefits are described in Table 3.2. Most are unchanged to the present day.

Table 3.2 Labour insurance schemes in the PRC

---

1 Workers and employees injured as a result of their work are to be provided with all necessary medical expenses, hospital fees and costs for food during hospitalisation, all these expenses to be borne by the state factory management or owners of private enterprise. Full wages are to be paid for the whole period of convalescence.

2 Workers and employees injured as a result of their work and so disabled that they are unable to work are to receive disability pensions from the labour insurance fund according to the degree of disability. The amount of the pension ranges from 60 to 75 per cent of their regular wages. This pension is to continue until the worker recovers, or, if the worker or employee is totally disabled, for the rest of the worker's or employee's life.

3 Workers and employees who become sick or suffer from non-

occupational injuries are to have part of their necessary medical expenses paid by the factory management or owners Besides them, they will receive all or part of their regular wages during the period of convalescence. Such wage payments shall continue for a period of no more than three months. If workers or employees are sick for longer than a three-month period, or are so disabled that they can no longer work, they are to receive disability pensions from the labour insurance fund, the amount to be equivalent to between 20 and 30 per cent of their regular wages. Payments of such pensions also are to continue for the rest of the worker's or employee's life or until recovery.

4 The state factory management or owners of private enterprises are to bear all funeral expenses for workers and employees whose death is due to their occupation. In addition to this, the trade unions concerned will issue monthly pensions from the labour insurance fund to the direct dependents of the deceased worker or employee as long as necessary, the amount to be equivalent to between 25 to 50 per cent of his or her regular wages.

5 For workers and employees who die of disease or non-occupational injuries, subsidies shall be paid out from the labour insurance funds to cover part of their funeral expenses and their dependents are entitled to varying sums of relief payments.

6 Retirement pensions of between 35 to 60 per cent of their regular wages are paid to male workers over the age of sixty and women workers over the age of fifty from the labour insurance fund. To qualify for a retirement pension a worker must have worked for twenty-five years and have a ten-year record in the enterprise or factory from which he retires. In the case of a woman worker, the qualifying periods are twenty years and ten years respectively.

7 A paid maternity leave of fifty-six days is to be given to women workers and employees and a maternity allowance is to be paid from the labour insurance fund.

8 Apart from individual benefits workers and employees are entitled to admission to institutions financed by the labour insurance funds, such as rest houses, sanitoria, houses for the disabled and old age. In the event of a worker's or employee's death, his or her children have the right to enter orphanages.

The expenditure was divided into two funds. The first-category benefits such as maternity leave and medical expenses, are to be paid directly to the workers by the management. The amount will vary from unit to unit. The second is the labour insurance fund, which is paid monthly into the trade union organisations by the state factory management or owners of private enterprises. The amount was equivalent to 3 per cent of the total payroll. Seventy per cent of this fund is allocated

to the various factory trade union organisations for payments
such as retirement pensions, disability pension and pension to
dependents. The remaining 30 per cent is allocated to the All
China Federation of Labour, for the purpose of financing collective labour insurance institutions.(39)

These regulations applied to factories employing more than
one hundred workers whether state or privately owned. The
main reason for this was that both the management and trade
unions of the larger organisation were better organised and
would be able to cope with the regulations. The framework for
these schemes was based on the Soviet model, although because
of the stage of development of Chinese industry there was a
lower level of contribution and benefit.

*Factory hospitals and health centres*
The significance of this radical welfare legislation was that it
now covered 3.3 million workers for at least partial medical
expenses. By 1953 this number had increased to 4.8 million.(40)
With increasing aspirations and demand new facilities and health
services had to be supplied in factories and urban areas. In
1952 the insurance scheme was extended to government employees, e.g. civil servants and teachers, which increased urban
demand for health care still further. One report in 1954 noted
that nearly every factory and mine with over one hundred
workers had its own medical centre. In addition, there were
38,000 beds in the workers' hospitals and sanatoria of major
industrial enterprises like mining and railways. These industries also ran their own medical schools to provide medical staff
for the workers.(41) These industrial enterprises were outside
direct Ministry of Health control and were a response to the
need and pressure on managements based on the Labour Insurance Act. One report in 1952 spoke of an average of one doctor
for 880 workers in Chinese industry.(42) If this is a realistic
figure then it demonstrates the relative privilege of the urban
factory worker at a time when the ratio per Western trained
doctor was of the order of 1:10,000-20,000.(43) By 1958 there
were 13.7 million workers covered by Labour Insurance and
6.8 million eligible for free medical care.(44) Thus there emerged
a semi-independent sector within the health service based on
factories or industries.

*Industrial health and safety*
As soon as the new government came to power, the safety
regulations for coalmines were published in 1950. Health and
safety committees were to be established in every pit. Proper
rest periods were to be observed by workers, and the committees were to ensure healthy working conditions.(45) In the
docks, safety coverings were put on lathes and protection nets
over bridgeways.(46) Part of the incentive was due to the large
number of mining and other accidents. The Xinbo colliery in
Shandong reported eighteen accidents within twenty days.(47)

In the Quingdao Construction company, 107 accidents took place in one month, 5 of them serious. (48)

The new regulations had their effect, with mining accidents falling by 57 per cent in two years and fatal accidents by 58 per cent. (49)

It was not only industrial injury but industrial disease which received attention, and by 1953 specialists were encouraged to pay extensive visits to factories to diagnose difficult and dangerous diseases. (50)

Attention to workers' health would, it was hoped, cut down absenteeism and increase production. Air conditioning, dust extraction, adequate lighting and food improvements were all promoted, but these remedial measures could not take the place of close attention to sanitary practices. In 1953 the Ministries of Labour and Health issued a joint directive to change the emphasis on treatment rather than prevention to 'emphasis on prevention rather than treatment'. (51)

By 1954 factories with low or accident-free records were being publicly praised; the level of industrial safety which the government was hoping to improve can be gauged from their report on three coal mines which 'have had no cases of accidental death... from February 1953 to March 1954'. (52)

Conditions in private enterprises were sometimes below standard. In 1954 in Shanghai the proprietors of six private factories were sentenced to terms of hard labour 'for violation of labour protection laws which had resulted in the death or injury of some workers'. (53)

However, some of these proprietors received suspended sentences. The authorities were not always willing to prosecute, and although regulations were set up, they were not always enforced. The first Five-Year Plan committed the Party and government to the development of heavy industry. This meant a new pace and type of industrial work, and health and safety regulations were often combined with 'labour discipline' regulations. Although absenteeism through ill health threatened production, increased production was often bad for workers' health. A 'People's Daily' editorial in May 1956 complained of the high rate of accidents in factories, mines and construction units since the beginning of the year:

> higher than it had been in the corresponding period of 1955. The main reason was the use of shock methods by some cadres, involving the working of extra shifts. As a result the workers became tired, there are many accidents and State plans are not fulfilled. (54)

The writer ended by insisting that outstanding production invariably went with a good safety record.

Although the Party and state organs were keen to produce better industrial conditions, local cadres and managers often felt the need to fulfil or overfulfil quota responsibilities. Such a practice was almost built into the system and difficult to eradicate. The health organs of factories, mines, and railways, too, tended to concentrate their health efforts on the building of sanatoria and hospitals rather than the mundane work of prevention, although the need for the latter was continually stressed.

State Council regulations on safety and hygiene in factories were passed on 25 May 1956, and applied to all factories employing more than sixteen workers or workshops with more than thirty-one craftsmen.(55) In a strongly worded statement the Zhejiang People's Council supplemented this with a warning that those units which disobeyed 'could be suspended, even if the original production plans were hampered',(56) and the attempt by one metallurgical works to cut production costs by reducing health facilities was criticised for increasing sickness among the workers.(57)

The 'People's Daily' was critical of the practice of cash incentives for extra work, which, it said, was injurious to the people's health: 'workers could not be compelled to work endless extra shifts with little or no attention to their health in violation of the labour protection regulations'.(58)

During the Great Leap Forward, with its emphasis on huge increases in industrial production, one foreign witness reported that workers fainted from exhaustion, and women workers stopped menstruating.(59) The 'People's Daily' was still maintaining that 'safety in production is one of the most important conditions for achieving tremendous leaps in production', but remarked that 'a number of enterprises had neglected this matter, causing unnecessary losses'.(60)

The link between health work and the new emphasis on productivity was stressed:

> Health work must proceed with a view to developing production. The more intense the production, the more attention we must pay to health work; the better the health work is done, the higher will be the production level.(61)

Progress was made in the 'ten great years' to deal with some of the worst and most dangerous aspects of industrial production, but the tension between industrial growth and industrial safety was by no means resolved. A new emphasis on the link between increased production and safety was made during the Great Leap Forward, but since no central government department carried responsibility for industrial health, regulations were extremely difficult to enforce.

*Pharmaceuticals*
The pharmaceutical industry was not well developed in China in 1949. The vast majority of drugs had to be imported and 'the industry was still in a backward state because it was more

concerned with the production of patent medicines than with
the manufacture of essential pharmaceuticals'.(62) Private
ownership predominated and there was real concern about the
quality of the products, chaos in nomenclature and irrational
production of patent medicines rather than basic drugs. As
in other sectors of the economy the new government nationalised
part of the industry, formed public-private agreements with
others and left a wholly private sector. In 1952 and 1955 the
relative proportions were as shown in Table 3.3:

Table 3.3   Relative percentages of state, joint and private
ownership in the pharmaceutical industry

|  | 1952 % | 1955 % |
|---|---|---|
| State and local state | 43.5 | 42.0 |
| Public-private | 6.1 | 22.2 |
| Privately operated | 50.4 | 35.7 |

Source: 'Joint Publications Research Service', 672, 28 August
1955.

The production of penicillin started in 1952 and other drugs
such as sulphathiazole, sulphaguanidine, glucose, ephedrine
and calcium were to follow. The import figures for 1953 represented 38.5 per cent of the national consumption value and the
plan was to decrease this as China became more self-reliant.(63)
Despite increased state intervention, private production was
still predominant even by 1955, and

There was no denying the fact that the existence of private
enterprise impeded the development of state plans relative
to the fixing of prices, the control of quality and the readjustment of the pharmaceutical industry as a whole.(64)

Quality control was difficult and there were stories of blem-
ished tablets and precipitates in ampoules. One private company
in Shanghai had 76 per cent of their quinine dihydrochloride
declared 'unfit for sale' and a Beijing firm had its distilled water
discarded because of impurities.(65) One private producer was
alleged to have said: 'absence of reaction after the administering of an injection' should be accepted as the standard'.(66)
Medical supplies could not match demand, and the volume of
imported medicines in 1956 was 44 per cent greater than in
1955. Imports of injections increased by 36.5 per cent, pills
by 40 per cent, penicillin by 36 per cent, glucose by 108 per
cent and X-ray films by 54 per cent.(67)

The industry was also rather backward in the production of
Chinese herbal and other traditional drugs. The management
of the Chinese National Native Drug Corporation lay with the

Ministry of Commerce, whereas the Pharmaceutical Industry
came under the Ministry of Chemical Industry so there was no
unified policy.(68) Yet home grown herbal treatments were
cheaper than the expensive imported Western medicines and
this was crucial to reduce expenditure on health care, for low
cost medicines could be offered, although these economies
reduced the economic surplus of other Ministries. The State
trading company had to try to stimulate rural production,
especially as over 80 per cent of Chinese took herbal medicines.(69) In 1957 the sale and distribution of drugs was
brought under the control of the Ministry of Health. The Ministry also planned to cut health funds by 52 per cent compared
with 1956.(70) Both these changes were attempts to unify control and cut expenditure.

Attempts to rationalise pharmaceutical production were
hampered by the fact that demand for drugs was high. The
increased availability of health care to urban workers and
cadres under labour insurance legislation meant that they took
advantage of the opportunities offered. This made planning
difficult, particularly if Western drugs were demanded, or if
drugs were used wastefully by those entitled to free medical
care: 'Young cadres students and workers... each year on
average visit a clinic twelve or thirteen times.'(71)

*National minorities*
Another important question was the special health problems of
the minorities, of which there are fifty-six in China, although
the Han Chinese make up 94 per cent of the population.(72)
Although relatively small in number the minority peoples are
strategically important as they occupy large areas of the country
and particularly the sparsely populated border areas. Mao
pointed out in 1956 that they occupy 50 to 60 per cent of China's
total territory, and compared to the Han majority it is the minority nationalities whose territory is vast and whose resources
are rich.(73) The Long March and guerilla-base experience
had impressed the Communist leadership of the need for a
comprehensive nationalities policy. The aim was to preserve
local autonomy, language and culture and permit religious
activity. Laws were promulgated to this effect in 1949 by the
People's Political Consultative Conference in September 1949.(74)
At this time most of the minority peoples lived under a feudalist
system (the Zhuang, Mongolians, Hui and the Uygur); some
under feudal serfdom (for example the Tibetans), and the Yi
People were still a slave society. The peoples of Inner Mongolia
and Xinjiang were nomadic pastoralists. Different religious
beliefs also existed; the Hui, Uzbek, Kazakh and Uygur were
Moslems while the Tibetans, Mongolians and Dai were Budd-
hists.(75) Tibetans and Mongolians also had their own quite
distinct medical traditions while the Moslem cultures retained
a strong Arabic influence in their medical practice.

In health terms the fate of the minorities was showing the

all-too-common signs of an indigenous people being decimated
by the new diseases spread by war and invasion. In Inner
Mongolia the Ikechao League, whose population in the seventeenth century was approximately 400,000, had declined to
about 80,000 by 1949.(76) The Hulunbeir League of the
Dongxingba Banner had a population of 10,368 in 1933 and
only 7,670 in 1950. One investigation in the early 1950s of
2,334 nomadic families showed that 58 per cent had no children.
The Inner Mongolian Chenbaerhu Banner before 1949 had a
death rate in excess of birth rate but this was reversed by
1954.(77) Sexually transmitted diseases were an important
cause of infertility and population decline:

Table 3.4  Syphilitic infection in national minorities

|  | No. | Syphilis sero-positive | % |
|---|---|---|---|
| Inner Mongolia (Mongolian Nomadic) 1950-3 | 163,301 | 78,337 | 48.0 |
| Ganzi, Sichuan (Tibetan) 1952-3 | 32,170 | 9,416 | 29.3 |
| Milleh, Yunnan (Axi) 1957 | 4,814 | 1,348 | 28.0 |
| Hainan Island (Li) 1958 | 7,310 | 1,588 | 21.7 |
| Guangxi (Zhuang) 1959 | 3,302 | 332 | 10.0 |

Source: 'China's Medicine' 1, October 1966.

The highly effective 'mass line' approach to the eradication
of sexually transmitted diseases had by the early 1960s been
successful (see chapter 6).

Among the Walatechien Banner a ten-year follow-up survey
of the 1952 syphilis eradication campaign showed not a single
case of early infectious syphilis in 3,158 persons examined
in 1962. The same Banner had had an incidence of nearly
50 per cent during the first survey in 1952. Another recent
ten-year re-survey of the Jerimu League, Djarod Banner,
in 1965 showed no new cases of infectious syphilis or congenital syphilis in the 3,343 persons examined (97 per cent
of the whole population). Seropositivity of this area in 1952
had been around 35 per cent.(78)

This particular policy had improved the health of national minor
ities. The organisation of a comprehensive system of health
care for national minorities was not made a priority, however,
and received little attention during these ten years. However,
during the Great Leap Forward, medical schools were opened
among minority nationalities, and minority graduates numbered
some 3,600 from intermediate colleges.(79)

THE PARTY AND THE MINISTRY - ISSUES IN THE DEVELOP-
MENT OF HEALTH CARE 1950-9

Developments in the 1950s offer a good example of the close
relationship that obtains between economic growth and health
service development. The First Five-Year Plan laid emphasis on
the need to develop an industrial infrastructure and particularly
stressed heavy industrial plant. Thus the mining, steel and
machine-tool sectors were prioritised in the first plans for the
1953-7 period. However by the 1956 period, with a decline in
Soviet aid, the Twelve-Year Plan for Agricultural Development
showed different Party perspectives appearing. Mao had always
stressed the importance of the peasantry in China's revolution.
Economic development in the rural areas was thus a prominent
political objective. The new 1956 plan made agricultural development the first priority, followed by light industry and then
heavy industry. The National Programme for Agricultural
Development introduced new instructions on health work and
the relationship between health and production was stressed.
    These health policies emphasised that the delivery of health
care should be at the point of production and should seek to
minimise disruption to production. Preventive work was to be
linked to economic developments such as anti-snail drives with
irrigation projects. A typical slogan was 'five-to-the-fields',
which meant that health workers should carry out propaganda,
conduct investigations, provide medicines, give treatment, and
themselves work in the fields.(80)

*Organisational and financial problems*
After the initial honeymoon in the early 1950s some fundamental
problems in the relationships between the Party, Ministry of
Health and medical profession became apparent. One complaint
was that the Ministry of Public Health had 'become divorced
from Party Leadership': 'The most important [problem] is that
numerous health departments to varying degrees have come
under the influence of bourgeois thinking and disregard
political leadership'.(81)
    There was obviously concern at the Party centre that the
Ministry of Public Health was politically suspect, being heavily
influenced by Western trained doctors, and could not be relied
upon to implement Party policy. Two developments examined in
detail in chapter 10 show how, firstly, Mao criticised the
Ministry for its policy on traditional medicine, singling out two
senior officials. Wang Bu, head of the north-east Public Health
Bureau, was alleged to have regarded traditional medicine as
'feudal', and He Cheng, the Vice-Minister of Health, who had a
revolutionary pedigree going back to the Jiangxi Soviet in the
1930s, was relieved of his position for 'being divorced from
Party leadership'. He later admitted publicly to having been
opposed to traditional medicine.(82) Secondly, in 1955 the Party
removed parasite work from Ministry control and formed a

'Nine Man Committee' to take responsibility for it.(83) The feeling was that the professionals had been too cautious and had
dragged their feet on this important area that in the Party's
view would best be implemented by a 'mass line'. The appointees
of the new Committee were mostly political rather than professional and were under the direct supervision of the Party
Central Committee.

*The 'Hundred Flowers' Movement*
With the economic deterioration in 1956 and the disillusionment
with Soviet-style policies that appeared to favour urban development, the leadership looked for a unique Chinese solution.
This was the time of 'destalinisation' in the Soviet Union, and
in China the 'Hundred Flowers' movement of 1957 was designed
to release some of the frustrations felt by the intellectuals. A
number of eminent intellectuals took the opportunity to criticise
the workings of the Party and the Health Ministry. One senior
physician of the China Union Medical College (previously PUMC)
said:

> The quality of the work of Union College has deteriorated.
> It will take Union College a certain period of time to repair
> the damage, the whole of the Union College is in chaos; the
> Party Committees are simply hopeless.(84)

Much of the criticism concerned standards and the need for
quality in education research, pharmaceuticals and medical
equipment.
  Most importantly, these speeches demonstrated the conflict
between the medical profession, with a highly conservative
approach, the Party, who from a lay and political perspective
placed revolutionary objectives first, and the Ministry, which
while serving broad political objectives was organised bureau-
cratically and harnessed to the opposing objectives of health
care expansion, especially rural health, and cost control.
Attempts to resolve some of these difficulties are outlined below.

*Rural health services 1949-58*
Economic priorities geared to agriculture made the expansion of
rural health services a rational objective. Rural health services
had changed relatively little since 1949. The united clinics which
had been formed in the early 1950s were still by 1958 the main
source of medical care. The doctors in these clinics were largely
traditional practitioners and the system remained as 'fee for
service'. Although there were some 30,000 united clinics in the
countryside, many were in a precarious financial state.(85) Inequality in the provision of health care between urban and rural
areas contributed to the pressure for migration to the cities.

*The Great Leap Forward in health care 1958-9*
Considerable progress had been made in the early 1950s in land

reform, thus transforming social relations in the countryside. The feudal relationship of peasant-landlord had been altered stepwise, through the development of mutual aid teams, to elementary and then advanced agricultural co-operatives. These important changes had created the conditions for an economic surplus from which it was possible to develop collective social services. The Great Leap Forward in 1958 sought to take these developments further, by the formation of larger communes which could fund commune hospitals, clinics and pay for medical staff. The Beidahe Conference in August 1958 approved the mass movement to establish the People's Communes. Mao was the key leader behind the movement and it displayed characteristics typical of his political 'style'. The attempt was to promote a bold revolutionary programme that used the peculiarly Chinese 'mass line', to urge the formation of the communes, and create the economic infrastructure for a new collective health service. Since agriculture was to be an important focus of economic development the health needs of the peasants were of paramount importance. The health and welfare services were to be part of the benefits offered to the peasantry.

The commune clinics were locally funded and were not the responsibility of the Ministry of Health organisations. Their survival depended on an increasing agricultural surplus and luckily the 1958 harvest was a bumper one that encouraged their development. By the middle of 1959 Minister Li Dequan noted that half of the national communes had functioning medical facilities.(86) Many of course were united clinics that had been renamed and for which the commune now took financial responsibility.

*National plans*
In addition to the commune-level services, a twelve-year rural health plan was developed nationwide, operating at the provincial level. The main areas of planned change were:

increase in number of medical students (especially at the middle level);
increase in auxiliary health workers;
increase in commune clinics;
promoting collective insurance schemes in rural areas;
promoting traditional medicine;
medical students to undertake manual labour in rural areas;
mobile medical teams to do rural tours;
improved service to patients, e.g. 24-hour out-patient departments;
reducing costs of drugs;
encouraging Western doctors to undertake traditional medicine courses.

*Manpower changes*
By the end of 1959 there were said to be 800 higher and

secondary medical schools with approximately 240,000 students,
of which 5,000 were students of traditional medicine.(87) However, the main expansion was in the secondary or middle medical
schools. Paramedical health personnel peaked at 2.16 million in
1958.(88) The so-called key schools maintained rigid entry
requirements, however. The Academy of Medical Sciences and
other prestigious institutions were also permitted to continue
their work. Another important change was the development of
'spare-time' medical schools where students who were mainly
medical aides or nurses spent two evenings per week undertaking a three- to five-year course.(89)

*Collective welfare*
The attempt at developing collective medical insurance schemes
was a precursor to those developed during the Cultural Revolution. One scheme in Yangzi Xiang (Gan county, Jiangsu
province) with a population of 18,000, had the agricultural
producers' co-operative contribute Y1,000 to establish a ten-
bedded hospital. The peasants each paid an annual subscription
of Y0.20 which entitled them to free treatment.(90) The deficit
was met from the collective welfare fund. Another example was
in a commune in Huangbo county in Hubei province. Everyone
benefiting from the scheme paid Y1.50 annually to be advanced
by the agricultural co-operative and then deducted after the
autumn harvest. The co-operative put aside Y3.00 per family
for the welfare fund for health care.(91) Unfortunately these
progressive schemes were to falter when their economic basis
was undermined by the drought and economic chaos.

*Traditional medicine*
One of the slogans of the Great Leap was that of 'walking on
two legs' which in health care referred to the need to use both
traditional medicine and modern scientific methods. As the
Minister of Health put it:

> We are opposed to either the ideas of national nihilism
> which ignored the treasury of the medical science of the
> motherland, or the conservative ideas which tended to
> follow the old pattern and restrict progress.(92)

The integration of Chinese and Western medicine was stressed
and there was a seventeen-day conference in Baoding, Hebei,
in 1958 to review past work and to expedite integration.(93)
Full-time classes in traditional medicine for Western style
doctors increased from six before 1957 to thirty and the enrolment from 300 to 2,000. Traditional medicine was part of the
course for all medical students and district traditional medical
schools had more than 3,200 students with about 52,000 apprentices throughout the country.(94)
The most commonly heard slogan was Mao Zedong's urge to
produce 'more, faster, better and more economically'.(95) In

health care the close association between production and physical well being was made clear. The 'Southern Daily' had this to say: 'The most basic guideline in our health work should be the strengthening of the physique of the labouring people and the promotion of production.'(96)

Some of the main health care themes of the Great Leap were summarised in the 'three combinations':

1 Medical education and productive labour, mass campaigns, and traditional medicine.
2 Leading functionaries, teachers and students under Party leadership.
3 Teaching, scientific research and treatment with prevention.(97)

Of the mobile medical teams that were sent out one report speaks of 30,000 medical workers in Hubei province who were sent to the production brigades.(98) Similarly students were required to do at least two months' manual labour in the countryside.

Commune health services were developed. The model Wang-ssu People's Commune received much publicity. It had 50,543 inhabitants. The commune was divided into eleven administrative districts (zhu) with thirty-four production teams. In 1958 the average annual per capita income was 38.44 yuan and after the bumper harvest of 1958 this reached 72.34 yuan. The health service consisted of a small hospital with twenty beds and eleven health clinics. These facilities were staffed by thirty-four traditional practitioners and five Western trained doctors. In 1958 the Party Committee decided to put into effect a socialised health scheme.

There was an immediate rush for treatment. For the two months prior to the implementation the number of medical calls was 0.16 calls per person per month. In the two months after implementation there was a marked increase:

Table 3.5 Response to the introduction of socialised health care in the Wang-ssu People's Commune

|  | No. calls | Call/person/month |
| --- | --- | --- |
| August-September 1958 | 8,110 | 0.16 |
| October-November 1958 | 29,603 | 0.58 |
| January 1959 | 19,768 | 0.39 |

At this peak time doctors were being asked to attend to eighty to ninety calls per day. In response to the excessive demand it was decided to charge for visits to the hospital, outside calls, hospitalisation and excessive medical expenses. The conclusion was that:

there was a great unmet need that had been exposed;
there was an incorrect attitude to the scheme, i.e. since
   it was free people got what they could. There were cases
   of hoarding medicine;
some people feigned sickness to avoid work.

In response to this the leadership organised public campaigns
on the subject of 'not worth the money' or 'getting our money's
worth' and an example was made of malingerers. Despite the
individual fees the scheme was kept intact.(99)
'The Hsinlitsun People's Commune with more than 115,000
members consisted of ninety-one villages, twenty-six rural
medical and public health centres with a staff of over 120. All
the production teams are provided with a commune health centre,
health stations and maternity centres. In addition to the medical
workers there are contingents of part-time assistants and health
workers drawn from among the people. Many doctors spend
half their time attending patients and the other half out among
the people doing health publicity and instruction.'(100) These
were in fact early examples of the 'barefoot doctor' who became
more popularised during the Cultural Revolution.
   The optimism of 1958 and 1959, after the 'ten great years', was
dampened by economic disasters which followed the Great Leap
Forward. These produced many changes in the organisation of
medical care, as we shall see in the next chapter.

## NOTES

1 UNRRA in China 1945-1947, 'Operational Analysis Papers'
   no. 53, April 1948, p. 168.
2 A.P. Blaustein (ed.), 'Fundamental Legal Documents of
   Communist China', 1962, p. 51, quoted by Hsia Tao-tai,
   Laws on public health, in J. Quinn (ed.), 'Medicine and
   Public Health in the People's Republic of China', Washington,
   John Fogarty Center, 1972.
3 National Health Conference, New China News Agency
   (NCNA), 22 August 1950.
4 J. Schuman, 'Assignment China - an American journalist's
   report of four years in Red China', New York, Whittier,
   1956, p. 113.
5 Li Teh-chuan (Li Dequan), Health work in New China,
   'People's China', vol. II, no. 7, 1 October 1950, p. 11.
6 Ibid., pp. 9 and 11.
7 Li Teh-chuan, Two years of health work in China, 'People's
   China', vol. II, 16 January 1952, p. 8.
8 R. Lapwood and N. Lapwood, 'Through the Chinese Revolution', People's Books Co-operative Society, private publication, USA, 1954, p. 71.
9 Yen Ching-ch'ing (Director of the Health Department of
   Peking) in Appendix P.P. of 'International Scientific

Commission for the Investigation of the facts concerning bacterial warfare in Korea and China, Peking', 1952.

10 Lapwood and Lapwood, op. cit., p. 67.

11 Ibid., p. 68.

12 P.Z. King, Epidemic Prevention and Control in China, 'CMJ', 61, January-March 1943, p. 2.

13 'Report of the International Scientific Commission for the Investigation of the facts concerning bacterial warfare in Korea and China', Peking, 1952.

14 Ibid., pp. 233-4.

15 Ibid., pp. 615.

16 'People's China', vol. II, 14, 1952, p. 30.

17 Hsia Tao-tai, Laws on public health, in J. Quinn (ed.), 'Medicine and Public Health in the People's Republic of China', Washington, John Fogarty Centre, 1972.

18 P. Wilenski, 'The delivery of health services in the People's Republic of China', Ottawa, International Research Development Centre, Ottawa, 1976, p. 20.

19 Ibid., p. 21.

20 S. Shapiro, 'An American in China: Thirty Years in the People's Republic', Los Angeles, Meridian Press, 1979, p. 154.

21 S. Chandrasekhar, 'China's population. Census and Vital Statistics', Hong Kong University Press, 1959, pp. 53-64.

22 'Report of the International Scientific Commission', op. cit., p. 612.

23 'People's China', vol. 2, 16 January 1952, p. 8.

24 Ibid.

25 Editorial, 'CMJ', 67, no. 7, July 1949.

26 Association News, ibid.

27 Fu Lien-chang Association News, 'CMJ', 69, September-October 1951, p. 462.

28 R. Croizier, 'Traditional Medicine in Modern China', Cambridge, Mass., Harvard University Press, 1968, p. 249.

29 J.E. Bowers and Purcell, 'Medicine and Society in China', New York, Josiah Macy Jr Foundation, 1974, p. 135, and 'Ch'uan wu-ti' (Invincible), no. 17, 26 June 1967, p. 2.

30 Presidential Address, 'CMJ', 74, no. 5, September-October 1956, p. 414.

31 Fu Lien-chang Association News, Learning from advanced Soviet medicine, 'CMJ', 71, no. 4, July-August 1953, p. 246.

32 Li Teh-chuan, Two years of health work in China, 'People's China', vol. II, 16 January 1952, p. 9.

33 'First Five-Year Plan for Developing of the National Economy of the PRC in 1953-57', Peking, Foreign Languages Press, 1956.

34 Ma Hai-teh, personal communication, August 1981.

35 S. Schram, 'Mao Tse Tung Unrehearsed', Harmondsworth, Penguin, 1974, p. 98 (from Talks at Chengtu: On the problem of Stalin, 1958).

36 Blaustein, op. cit., p. 120 (Directive of the Ministry of

Public Health regarding the 1950 medical administrative
work, 14 April 1950).

37 Ibid., p. 121 (Provisional regulations governing the management of hospitals and clinics approved January 19th
1951).

38 Chu Hsueh-fan, Labour insurance in New China, 'People's
China', vol. III, 9, 1 May 1951, p. 6.

39 Ibid., pp. 6-7.

40 A. Donnithorne, 'China's Economic System', New York,
Praeger, 1967, p. 213, quoted in D. Lampton, 'The Politics
of Medicine in China',Folkestone, Dawson, 1979, pp. 25, 26.

41 Workers' welfare, 'New China News Agency', 5 October
1954.

42 Li Teh-chuan, op. cit., pp. 8-9.

43 Taking the number of Western trained doctors to be approximately 40,000 for a population of 450 million gives a ratio
of 1:11,000.

44 'Ten Great Years - statistics of the economic and cultural
achievements of the People's Republic of China', Peking,
Foreign Languages Press, February 1960.

45 'NCNA', 7 April 1950.

46 'NCNA', 27 March 1950.

47 'Tsinan Provincial Service', 10 August 1952.

48 'Tsinan Provincial Service', 12 September 1952.

49 'Peking Home Service', 6 June 1952.

50 'NCNA', 10 June 1953.

51 'Peking Home Service', 12 July 1953.

52 'NCNA', 14 May 1954.

53 'Shanghai City Service', 21 July 1954.

54 'NCNA', 7 May 1956.

55 'NCNA', 20 July 1956.

56 'Hangchow City Service', 20 July 1956.

57 'NCNA', 13 August 1956.

58 Editorial, 'People's Daily', 30 July 1956.

59 Marie Sieh, Medicine in China: Wealth for the State, I,
'Current Scene', vol. III, no. 5, 15 October 1964, p. 2.

60 Editorial, 'People's Daily', 17 June 1959.

61 Hsin Yun Pei, Advance the great work of protecting the
people's health, 'CMJ', 80 (5), May 1960, p. 409.

62 'China Light Industry', 28 August 1955, p. 15 in Joint
Publications Research Service (JPRS) Report no. 672,
New York, 25 August, p. 1.

63 Ibid., 28 December 1955, p. 12, in JPRS 672, p. 5.

64 Ibid., 20 December 1955, pp. 14-15 in JPRS 672, p. 3.

65 Ibid., 18 April 1955, p. 13 in JPRS 672, p. 22.

66 Ibid., 28 December 1955, pp. 14-15 in JPRS 672, p. 3.

67 Chien K'ang Pao (CKP), 'Health News', 12 March 1957.

68 Ibid., 22 March 1957.

69 Ibid., 26 March 1957.

70 Ibid., 25 February 1957.

71 Ibid., 7 May 1957.

72 'China - A general survey', 1979, Peking, Foreign Languages Press, 1979, p. 17.

73 Mao Tse-tung, On the Ten Major Relationships, (25 April 1956), from 'Selected Works vol. V', Peking, People's Publishing House, p. 295.

74 L. Jagan, China's national minorities, 'China Now', 95, March/April 1981, p. 2.

75 Ibid.

76 Ma Hai-teh, With Mao Tse-tung's thought as the compass for action in the control of venereal diseases in China, 'China's Medicine', 1, October 1966, pp. 52-68.

77 Ibid., p. 57.

78 Ibid., p. 56.

79 'CMJ', 1, January 1962, p. 64.

80 Ho-Piao, Health departments should take aid to agriculture as their primary task (Hung Ch'i (Red Flag), 18, 1960, pp. 12-20), in P. Wilenski, op. cit., p. 8.

81 'Nan-fang Jih-pao' (Southern Daily), 8 April 1954, in D. Lampton, op. cit., p. 46.

82 D. Lampton, op. cit.

83 Ibid., p. 48.

84 Li Tsung-en, 'People's Daily', 6 October 1956, in R. MacFarquhar, 'The Hundred Flowers', London, Stevens, 1960, p. 127.

85 Lampton, op. cit., p. 51.

86 Ibid., p. 107.

87 Li Teh-Chuan 2nd session of 2nd National People's Congress 4 April 1960, Survey of China Mainland Press, (SCMP) 2237, p. 18.

88 Cheng Chu-yuan, Health manpower: growth and distribution, in M. Wegman, *et al.* (eds), 'Public Health in the People's Republic of China', New York, Josiah Macy Jr Foundation, 1973, p. 144.

89 'NCNA', Medical workers graduate from part-time colleges, 1 November 1964.

90 News and Notes, 'CMJ', 77, 5 October 1958, p. 403.

91 News and Notes, 'CMJ', 77, 4 September 1958, p. 289.

92 'NCNA', 4 April 1960. Li Teh-chuan at 2nd session of National People's Congress.

93 Medical Activities in New China, National Conference on Traditional Chinese Medicine, News and Notes, 'CMJ', 78, January 1959, p. 100.

94 Hsu Yun-pei (Vice-Minister of Public Health), Co-operation between traditional Chinese and Western medicine to promote the people's health, 'CMJ', 79, December 1959, pp. 439-95.

95 MacFarquhar, op. cit., p. 30. He points out that in 1955 Mao used the slogan 'more, faster, better' and the more economical part was added in 1958.

96 Marie Sieh, Medicine in China: Wealth for the State, I, 'Current Scene', vol. III, no. 5, 15 October 1964, p. 1.

97 Li Teh-chuan, 2nd session of 2nd NPC, 'SCMP' 2237, p. 22.
98 Medical workers go to the countryside, News and Notes, 'CMJ', 80, June 1960, p. 595.
99 'Jen-min Pao-chien', vol. II, no. 5, Peking, May 1960, p. 278.
100 News and Notes, 'CMJ', 78, February 1959, p. 199.

# 4 THE 'THREE BITTER YEARS': OVERTURE TO THE CULTURAL REVOLUTION – FINANCIAL AND ORGANISATIONAL PERSPECTIVES, 1960–5

## S.M. Hillier

During the Great Leap Forward of 1958-9 huge increases in both agriculture and industrial production were reported, but by the summer of 1959 natural disasters of flood and drought led to a drastic revision of production data, with estimates for grain, steel and cotton being downgraded between 30 and 70 per cent.(1) Drought continued throughout 1960 and, in its wake, famine.

Sections of the leadership criticised Mao for the dramatic decline in economic and industrial fortunes, maintaining that the formation of People's Communes had contributed to the disasters. Thus from 1960 onwards there was a downward transference of ownership of land machinery and tools to the production teams, the lowest level of commune organisation and private plots were also allowed to develop.(2) Mao's prestige suffered and his leadership was temporarily eclipsed. Major policy decisions, which sought to comprehensively change the direction of Party policy, were put forward under the leadership of Deng Xiaoping, Liu Shaoqi and Zhou Enlai.

The changes in the economy had wrought their worst effects on the quality of life in rural China. Not only widespread famine and disruption, but rapid organisational changes during the formation of People's Communes had demoralised both rural population and rural party cadres. It was the latter, together with Mao, who bore the brunt of criticism for failures, rather than the higher echelons of the Party.

The consequences of economic disasters, policy modifications and the final struggle for power between Mao and sections of the Party leadership and State apparatus, were experienced in the field of health care organisation as elsewhere. As internal opposition to Mao increased during 1964 and 1965, Mao responded with a series of attacks on the workings of the Party and state bureaucracy, one of which concentrated on the inequalities in health care resources between town and countryside.

## HEALTH CARE IN THE COUNTRYSIDE

The Great Leap Forward had instituted innovations in both the organising and financing of health care. The aim was quite simply to improve health care for peasants and make communes self-reliant in this as in other aspects of rural life. A further objective was to reduce the dependence on hospitals in the county towns. These were often a long distance away, and provided expensive and time-consuming care.

The objective was to ensure some kind of basic facility in every People's Commune. Ideally, communes were to have a hospital and a number of smaller clinics throughout the commune. It was financed as follows:

Each commune member must pay a medical fee of one yuan per year and each of the commune's production teams must subsidize each member by one yuan every year out of public funds. The medical fees are to be collected and paid by the production teams to the commune in four annual instalments, and the commune turns over the fund to the health institute to defray the entire year's medical expenses to all the commune members. Staff wages were paid for by the commune, and the principle of 'whoever administers treatment is entitled to receive the fees' was abolished.(3)

Immediate results of the new system were: better quality health care, a decline in absenteeism(4) and a rush on services (in one commune demand almost quadrupled): 'each doctor had to attend to 80 or 90 calls a day which left him with little time for meals and visits to the toilet',(5) and abuse and overuse:

A few of the peasants felt that since the treatment is free they must get all their worth by paying visits to the hospital whether they are sick or not. An old lady... once obtained six different kinds of medicine to be hoarded at home... some commune members... pretended sickness or tried hard to avoid work under the pretext of sickness.(6)

In May 1961 People's Communes were reduced in size by about two thirds. The transference of the means of agricultural production down to production team level meant that decisions about the amount and organisation of health care resources were now made at a lower level, and health care was in direct competition for resources with agriculture.

Before 1961 when commune management was in control of welfare services, the members of richer, bigger and healthier production teams could support the poorer and sicker in other teams, since finances were pooled by the commune. Now, with resource control lying with the teams, finances for health became more difficult to generate. People still required health services, and continued to use them when required; when bills fell due, they often remained unpaid. Even in a model commune only 65 per cent of production teams paid their quarterly medical fees on time.(7) Wangsu People's Commune, estimated its annual medical expenses at Yuan 74,799 per annum, but had received Yuan 68,243.(8)

Attempts to keep the system solvent by reducing access

through increasing the proportion of individual contributions to be paid for 'hospitalisations, outside calls and hospital visits' met with little success.(9) This only hastened the decline of all collective forms of payment, for if people had to pay more at the time of sickness, why pay any contribution when they were not sick? In any case, during this period of economic crisis, people faced many demands on their pockets.

As a result peasants seeking health care obtained it in several different ways. If their commune was rich, or for some reason received a state subsidy, then they might have their own commune-based hospital and clinics, which offered partly subsidised treatments. In West Hubei, which seemed especially favoured, 'most of the rural People's Communes and production brigades have their own clinics'.(10) More likely they paid fees for service to doctors at their commune clinics. Otherwise, they could join and augment the queues at county hospitals, or seek treatment from public health clinics and sanitary stations primarily concerned with prevention. Or they could go without.

The economic difficulties of the state thus made themselves felt in the ability of many communes of reduced size to maintain free or partly subsidised health care.

During the Greap Leap Forward, the Ministry of Health had launched a programme of hospital expansion. In the countryside this had taken the form of some support for commune clinics and hospitals. In 1961 the Minister claimed that rural hospitals had doubled in number since 1958, but the word 'rural' covered both commune and county hospitals.(11) In 1962 the position was made clearer when it was claimed that the number of beds in *county* hospitals had doubled since 1958 and it was confirmed that the main organisational development in health care was to be at the county rather than the commune level (12) and that 'the establishment of county hospitals is the most important part of the health department's construction programme', (13) and by 1964, every one of China's 2,000 counties had a hospital.(14) Eight new hospitals were set up in West Hubei.(15) In Sichuan county hospital beds increased 138 per cent.(16) In Jiangsu, each one of the 60 counties had its own hospital.(17) The equipment of rural county hospitals was improved especially in national minority areas, and more money made available to them to buy drugs. In Hupei 85 per cent of the drugs manufactured in the province were bought by rural hospitals.(18) More manpower was also made available: 'In recent years most graduates of China's medical colleges and secondary schools have gone to staff xian (county) hospitals'.(19)

This new expansion, combined with decline at the commune level, meant that the county hospitals now took up the slack in patient care. At one county hospital

There were about one thousand outpatients daily from other nearby towns. If there were too many to deal with, the overflow could have temporary accommodation in the hospital at fifty cents a bed, but the patient had to bring his own rice coupon or rice to cover his food needs.(20)

Commune sanitary stations were also oversubscribed. A doctor at one station in 1959-60 remembered 'about two hundred patients per day, some [of these] were from neighbouring towns'.(21) The ten staff worked an eight-hour day, but found that the most serious problem was: 'vitamin deficiency, which affected nine out of the ten cases at my station. There wasn't much we could do except... try feeding them on a kind of brew of red dates and rice bran'.(22)

The whole emphasis in county hospital policy was to improve the service to rural areas; but if, as the health profile suggests problems of malnutrition and infectious and parasitic disease were still paramount in the rural areas, decisions to improve X-ray and surgical equipment and provide more hospital beds were really only part of the answer. Furthermore, these county hospitals, despite improvements, still did less well in terms of resources than their city counterparts. While the rationale for a policy which concentrates resources in a few units, rather than spreading them thinly over many, is easy to understand, whatever was done in terms of budgeting allocation could not solve a central problem of rural health service - that of 'accessibility'. The preferred solution of the Ministry - to place a proportion of its organisational and financial resources at county level - ensured greater direction from the centre, which could control waste and monitor facilities. But it was a long-term solution, in many cases an expensive one, and unless carried out nationally, would provide an inadequate and unequal standard of health care. As one peasant put it:

I took two hours to walk here and two hours to return home. I waited in a queue nearly all morning, yet the doctor examined me for five minutes and told me to return next day. I would have been better off resting at home.(23)

There were further problems. Although equipment grants had increased, the relatively inexperienced doctors sent to work in county hospitals were not always skilled enough to use the technology. Nor had they always the clinical expertise necessary to deal with the many illnesses presented. Cases which would be difficult or expensive to treat could be refused admission, hardly a satisfactory form of medical care.

## INEQUALITIES IN MONEY AND SKILLED PERSONNEL

In his declaration on the state of rural health care on 26 June 1965, Mao painted a picture of urban privilege set against rural deprivation. He criticised the 1964 health plan, claiming that:

> More than 90 per cent of higher level health workers, more than 70 per cent of the middle level health workers, more than 80 per cent of the health expenditures were concentrated in the *hsien* (county) and above the *hsien*, the cities. (24)

The figures are probably correct, although part of the discussion must take into consideration the fact that 'Xian' (county) hospitals were intended to serve as a focus for the health care needs of rural areas. The most politically sensitive resource was skilled manpower, a stock of which had been slowly built up since 1949.

Prior to 1966 C.Y. Cheng estimates that the physician population ratio in the urban areas was between one in 680 and one in 890, whereas in rural areas, where 85 per cent of the population lived, the ratio was somewhere between one in 8,000 and one in 15,400. (25) Even if one takes into account the fact that peasants near county towns and cities could use urban hospitals, the differences remain large.

In order to cope with the manpower needs of the expanding rural hospital service, new graduates, usually from secondary medical schools, had been assigned to work in county hospitals. (26) This meant that rural doctors were relatively junior and inexperienced. Another policy was to send mobile teams composed of doctors from urban hospitals, who would move from region to region for a few months and then return to the city. In 1960 about half a million health workers went to the countryside (27) but by 1962 some resistance from urban doctors was noted, since 'leading government and party organisations pay great attention to ideological education among those dispatched and efforts have been made to solve problems in their livelihood to heighten their enthusiasm'. (28)

The withdrawal of Soviet experts from China in 1960 had made the home-grown variety even more valuable; intellectuals felt able to speak out more on policies which they disliked, and work in the rural areas, where equipment was scarce and career prospects nil, was unpopular.

The teams continued to flow in a small but steady stream to the countryside, yet the effort remained on a minor scale, and urban dwellers still retained a doctor/patient ratio far superior to that of the countryside.

## EFFECTIVE DEMAND FOR HEALTH CARE

Not only were health care facilities more accessible in the cities, but there were two important groups there who were not constrained financially in their pursuit of demands for health care. The first group was composed of state employees – cadres and workers in state enterprises, who had always enjoyed the benefits of free health care. In the mid 1950s these benefits account for something between 19 and 25 per cent of the total health budget. While originally the measure was introduced with other benefits, to compensate cadres for not receiving a salary, when a new wage system was introduced in 1956 the benefits of free health care and schooling were retained.(29)

The second group were urban industrial workers whose welfare schemes included a free health insurance for themselves and a partial one for their dependants. The existence of both these groups was a factor in producing greater demand for health care in the cities, and this, allied with the historical distribution of health care facilities in the major towns and cities, lends support to the idea that a bias existed in favour of urban health care.

In 1962, for example, set against the rural facilities based on county towns, a city like Shanghai could boast over one thousand health care institutions,(30) and plans for building new hospitals in each district of major cities were under way in Beijing.(31) Later during the Cultural Revolution, Red Guards claimed that in Shanghai at least between 1957 and 1965 81 per cent of the health budget went to the urban areas, and only 19 per cent to suburban rural counties.(32)

## FACILITIES IN THE TOWNS

In the main, urban health care facilities were and continue to be arranged in three tiers – the neighbourhood health clinic and its counterpart the factory clinic, the district hospital, with somewhere between four and ten departments, 80-100 beds, and eight to ten medical staff, and the municipal hospitals with twenty or so departments, 500 beds and ninety medical staff. In addition some industrial factories owned and ran their own hospitals.(33)

## PROBLEMS IN URBAN HEALTH CARE

Despite this network of facilities, the urban health care system was less than ideal, and suffered from overcrowding, misuse and waste, and low staff morale.

*Overcrowding*
Overcrowding was an almost accepted feature of both 'Xian'

hospitals and city hospitals, since peasants close to a big city
would tend to use the latter, together with the urban population. Out-patient departments (OPD) regularly saw about one
thousand people per day, and throughout was often slow due
to inefficient registration procedures.(34) Clearly, also, overcrowding occurred because 'with free medical service and labour
protection provided by the State since Liberation chances for
the masses to receive medical attention in hospitals have greatly
increased'.(35) In addition

> the peasants who have implicit faith in medical treatment
> prefer to have minor diseases treated in the clinics of a
> large hospital. Although the Municipal Children's Hospital
> recently set up a branch OPD many parents would rather
> 'push into the crowd' at the Municipal OPD than bring their
> sick children to branch OPD.(36)

A survey carried out in Guangzhou No. 1 People's Hospital
showed that over half the patients in OPD could have received
treatment at basic level (i.e. factory and neighbourhood)
units.(37)

In an attempt to cope with overcrowding, hospitals increased
their hours of working, and conditions of employment for
doctors became harder. They usually worked a nine-hour day
with two days off a month.(38) In addition, an attempt was
made to improve health care in basic-level units by making each
municipal and district assume responsibility for health care
standards in sectors of the city. Beijing Second People's Hospital, for example, was responsible for training and supervising
the nearby maternity hospital, a neighbourhood hospital, six
branch health clinics and thirty-six health stations.(39) In
Tianjin and Beijing, doctors were required to visit factories
and neighbourhood stations.(40)

*Cadre privilege*
It was customary for special rooms in hospitals to be reserved
for cadres only,(41) which restricted the number of beds available, and there was also evidence of misuse and waste of facilities. In Guangzhou, admission procedures were tightened
up,(42) and the referral system strengthened to inhibit persons
suspected of malingering. Throughout the early 1960s the newspapers carried many examples of cadres and others with access
to free treatment misusing the service by demanding expensive
drugs and special consultations, 'on the excuse of illness, some
cadres ask doctors to write certificates of sick leave. This way
they may take rest.'(43)

> Dr Ts'ai earnestly told the woman cadre: 'Penicillin is not
> a drug to be used in your case'. At this the woman angrily
> threw the prescription at his feet and shouted: 'What is the
> use of your damnable medical service? If this were not

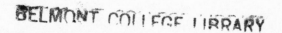

the appointed hospital, I should not have come!'(44)

Sometimes they prescribed placebos for symptomless cases, or suggested a mental hospital admission to the patient(45) as a means of reducing the number of unnecessary consultations and expensive prescriptions.

*Low morale*
Morale amongst ordinary medical and nursing staff was often poor, and reflected in their treatment of patients.

> Some nurses... take the wrong view that waiting on patients is a low and worthless job. At the dictate of personal whims they rudely deal with patients. A nurse whose attitude towards service is bad retorted 'Criticise me as much as you like, I shall soon cease to be a miserable nurse'. Some doctors take the wrong viewpoint and 'live on their ability' saying 'it is you who have come to beg favours of me'... they are careless and perfunctory in their work and deal with patients in an overbearing manner.(46)

The changing status of intellectuals did however bring improvements for those doctors at the top of the profession. In the early 1960s an increase in the number of academic conferences and more pure research articles were published.(47) The world's first limb reattachment was performed in Shanghai,(48) open heart surgery and pacemakers were developed,(49 and there were advances in traumatic and urological surgery.(50

CONCLUSION

Despite severe economic difficulties, the health care system survived the 'three bitter years'. The collapse of commune-centred schemes enabled the Ministry of Health to pursue its preferred policy of basing rural health care resources on the county hospital, and there were attempts to consolidate this into a rural network. In the cities too, the existing hospital infrastructure was built upon and increased. By 1965 hospital beds had increased to 340,000 as compared to 50,000 in 1954. The modest groundwork to fulfil long-term objectives was undertaken. An improvement in the national economy from mid 1962 onwards when output rose again to its 1958 level(51) made such developments possible. Still, both rural and urban hospitals suffered severe shortages of equipment and personnel, basic-level health care in the countryside and to a lesser extent in the towns was neglected and the gap between what was available for the rural peasantry compared with the urban worker or political cadre, remained wide.

By the mid 1960s, it was no longer possible to ignore rural-urban inequalities. Officials of the Ministry of Health may have thought their programme would be a long-term success, given sufficient time and resources, and would be 'a step in the direction of *gradually* obliterating the difference between city and countryside'.(52) Sections of the Politburo, principally Mao and his supporters, were doubtful about the long-run effectiveness of the strategy, and disturbed by the short-run consequences. While the Ministry officials might present themselves as having performed a successful salvage operation from the wreckage of the Great Leap Forward, an alternative perspective would regard developments in health care as symptomatic of an overall political strategy to change the style of government in China, and to curb the innovative but disruptive Mao Zedong.

NOTES

1 Chou En-lai, Report on adjusting the major targets of the 1959 National Economic Plan, in Jurgen Domes, 'The Internal Politics of China 1949-72', London, Hurst, 1973, p. 113.
2 Domes, ibid., p. 118.
3 'Jen-min Pao-chien', vol. II, no. 7, July 1960, pp. 384-7, in 'JPRS', 4340.
4 Ibid.
5 'Jen-min Pao-chien', vol. II, no. 5, May 1960, pp. 278-80, in 'JPRS', 4340, op. cit.
6 Ibid.
7 Ibid.
8 Ibid.
9 Ibid.
10 'Summary of World Broadcasts (SWB)' (Far East), 19 March 1963, ('SWB'/FE/W203/B).
11 Speech by Li Teh-chuan, 'People's Daily', Editorial, 1 November 1961 ('SWB'/FE/W82*A*2).
12 'SWB'/FE/W207/B, 26 March 1963.
13 Progress of rural medical work, 'NCNA', 8 January 1963 ('SWB'/FE/195/B).
14 China's hospital and health network, 'Survey of Mainland China Press' ('SMCP'), 3309, 27 September 1964.
15 'SWB'/FE/W203/B. 'NCNA', 19 March 1963.
16 Progress of rural medical work, op. cit.
17 'SWB'/FE/W207/B/13, 26 March 1963.
18 'SWB'/FE/W192/B27, 14 December 1962.
19 China's hospital and health network, 'SWB'/FE/W266/B/6, 27 September 1964.
20 Interview with Chinese medical doctor, 'Current Scene', vol. 1, no. 3, 12 June 1961, pp. 1-12.
21 Ibid., p. 2.
22 Ibid., p. 11.
23 Marie Sieh, 'Medicine in China: Wealth for the State, II, Current Scene', vol. III, no. 6, 1 November 1964, p. 6.
24 'Ch-uan-wu-ti (Invincible)', no. 17, suppl. 'SCMP' 209.

25 C.Y. Cheng, Health manpower: growth and distribution, in M. Wegman *et al.*, 'Public Health in the People's Republic of China', ed. New York, Josiah Macy Jr Foundation, 1973, pp. 139-57.
26 'SWB'/FE/W94/B/7, 11 January 1961.
27 Ibid., B/26.
28 'NCNA', 17 April 1962.
29 Chen Pi-chao, Population and health policy in the People's Republic of China, 'IPC Work Agreement report No. 9', Washington, Smithsonian Institution, 1974, pp. 25-8.
30 'NCNA', 3 March 1962 ('SWB'/FE/W152/B/23).
31 Work in Peking hospital, 'NCNA', 17 March 1962 ('SWB'/FE/W154/B/19).
32 The Mao-Liu controversy over rural public health, editorial, 'Current Scene', vol. VII, no. 12, 15 June 1969, pp. 1-18.
33 S.M. Hillier, Travel Notes, March 1978.
34 Canton 'Yang-ch'eng Wan-pao', 5 December 1962, Suppl. 'SCMP', 105, p. 29.
35 Ibid.
36 Ibid.
37 Ibid.
38 Sieh, op. cit., p. 2.
39 'Jen-min Pao-chien', vol. II, no. 7, July 1960, p. 386; 'JPRS', 4340, pp. 1-12.
40 Work in a Peking hospital, 'SWB'/FE/W154/B19, 17 March 1962.
41 Interview with a Chinese medical doctor, 'Current Scene', op. cit.
42 Canton 'Yang-ch'eng Wan-pao', suppl. 'Survey of Mainland China Magazines', 16 September 1965 ('SCMM'), 138, p. 33.
43 Shanghai 'Wen-hui Pao', 13 January 1965.
44 Shanghai 'Hsin-min Wan-pao', 10 January 1965, Suppl. 'SCMM', 138, p. 18.
45 Sieh, op. cit., pp. 4-5.
46 Canton 'Yang-ch'eng Wan-pao', 5 December 1962.
47 D. Lampton, 'The Politics of Medicine in China', Folkestone, Dawson, 1979, p. 170.
48 Peking 'Jen-min Jih-pao (People's Daily)', 6 August 1963, 'SCMP', 3044, p. 12.
49 'SWB'/FE/W227/B/17, 17 August 1963.
50 'SWB'/FE/W232/B/22, 20 September 1963.
51 Domes, op. cit., p. 135.
52 Ch'ien Hsin-chung, Prelude to the Great March of orienting health work towards rural areas, 'CMJ', 85, 4, April 1966, p. 212.

# 5 THE CULTURAL REVOLUTION AND AFTER – HEALTH CARE, 1965–82

S.M. Hillier

## A. HEALTH CARE ORGANISATION AND FINANCING DURING THE CULTURAL REVOLUTION 1965-70

### POLITICAL BACKGROUND

Criticism of Mao Zedong's policies led to a split in the leadership of the Chinese Communist Party, and a struggle emerged over who should hold power, and what the goals of development should be. Liu Shaoqi, the no. 2 in the leadership, and his supporters emerged as Mao's principal opponents. Mao's response was to launch an attack on both the Party and state institutions. As early as June 1965, Mao had expressed his opinions on the working of the health care system:

Tell the Ministry of Health that it only works for 15 per cent of the total population of the country and this 15 per cent is composed mainly of gentlemen while the broad masses do not get any medical treatment. First, they don't have any doctors. Second they don't have any medicine. The Ministry of Public Health is not a Ministry for the people, so why not change its name to the Ministry of Urban Health, the Ministry of Gentlemen's Health, or the Ministry of Urban Gentlemen's Health? In medical and health work, put the stress on rural areas.(1)

Mao condemned what he believed to be the Ministry's concentration on high-level research, the growth of urban hospitals and cadre privilege in health care. Whatever policy decisions had been made at a time of economic shortage he felt should be altered when economic recovery took place, but health care policies, he argued, showed no sign of changing their direction, and concentrating on bringing up the standard of basic health. Health care policy was neither the main, nor the only, area singled out for attack by Mao, but it was an area of controversy, and the effects of Mao's assault were felt throughout the health care system. The Ministry of Health tried first to deny allegations, to delay changes in policy, then to undertake actions which would assuage criticism(2) without radically altering anything, and finally to lay the blame on both the lower levels of administration and central government, accusing the former of inefficient bureaucracy and the latter of stinginess in the allocation of resources for health care.

All these attempts at self-preservation came to nothing. Along with other senior Party officials, the Minister of Health was purged in 1967, and the Ministry itself virtually ceased to function. As in other areas of administration, power became centralised in the hands of Mao and his supporters. During 1966-8 factional fighting among the young Red Guards was violent and bloody. Many people died, schools and universities were closed, and a chaotic situation existed. By 1968, at Mao's request, the People's Liberation Army restored a measure of public order at the expense of the more extreme left elements among the Red Guards. In October 1969 the first attempts to rebuild the Communist Party began. In the new leadership Mao's previous opponents were missing. Half the members of the Central Committee were army men. The ruling Politburo presented a coalition of army commanders, notably Lin Biao, the remaining fragments of the state apparatus, and members who were at the 'Maoist left'. In all the new Party and regional committees being set up, the army had a dominant role.

By 1968 a new system of administration which had been evolving slowly since 1967 based on revolutionary committees at every level, gave a considerable measure of responsibility to local and basic-level units. In the communes, much of the responsibility for initiating and operating health and welfare systems devolved to the production brigade revolutionary committees which were usually composed of revolutionary cadres, members of the militia (at higher levels, the army) and representatives of the poor and lower middle peasants.


RURAL HEALTH CARE 1965-70

In the rural areas, initially the previous policies of health care were intensified. The emphasis was on promoting the technical skills of rural health workers, in particular the 'part farming part practising' rural doctors (immediate forerunners of the barefoot doctors), and stressing the importance of preventive health work. Greater efforts were made to make county hospitals responsible to the needs of the peasantry, which included recruiting small mobile teams of doctors from county hospitals to visit villages,(3) and extending hospital opening hours.

The problems from which these hospitals and their patients had suffered during the Three Bitter Years left a legacy of poor health care, which it was now hoped to overcome. Hospital staff were urged to serve the people and surrender the unhelpful attitudes or 'four refusals':

> refusing to treat illness on credit for fear of bad debts, refusal to make a call before receiving payment, refusal to treat patients in foul weather and at night, refusal to cure illness for fear of serious responsibility.(4)

A rapid transfer of qualified medical staff to the Guangdong countryside in late 1965 signalled that real attempts were being made to meet criticisms of the imbalance in care. The new emphasis in health departments was on training qualified doctors for the rural areas. Guangdong health department announced its plans:

It will especially train for the countryside 10,000 graduates from university special courses, 20,000 peasant doctors, and 300,000 health workers who are not separated from production. Thus the health clinic of every commune can be staffed with six or seven graduates of medical colleges capable of treating diseases related to internal medicine, surgery, paediatrics, eyes and teeth, etc., and performing general operations. Every production brigade can be staffed with one peasant doctor and one midwife, and every production team with one health worker.(5)

## ORGANISATION OF THE RURAL HEALTH CARE SYSTEM

*Hospitals and clinics*
The model rural network quoted for Guangdong province was to become the major policy objective. This definite switch was demonstrated in late 1965, when it was claimed that 'the gradual establishment of a comprehensive medical network with the *commune* as its nuclei',(6) should replace previous emphasis on county hospitals. The problems of rural health care were, however, still enormous. First, even the county hospitals suffered from lack of equipment and resources; second, commune clinics, which had once existed in most communes in some form, were usually defunct; third, funds for medicine and equipment were not readily forthcoming from the state, and no system had been organised for generating finance; fourth, there was a chronic shortage of health personnel.

It is not known how many new clinics were actually built in the communes. Press reports often cited model clinics built in the 1950s or in the early 1960s(7) which were now revamped. Qian Xinzhong was later accused by Red Guards of having sought to assuage criticisms of his rural health care policies by setting up some expensive rural showpieces.(8) Many more reports stressed the excellence of clinical work carried out in dilapidated or poorly equipped commune clinics, stressing that the key to improving rural medical work lay not so much in the improvement of facilities by greater expense but by the correct political attitude - by putting politics in command. In one rural area

they built a new hospital from scratch. They borrowed some stools and boards to make some beds and fetched water from a well half a kilometre away. The operating table was only a

bed of boards... a washbasin was used as a steriliser. They
did not spend a single penny of State funds... it was in this
operating room that had no operating table, no shadowless
lamp, no blood bank, no oxygen and no running water, that
the comrades performed... numerous major operations by
kerosene lamp and flashlight.(9)

Although writers on the Cultural Revolution have viewed the
attack on expertise and technique characteristic of the period
as a fundamental assault on concepts of bourgeois science, a
more mundane corrective is that ideology and rhetoric inspired
medical workers to act irrespective of the difficulties they
encountered in the far-from-perfect situations of practice, to
abandon inappropriate notions of specialisation, and expensive
forms of treatment unsuitable to the rural economy. 'In so far
as the broad peasant masses are concerned, for them the prime
need is not "more flowers on the brocade", but "fuel in snowy
weather". In present conditions therefore, popularisation is
the more pressing task'(10) said Minister Qian Xinzhong.

Doctors and nurses have set themselves the task of being
'expert in one field and competent in many'.(11)

Staff at all levels were continuously urged to 'dare to treat'
cases which appeared doubtful or difficult, rather than refer
them upwards. This message applied particularly to workers in
commune clinics and below. In one example a model barefoot
doctor was praised for having opposed the decision of a medically qualified doctor who had said: 'How can such a poorly
equipped clinic treat disease? You will be held responsible if
something goes wrong'(12) and reports of difficult surgery
carried out successfully despite the lack of facilities abounded.
Political opponents who had claimed 'hospitals are not academies
of Marxism-Leninism. Technique is needed in operations. They
can't be done just anyhow' were strongly criticised.(13)

By 1968 moves to consolidate the system of rural care were
under way, and reports were made of advanced units with one
or two barefoot doctors to every production team (about 500
people), a small clinic in every production brigade (serving
about 2,500 people), and clinic or hospital in every commune
(serving anywhere between 20,000 and 50,000 people).(14)

The picture of facilities in the countryside which emerged
during 1968-70 was by no means a uniform one. While some production teams had 'one or two health workers' or in some cases
trained midwives, others had one or two barefoot doctors per
production brigade.(15) Some commune clinics had twenty or
thirty medical staff, others less than ten. It is interesting to
note that no directives were given which exactly specified
what the ratio should be. Since the governmental emphasis was
upon decentralisation, local units were largely left to develop
their own clinics and hospitals within the terms allowed by their

wn budget. Commune and brigade cadres therefore carried
considerable responsibility in the distribution of health care
resources. At county level, staff salaries, control, and health
policy was in the hands of the local county revolutionary committee, and the bureau of public health.

## MANPOWER

### Mobile medical teams

These teams whose job was to tour the rural areas offering
medical assistance went through a number of changes during
the Cultural Revolution. At first in 1965-6 they were composed
of doctors from city hospitals and from county hospitals. The
transference of the first group in particular was seen as temporary. Their tasks were curative, preventive and educational
they were supposed to train personnel at county hospitals
or work at the basic level. Mao had asked that one half of the
staff of urban hospitals be transferred to the countryside but
by 1968 probably about one third of urban hospital staff, some
50,000, had been on tours of duty.(16) As the Red Guards
complained:

> Hospitals held fast to the backbone technical staff. Even
> when a few specialists and professors were added they
> constituted no more than a decoration.... Some units...
> even resorted to conferring the title of 'doctor' on their
> administrative personnel: [they] were asked 'to keep this
> secret' from the peasants.(17)

By 1970 it was suggested that members of these mobile teams
should settle permanently in the countryside and leave the
cities altogether. How far this later decision was a response to
the demands of rural areas for more personnel, and how far it
represented a method of political exile for doctors who had been
criticised, is unknown. This writer met some doctors who had
done a six-week tour of the countryside, others who had completed several, and yet others who had stayed in the countryside for up to eight years.(18)
The transference of skilled medical personnel represented a
health care subsidy to county services, for doctors still received
their salaries. Doctors at commune and brigade level were
supported by communes and brigades on a work points system
to approximate the standard of living of middle peasants.(19)
These teams undoubtedly brought a higher standard of health
care to the peasants. The skill ability and dedication of experts
was praised when the teams first went out in 1965-6. In later
1968-9) teams, stress was laid on the inappropriate nature of
their training for dealing with the diseases which peasants had
which hints at the strain mobile teams were under. Only doctors
whose political attitude was correct, it was held, could effec-

tively deal with peasant ailments, since, in their desire to serve
the peasantry, they ingeniously adapted their training to the
hardships and scarcities of rural life.

In effect, doctors were blamed for their inability to provide a
solution for rural health care problems, but the reasons for this
were far more complex, and reflected the inadequate facilities
and disease burden in the countryside, and lack of enough doctors to satisfy both cities and rural areas.

*Barefoot doctors*
These health care workers will be discussed in detail elsewhere. Although earliest plans originating from the Ministry of
Health envisaged two levels of 'barefoot doctor' - a part-time
trained assistant doctor, and a part-time health worker, the
former to deal with acute illness, and the latter to undertake
preventive work - the distinction gradually disappeared. Decen
tralised control meant that the members, distribution and type
of training of barefoot doctors varied. Their presence as a
'backbone force' in rural health care would, it was thought,
provide greater accessibility to health care for the peasants,
and drive out private practice which had flourished in the early
sixties. By 1970 there was an estimated 1.08 million barefoot
doctors, (20) a ratio of one in 760 of the rural population. It
must be remembered however that the barefoot doctor was a
part-time worker, allotting roughly one third of his/her time to
medical work, but even taking this into account, which might
produce a hypothetical ratio of one in 2,280, the change from th
pre-1966 figure is dramatic, particularly if it is remembered tha
barefoot doctors are supported by public health workers and
'sanitarians', of whom there were an estimated 3,120,000 in
1970.(21)

Numerous examples of the cost effectiveness of barefoot doctors, who according to 'Red Flag' were able to treat the common
illnesses which in any case formed 95 per cent of the peasant
burden of disease, (22) were cited in 1970 and subsequent years
Hu gives a telling example quoted from 'Red Flag' of Zhunxing
brigade, Cugon xian, Guangdong province. The brigade has a
population of 2,900 of whom 1,139 are active workers. If the
peasants sought treatment at the commune hospital they would
have to walk three miles to the hospital and three miles back.
Together with waiting time at the hospital about one day's work
would be lost. Because services were provided at brigade level,
6,000 man days had been saved in 1968, representing a saving
to the brigade of Y4,750.(23)


FINANCING RURAL HEALTH SERVICES

*State finance*
The hospitals and public health bureaux at county level were
financed from provincial funds. Prior to 1968, expenditure on

health care at county hospitals had resulted in deficits, since peasants and their brigades would contract for services and then not settle their bills. Hospitals responded by refusing treatments for defaulters, or demanding cash before treatment,(24) but more often expenses were simply not covered, and county hospital finance suffered. Attempts were now made to alter the balance of expenditures within provinces and counties between urban and rural facilities and give the county hospitals more money from state funds. One model county, Dexing county in Jiangxi province, sent two thirds of its medical equipment to the rural areas.(25) Sixty per cent of the town's medical personnel were sent to the countryside, and the number of college trained doctors working in the countryside increased from 81 in 1965 to 265 in 1968. Eighty per cent of the health budget was spent in the rural areas.(26) In both Guangdong and Hebei provinces a similar pattern in favour of the rural areas was reported.

State expenditures were allocated in two main ways. Firstly, they would go in providing equipment for county hospitals and paying wages and salaries for county hospital employees. Secondly, they could be used in providing funds to set up and equip commune hospitals, the running costs of which would then be taken over by the communes.(27)

*Co-operative medical service*
While the balance of state expenditure appeared to be shifted in the direction of the rural areas (and evidence is only available from a few sources that this was the case) the major part of health care funding for basic rural health care was generated by the co-operative medical service, which came into existence nationally in 1968. It was not, and is not, uniform throughout China. Under the system, each commune or brigade member paid a standard fee which then went into a collective pool out of which medicines, a portion of hospital costs, equipment and barefoot doctors' workpoint remuneration were paid for.

The aim of the co-operative medical service was to make it possible for peasants to afford treatment. Using this method it was possible to finance local health care facilities, thus removing the treatment burden on county hospitals, and saving money for the brigade or commune through days lost either by sickness absence or by time spent seeking treatment. The system also satisfied socialist objectives by providing for the needs of some by the collective labour of everyone and maximising community participation and investment. Being locally based, and composed of individual contributions, it was possible to control waste, since people would be sensitive to overuse and misuse of services. The barefoot doctors employed by the co-operative medical service, using locally grown and compiled remedies, could produce cheaper remedies and provide effective competition for private practice.

The child of a poor peasant in the Hsinglung production
brigade was ill and was first 'attended' by a 'bad egg'
who had come from elsewhere. By trickery, he charged
over ten Yuan. A barefoot doctor came and carefully attended the child. The child was cured and the patient's family
paid little over three Yuan.(28)

Methods of coverage and payment varied. Some systems,
like that of Dengbu commune, were based on the whole commune, others were based on the production brigade or a collection of brigades, such as Duayang production brigade in Liang-
xiang People's Commune.(29) The amount paid by members of
the scheme varied from place to place, from Y1.50 to about
Y3.50 (Y3.30 = £1 sterling) per person, per annum. In addition
a small registration fee of about ten Fen (about two pence)
would be required on seeking treatment. In some brigades a
matching sum was set aside from the welfare fund. Although
these amounts seem small compared with the amount a family in
the West might spend on health care, relatively speaking they
amount to about 1.5 per cent to 3 per cent of disposable income
to cover a family of two workers, and two or three children.(30)
The cost of the co-operative medical service was by no means
cheap; and its inception depended upon a relatively better
economic position in China by the late 1960s; when versions of
the scheme had been originally tried out in the Great Leap
Forward and early 1960s they had failed due to economic circumstances. However, it should be remembered that medical costs
prior to the introduction of the co-operative system were heavy.
As one peasant said:

A member of a production team became ill in 1964. Failure
to get prompt medical care caused peritonitis. She would
have had to pay 180 Yuan just to get into hospital... the
commune had to come to her aid. She was in hospital for 80
days and the cost was Y306. In another similar case prompt
treatment was given under the united system and the patient
recovered within a week.(31)

The co-operative funds were to be used to pay costs of treatment within the commune, and hospital costs incurred outside
the commune. It was made clear to members that if adequate
treatment was available for them at commune level, they would
be expected to accept treatment from their local facility. Even
where treatment necessitated a visit to a county or provincial
hospital, costs greater than a fixed sum or, in some communes,
50 per cent of costs, should be met by the patient. Frivolous
or cosmetic treatment would not be paid for by the co-operative
medical service.
When treated in hospital, the patient would apply to the co-
operative medical fund for money which he/she would then be
responsible for paying to the hospital. Treatment on credit was

ended, thus strengthening the previously precarious accounting
of the county hospitals. Applications for expenses were to be
subject to review by the production brigade to ensure that no
waste or misuse of funds occurred.

This method of payment for rural health care thus shifted the
balance of financial provision to the communes and brigades,
following the principle of 'self-reliance'. It could not be said to
amount to a large-scale redistribution of resources from town
to countryside, although in some ways it would represent a
redistribution of resources within communes and brigades.

The co-operative medical system carried a number of disadvantages, which were discussed in 1968: 'Some of the masses with
relatively strong labour power and living comparatively well were
afraid they might lose something.'(32) Richer peasants were
sometimes reluctant to pay for poorer ones. Healthier people
thought the investment not worth it. While richer brigades
could perhaps afford a co-operative system, poorer ones were
less likely to, and within brigades, poorer peasants and the
older and sicker would have less funds to pay in to the co-
operative service. The latter, probably the more vulnerable,
would have to ask for funds perhaps at a time when they felt
least able to do so or might require constant medication.

Co-operative medical services might have insufficient funds
to cope with the demands on them. This appears to have been
the case at the beginning and the small registration fee was
introduced to reduce demand. Finally, participation in the co-
operative medical service was not open to all. Certain groups -
ex-landlords, rich peasants and those who had committed
political errors - were specifically excluded from many brigade
schemes, although through their contributions to the brigade
surplus, a proportion of which was allotted to health care, they
made a contribution to the financing of health care.

Nevertheless, in the better economic climate of the late 1960s,
the co-operative medical service can be seen as an efficient
solution to providing low-cost services to the rural areas,
removing economic barriers to treatment, and redistributing
income in accordance with socialist principles.


URBAN HEALTH CARE DURING THE CULTURAL REVOLUTION

*Hospital services*
The net effect of changes in the distribution of health personnel
from the cities to the countryside was to reduce the number
of doctors working in urban hospitals. The urban demand for
medical care was still high, however, and in order to cope with
it hours of hospital opening were lengthened, many 'unreasonable rules and regulations' were abolished, and departments
merged - for example ophthalmic and ENT departments. The
functions of doctors, nurses and administrative staff became
less clearly differentiated. At Shanghai Children's Hospital

'workers perform nursing tasks, administrators help in the out-patient department'.(33) At Linfen District Hospital in Shaanxi province 'doctors have undertaken some nursing tasks and nurses take part in the medical treatment of patients'.(34)

In Shanghai, in July 1967, patients had occupied the hospitals demanding changes in organisation and better facilities, and the Shanghai Municipal Revolutionary Committee had been forced to issue a directive saying: 'The masses of outside units must not interfere in the hospitals' great Cultural Revolution so as to safeguard the smooth progress of medical work.'(35)

The response to the crisis in urban health care was threefold. Firstly, great attention was paid to the political attitude of doctors. There were two kinds of medical attitudes held to be in need of correction, one of which was the reluctance, with shortages of skilled staff, to undertake treatment of serious conditions. Thus, there was much criticism of those doctors who placed reliance on 'experts', and examples were broadcast of the successes of those medical workers who took as their guiding philosophy the need to serve workers, soldiers and peasants, and to learn from them:

> By combining revolutionary bearing with truth seeking spirit, the broad masses of medical personnel have performed one miracle after another... despite crude equipment and inadequate experience, they have successfully removed a big tumour - an incurable ailment according to bourgeois 'experts'.(36)

Another attitude which was criticised was the erroneous emphasis on 'technique first'. 'An ideologically reactionary fellow spread hearsay and announced "a clumsy hand is incompetent to handle an operating knife".'(37)

Hospital staff held 'struggle-criticism-transformation' meetings at which these topics were discussed, and staff members who were held to have a wrong political viewpoint were criticised. Those who had previously held relatively lowly positions in the hospital often initiated criticisms of those who had held high positions. In some cases, senior doctors were not allowed to practice, or were given menial tasks to perform in order to re-educate(38) them. 'It is a misfortune to be a doctor', was the response of some sections of the medical profession to the changes in work circumstances.

The second development in response to the urban health crisis was equivalent to the rural mobile teams. Hospital doctors were sent to basic-level clinics in neighbourhoods and factories to work for periods of time. A team from Sichuan Medical College Hospital in the capital Chengdu:

> Working in close co-operation with local clinics... carried out a thorough physical check-up in the area [southern part of the city] recording the health conditions and ailments

of every family and individual... where it is difficult for patients to go for regular treatment to OPD, the doctors and nurses visit them at home... preventive inoculations were given to over 200 children... medicines are charged at the same low prices as at the city's hospital.(39)

The 'revolution in urban hospitals' particularly affected the cities of Tianjin, Harbin, Nanjing, Jinan, Guangzhou and Chonqing,(40) and later hospitals in Shanghai and Beijing would also adopt similar methods of working.

A further attempt to improve urban health care was by the development of a basic-level health worker, the 'Red Medical Worker's' equivalent to the rural barefoot doctor. These health workers received far less publicity, and were sometimes counted with public health volunteers or employees. Since the 1950s a corps of part-time health workers had been available for epidemic prevention work and in many cases the roles of exis- tent paramedical workers were probably expanded to include simple curative work in neighbourhood or factory clinics. In Chengdu, 10,000 were trained,(41) but figures on the total number of urban basic-level health workers are hard to come by.

A description of urban health services in Chengdu in 1966 shows:

a network of three hundred hospitals and health centres, linked together in a close-knit system of comprehensive and specialised hospitals, with clinics in all localities, and in factories, government institutions, schools and 'suburban' people's communes. In addition there are Red Cross Stations and an army of voluntary health workers.(42)

This was the ideal pattern of an urban health service, which would be emulated, with minor differences, throughout China's cities.


CONCLUSIONS

Health care policies during the Cultural Revolution put a new emphasis on reviving and developing a comprehensive system for rural areas. In cities, too, there was development of basic- level units and the role of out-patient care at the hospitals was diminished, as a more accessible system, based on neighbour- hood and workplace, evolved. The foundations of a more extensive, fairer and more accessible system of health care were thus strengthened, and great attempts were made to overcome difficulties in shortage of personnel, equipment and buildings. Although developments were patchy, there is no doubt that efforts which were made, especially after 1968, when the Central Committee of the Communist Party under Mao con- trolled the overall policy for health care, produced substantial

improvement in the level of health care available to the Chinese
people.

The decision to 'lay the stress on rural areas' made sense in
several ways. In the first place, attempts to even out the
balance of resources between town and countryside satisfied
fundamental socialist objectives of equality; secondly, by
improving the quality of life of the peasantry, the tendency
often observed in Third World countries of wholesale immigra-
tion to the cities was avoided. Thirdly, by linking health care
with improved economic production in agriculture; the policy
underscored beliefs that a prosperous and stable peasantry wa
basic for the maintenance of a healthy and successful socialist
state.

## B. HEALTH CARE POLICIES 1970-6

### POLITICAL BACKGROUND

The Ninth Party Congress in April 1969 saw Mao apparently at
the height of his power. With army support he controlled Chin€
and his allies held influence in the new Central Committee of
the Chinese Communist Party. His second in command, Marshal
Lin Biao, also held enormous power. His role as commander of
China's military forces made him a 'natural successor' to Mao,
until they clashed over foreign policy issues. In September
1971 Lin apparently died in a plane crash in Mongolia while see
ing asylum in the Soviet Union after an abortive coup against
Mao. Mao then purged Lin's supporters from positions of powel
and sought to reduce army influence.

From this time on the polarisation of the leadership between
radicals and moderates became more dramatic. Radicals like
Jiang Qing (Mao's wife), Wang Hongwen (mentioned as Mao's
successor), and Zhang Chunqiao still maintained the momentum
of the Cultural Revolution. In the early 1970s, however, a
growing feeling against the Great Proletarian Cultural Revolution, a negative assessment of its achievements and methods,
had led, particularly in educational matters, to more conservative policies. The disgrace of Lin, who had been associated wit
the Cultural Revolution, fuelled criticisms, as did the replace-
ment of his supporters by rehabilitated cadres. By 1973 Deng
Xiaoping, who had been called 'the second top capitalist roadel
in the Party' and had been purged in 1966, was back in public
life. His reappearance was the signal for renewed efforts by
the radicals to implement their policies against what they saw
as his efforts at 'capitalist restoration', and this heralded a
period of severe factional struggle in the Party. Zhou En-lai,
his major protector in the leadership, was the subject of thinly
veiled criticism in the Anti-Lin Anti-Confucius campaign of 197

In 1976, when Zhou died, and Deng looked to take over as Premier, the radical faction, with Mao's assistance, had him dismissed from all Party posts. Further actions by the radicals were prevented by Mao's death in September 1976. Within a month the balance of power changed dramatically in favour of the conservative forces. Wang Hongwen, Jiang Qing, Yao Wenyuan and Zhang Chunqiao, Mao's radical protégés, later known as the Gang of Four, were arrested. With their arrest the radicals' hold on leading positions of power in China was removed, but a radical influence in China's policy still remained in those members of the Communist Party who were admitted during and after the Cultural Revolution.

## HEALTH CARE POLICIES

The direction of health care policies mirrored the struggles occurring in the politics of the Central Committee. It must be remembered, however, that the relationship between the Central Committee and the local health services was by no means a simple chain of command. Decentralisation left a lot of organisational power and responsibility in the hands of local cadres, and although the centre had power to issue directives, in the early 1970s at least the organisational machinery did not always exist to ensure that they were efficiently carried out. Pressures for action were exerted through political rather than bureaucratic channels. The Ministry of Health was slowly being rebuilt, but its organisational role was severely limited, as witness the small numbers of public conferences and directives emanating from there between 1970 and 1975. The disgraced Minister of Health Qian Xinzhong (Ch'ien Hsin-chung) was rehabilitated as Vice-Minister in 1973, but the Minister of Health was herself a radical, who tried to ensure that Cultural Revolution policies in health care continued to be promoted.

## POLICIES IN RURAL HEALTH CARE

*Settlement of urban medical workers*
The first of these policies related to 'xiafang' the sending of urban medical workers to settle in the countryside. This policy was an extension of the earlier mobile medical teams. Its objectives were twofold. First, the settlers would carry out the functions of the mobile teams' curative work, prevention, and training of barefoot doctors, but second, they would themselves settle and be re-educated into a life of service to the deprived areas. As one doctor put it:

I mistakenly thought that after having worked many years in the city, going to the countryside would mean laying aside my speciality and burying my talents in an unimportant

post.... The commune hospital's poor facilities made me feel
more depressed.

Later:

after several years' work in the countryside, a number of
people said to me: 'Old Yuan, you've been in the countryside several years and made great progress ideologically.
You could now return to the city.' This made me waver in
my determination.

When this doctor was ill himself, an old peasant woman came
to see him to comfort him:

The poor and lower middle peasants work hard year in and
year out to win harvests for the revolution, and here they
are, concerned about my health too. Afterwards, I determined to spend the rest of my life in the countryside.(43)

Although this is a 'model' story, doctors interviewed by the
authors agreed that their time in the countryside had awakened
them to the enormous hardships of rural life. The xiafang
movement had many facets. One was the rustication of youths
who had been Red Guards. Another was the punishment by
exile of disgraced intellectuals, including doctors, but in the
field of health at least some practical benefits ensued from
adding to the numbers of medical personnel in the countryside.
   In 1973 it was claimed that ten thousand of the one million
urban medical workers who had visited the countryside had
settled there permanently, and the same figure was again
quoted in 1976.(44) There appears to have been a dispute over
the length of settlement: whether for a lifetime, a year, or
a period of years. Uncertainty in this matter suggests that
there was resistance from doctors, and from more conservative
opinion to the idea of permanent rustication. Isolated figures
from provincial sources seem to support this. Thus in Hubei
in 1972 'many medical workers' settled down. In Yunnan in
1970, 2,000, in Jiangxi 4,000; in Gansu 4,600, in Jilin in 1973,
8,000.(45) Certainly the final numbers quoted - one tenth of
the total - does not represent a huge transfer of medical person
nel. The million plus figures quoted in 1970 amount to more than
the total numbers of college or intermediate level trained staff
for China as a whole, therefore many health personnel who were
not doctors must have, as we know and this figure suggests,
gone to the countryside. The figures for those settling down
give no estimate of what proportion were trained medical doctors
and how many were other types of personnel such as nurses,
pharmacists, dentists or medical auxiliaries.
   In 1975, when figures were quoted for a total number reset-
tled, the struggle between conservative forces represented by
Deng and the Cultural Revolution radicals was reaching its

height. In the health field, the conflict was clearly apparent in the number of articles appearing criticising:

> some comrades who say 'We've already worked in the countryside for many years, it's about time we switched over to the cities.' In other words to do a good job in urban health work, they must abandon the countryside as the key point.(46)

But by 1975 even amongst the most radical was a recognition that good rural health care was 'not simply a matter of trans-erring manpower, material and financial resources to the countryside... the important thing is to mobilise the broad masses of people in the countryside to run their own clinics'.(47) In order for this to take place, two other important planks of rural health care, the barefoot doctors and the co-operative medical service, had to be sustained.

## Barefoot doctors

The employment of barefoot doctors was intimately tied to the financing of the rural medical system by the co-operative medi-al service, which in turn depended to a large degree on the general income of the commune or brigade. This was because the level of income in households, together with brigade or commune surplus, was used to finance them. This distribution of barefoot doctors per head of population varied throughout China with the ratio of population to barefoot doctor ranging from one in 340 in Jiangxi to one in 1,600 in Heilongjiang.(48)

At their inception, it was claimed that barefoot doctors created 87 per cent of illness, and 90 per cent of patients,(49) but by the mid 1970s attacks were made on their competence. The response to these attacks was to re-emphasise the superi-ority of this 'socialist new thing' both in medical skill and revolutionary feeling.

Without doubt the employment of barefoot doctors had been associated with some problems, of which difficulties over skills were a major part. The initial short training courses for bare-foot doctors were probably not adequate for all requirements. The original plan had been that doctors should go for refresher courses and gradually improve the longer they did the job. Unfortunately their clients, the rural peasantry, were not always willing to wait for the improvements in skill; re-training also posed the problem of who should fill the gap while the barefoot doctor was away. Further, who should pay for the re-training. Essentially, communes and brigades required a strong political commitment to the notion of barefoot doctors to foot the bill for their absence. At county level, too, county hospitals had service obligations to fulfil with scarce resources, as well as running training courses for barefoot doctors. For this reason Deng Xiaoping's attack on the skill levels of bare-foot doctors was regarded by the radicals as a serious attempt

to undermine rural health care. However, they were forced to
admit problems and institute training classes for barefoot
doctors,(50) if only to stave off the possibility of peasants by-
passing commune-level health care, and using the county hospitals instead, thereby increasing demand on these facilities.

The barefoot doctors' medical treatments utilised much of
traditional Chinese medicine but also Western medicine. While
some Western drugs were expensive, and contributed to brigade
insolvency, traditional herbs cultivated on site, or acupuncture
although cheaper, required time and skill. There were also
problems of quality control of home-made drugs. Often barefoot
doctors 'preferred to buy Western drugs' despite costs to the
brigade, but by so doing undermined the delicate balance of
co-operative medical service finance.(51)

The original conception of barefoot doctors would be that
they would be 'part peasant part doctor'. They would treat peasants in the fields or their homes, and by bringing the medicine
to the patient solve the problems of the accessibility of treatment. Except for 'model' cases cited in the news, the idea of
the barefoot doctor as a mobile practitioner seems to be somewhat inaccurate. As one editorial remarked: 'Some barefoot
doctors did not go to the patient to provide medical service but
sat idle indoors waiting for patients to come to them',(52) and
several sources have remarked on the fact that the barefoot
doctors' workload depended upon the degree to which they
chose to 'look for' patients. In one commune near Xian 'the
barefoot doctors were usually the daughters of the party cadres
who sat around and did nothing all day. It was easier than
working in the fields.'(53) If underuse was a problem, however
so was overuse, particularly where barefoot doctors were sparse
in number.

> Over the last two years, more patients came to see me. They
> came not only from my own brigade, but from other communes
> and brigades. At times, because I could not really deal with
> them all, I neglected some and the quality of medical treat-
> ment was also lowered... my failure to deliver them quickly
> from their illnesses often made me feel ill at ease.(54)

In other words, barefoot doctors often worked without supervision or support. Their existence, and indeed the whole rural
infrastructure of health care, depended upon a political ideolog:
While this was clearly effective in bringing barefoot doctors into
existence, it was less useful in maintaining them as a viable
rural medical force. For the latter, organisational and financial
factors were paramount.

Hu Teh-wei, in a cost-benefit analysis of four commune medical services, had concluded that the costs of the barefoot docto
system in terms of their training and the services provided,
are less than the benefits accruing to peasants as a result of
the provision of a cheap, basic and accessible service,(55) but

admits that the effectiveness and acceptability of such a
service is far more difficult to calculate. Policies during the
1970s sought to preserve the rural medical system and its
barefoot doctors, and strong political pressures from the radical centre were no doubt extremely important in keeping the
system going. At the 1975 conference on public health work the
Minister criticised local public health administrations for insufficient support of the barefoot doctors and co-operative medical services, claiming that this was due to their being influenced
by the wrong political line.(56) What is more likely, however,
is that practical questions of skill, and remuneration of barefoot
doctors, were causing difficulties.

In the early 1970s the amount of time spent working as a barefoot doctor was credited with work points, and the remainder
of the income was derived from participation in the agricultural
work of the commune. The amount of time spent in such work
varied according to local needs and conditions. In some brigades
the health centre closed completely during the harvest season
(i.e. for about two months of the year). In two model counties
barefoot doctors worked 253 days per year in collective productive labour.(57) However, barefoot doctors complained of overwork and inadequate pay, commune members of poor levels of
skill and wastefulness. In 1975 the Ministry of Health, under
the control of the radicals, set the level of working in 'productive labour' at 180 days, or half a year, but dropped the
requirement of taking part in agricultural productive labour,
and did not specify that barefoot doctors should earn work
points.(58) In other words 'productive labour' could include
medical work. This was a departure from previous policy, which
in order to counter criticism of 'barefoot doctors in name only'
had held that 'barefoot doctors can take part in collective labour
and look after sick commune members *at the same time*'.(59)

Although no direct evidence is available, the change seemed
to indicate a desire to improve the working conditions and
remuneration of barefoot doctors in order to prevent wholesale
defections, and to organise a method of payment that did not
alienate peasants by being derived from the annual brigade
share-out. Later the Minister of Health, a 'trusted follower of
the Gang of Four' was accused of 'corrupting barefoot doctors'
by promising promotions and other favours,(60) but this probably amounted to an attempt to maintain barefoot doctors by
devising a more stable system of payment.

*Co-operative and state financing of rural health care*
The co-operative medical system was operating in 70 per cent
of China's brigades in 1973.(61) Provincial variations existed -
in Anhui it was 50 per cent of brigades, in Jiangxi 66 per cent,
in Hunan 90 per cent, in Guangdong 80 per cent.(62) Payment
schemes varied, as described above, as did the coverage and
accounting unit, which was sometimes the brigade, and sometimes the commune. Problems of overuse and bankruptcy

occurred in some schemes, disillusion in others, 'what is called co-operative medicine actually amounts to requiring everybody to foot the bills to enable a few to receive treatment'.(63) Lampton reports a variation in the number of brigades operating co-operative systems with the rise and fall of grain output.(64)

Provincial governments continued to devote substantial proportions of their budgets to the rural areas. Sometimes the amount of money was specified as being for buildings and equipment, but it is likely that co-operative medical schemes were also being supported. Tacit recognition came from a Hubei report:

> at the start, peasants did not pay to see the doctor... there was a great waste of medicine and most of the co-operative medical centres were exceeding their budget. Later, a system was introduced where people had to pay... thus some households in difficulties could not afford medical treatment... [under] a new scheme the expenses would mostly be met by the individual with assistance from the collective as secondary. *The State would provide suitable support.*(65)

Provincial budgetary figures were published which showed the extent of funds allocated to rural areas: in Hainan Island 72 per cent, Guangxi 90 per cent, Henan 75 per cent, Yunnan 80 per cent, Hebei 50 per cent.(66) It was claimed by 1973 that State funding supported one third of China's 50,000 clinics.(67)

Clearly funding from central and provincial government was as important in supporting China's basic-level health care as the co-operative medical service. The radical line in health care had gone as far as to attack Deng Xiaoping for suggesting that co-operative medical services should be run profitably,(68) but during the 1970s absolute costs of health care were rising, and increasing funds were being demanded from central government for rural support. By 1975 over 60 per cent of the budget for health care was being spent in the rural areas. In Anhui province 70 per cent of the total provincial budget was spent on health care compared with only 52 per cent in 1965. In Beijing in 1975 spending on rural health was double that of 1966.(69) The growth of the co-operative system kept pace, however, being in operation in 85 per cent of communes and brigades, a 15 per cent increase on 1973.(70)

Although data is sparse, arguments over allocations to the rural areas must have taken place, with radicals supporting the view that central government should bale out local brigades if necessary, and conservatives constantly questioning the quality and efficiency of the services on which money was being spent. Despite the factional struggles during which many public health officials lost their jobs the radical line in health care prevailed, and in 1975 it was possible to claim that:

China's vast rural areas are covered by a medical care network which includes the county hospitals, commune hospitals
and co-operative medical stations at production brigades. Now
half the hospital beds are in the rural medical network, which
is serviced by six million medical personnel including part-
time barefoot doctors and public health workers. This works
out at an average of eight to nine medical personnel per
thousand medical population.... With over half the country's
professional medical personnel working in the countryside,
the development and improvement of the hospitals at county
and commune levels have transformed the medical and health
work there.(71)

The effectiveness of the system was less frequently commented
on, but in one county, 'in 1973, the incidence of common
diseases and recurrent disease had declined by 47.6 per cent,
compared with 1966, and in 1974 it declined further by 43.5
per cent compared with 1973'.(72)

The rural health care system on the eve of Mao's death
approximated with reasonable closeness to his vision of an
adequate system, with a wide network of rural health care,
focused on the communes and supported by a referral system
to county and provincial hospitals. This was a convincing
achievement. The stress was laid on rural areas but, some
critics felt, at the expense of the cities.


URBAN HEALTH CARE

*Hospitals*
The standard of health care in China's urban hospitals was
undoubtedly affected by the removal of a proportion of its
staff, for mobile teams continued into the 1970s. However, the
use of less skilled manpower was supported by the slogan
'technique is bourgeois'. Fear of political unpopularity was a
potent factor in suppressing criticism of working conditions by
medical staff.

Hostile assessments of the period talk of the 'years of turmoil'
in hospitals where the division of labour was abolished and
doctors became known as 'doctor-nurse-attendants' all in one.
'Nurses and attendants were encouraged to doctor the sick and
even perform operations, while highly trained doctors were
told to take up the duties of nurses and attendants.'(73)

An intriguing use of hospitals came to light after the fall of
'The Gang'. Apparently they had been used as asylums by
veteran cadres seeking refuge from political persecution. It was
said of Madame Liu, Minister of Health and 'sworn follower of
the Gang of Four', that

she personally toured the Ministry affiliated hospitals, questioning how this veteran cadre had been admitted, or why

that one wasn't discharged, and ordered a hospital to
report to her every month the list of hospitalised veteran
cadres.(74)

In Canton after the fall of the Gang, the joke was of

'two empties'. Liquor stores were empty because the masses were celebrating so thirstily, and hospitals were empty
because malingerers who had checked in to escape the endless campaigns... were now flocking back to work.(75)

It was, however, possible to point to a number of spectacular
innovations in research, surgery and medicine. Developments
in acupuncture and combined therapy were particularly emphasised as were toe to finger transplants, work on cancer,
eye problems and limb reattachment. A limited number of spectacular surgical feats were published which showed that 'the
pinnacles' were within the scope of radical health care, and did
not depend upon a city-biased research-based elite system to
be carried through.

*Basic-level services*
The network of factory and neighbourhood services that had
been evolving throughout the 1960s was extended. It could be
argued that basic-level care in the towns benefited from the
dispatch of hospital staff to rural areas, since short staffing
necessitated the growth of local basic units.

*Financing urban medical care*
The welfare funds continued to pay for health care for the
urban workers covered by labour insurances, and for 50 per
cent of the cost of their dependants. It must be remembered
however that in China's cities there still remained many people
who were not covered by any scheme of health insurance. These
were the unemployed who had no welfare facilities, contract
workers, and workers in small co-operative enterprises. Neither
these nor their dependants were provided for. There has always
existed a basic welfare system to ensure against destitution,
the 'five guarantees', although it is a last rather than a first
resort for China's citizens.

*The 1970s - the solution of rural-urban inequalities?*
Traditionally health care in the urban areas had always been
more accessible, and of better quality, but during the 1970s
the attempts to alter the balance continued. The attempts to
improve rural health care meant that urban facilities suffered
some depredations, but it is likely that the former gained more
than the latter lost, partly because the cities had an inbuilt
bias in terms of capital, equipment, revenue and prestige.
Although damaged, partly by loss of manpower and by the
cessation of many research opportunities, the urban system

survived and even developed, although neither as fast, nor in the direction it would have, had no policy existed to make matters otherwise.

The Minister of Public Health Qian Xinzhong (Minister since 1979), speaking of the period in health care from 1970 to 1976, was very condemnatory. His comments are instructive for they point the direction of present policies as well as describing the past. His analysis and phraseology are remarkably similar to that which he used in 1965. Speaking of the radical's health policy, he said:

Under the slogan of putting the stress on the rural areas, medical and health work in cities, factories, and mines was weakened.

Under the slogan of criticising 'bourgeois intellectuals' large numbers of professionals were deprived of the right to engage in day-to-day work and scientific research.

Under the slogan of doing away with revisionist rules and regulations, the normal order of many hospitals was disturbed.

Under the slogan of tackling the common diseases, research work in sophisticated medical science and technology and basic theoretical studies was criticised or discriminated against, and dismissed as 'theories divorced from practice'.(76)

Clearly, with the experience of thirty years in health care organisation the Minister saw little to recommend in the policies of his predecessors.

## C. HEALTH CARE POLICIES IN THE POST-MAO PERIOD 1976 ONWARDS

### POLITICAL BACKGROUND

Political developments since the fall of the Gang of Four have been characterised by a strong emphasis on China's modernisation and economic advance. Commitment to new economic policies has led to an acceptance of a degree of material inequality in society where bonus incentives now exist, together with legitimate private agricultural plots. The Chinese Communist Party has resisted wholesale de-Maoisation, but has encouraged an attenuation of the Maoist image and scrapped many Maoist policies, especially those relating to education. At present the Communist Party seeks modernisation and is striving for unity and authority in order to achieve it. However, disagreement exists between those Chinese who regard ideology as a barrier to achieving modernisation but a strong Communist

Party as a necessity, others who regard socialist ideology as
an essential aspect of political and economic life, and those,
mostly young, who care for none of these things but want a
strong, modern and prosperous China.


## A CHANGE IN DIRECTION

The new Minister of Health, Jiang Yizhen, who was appointed
after the dismissal of his predecessor, a radical, was described
as a Red Army veteran and surgeon. He epitomised the breed
of senior cadres, who, it was claimed, had suffered persecution
at the hands of the Gang of Four. His deputy Minister of Public
Health was the rehabilitated Qian Xinzhong (Ch'ien Hsin-chung)
a man who, prior to being purged from the Ministry in 1967,
had been an important influence on health policy. In speeches
in 1978 both defined a new shift in China's health care policies.
The new direction was twofold; the first, and most obvious,
was a new emphasis on the importance of science and technology
in medicine, a sine qua non of which was the rehabilitation of
many doctors and medical scientists disgraced during the Cultural Revolution. The second was the re-emphasis on the health
needs of urban areas. Qian, speaking at National Science Conference in 1978, said 'great progress must be made in modernising China's medical pharmaceutical and public health work and
in raising the country's medical science to advanced levels by
the end of this century',(77) and Jiang Yizhen, interviewed
during the same conference, said: 'We will keep to the principle
of putting the stress on rural areas, and will at the same time
be conscientious in health work in factories, mines and urban
areas.'(78)


## SCIENCE AND TECHNOLOGY AND THE ROLE OF INTELLECTUALS

The last five years have seen further developments in heart
and kidney transplants, feet, arm and finger reattachments,
microsurgery, plastic surgery, the treatment of burns, com-
puter diagnosis and new drugs and equipment. A recent visit
revealed that both Beijing and Shanghai have several body
scanners in their hospitals and medical workers proudly display
the newest imported medical technology. The 'Chinese Medical
Journal' has carried no political editorials since 1978, but has
devoted increasing amounts of space to both basic and applied
research and experimental methods of treatment. There is little
on preventive or industrial medicine, and no mention of the
adaption of some of the more advanced treatments to the simpler
uses of the rural areas. Articles are written by clinicians in
major teaching hospitals, or researchers from research institutes.
A considerable number of conferences have been held in the
past few years, including several international ones, and the

Chinese Medical Association again enjoys power and prestige.
The new treatment of intellectuals is symbolised in their official
reassignment in political rhetoric from a 'bourgeois' category
to the status of 'mental workers' with designated time for research and abolition of the requirement to perform manual labour.
Great emphasis is laid on training of scientists and investment
in large numbers of well trained medical personnel: 'a huge
professional contingent'. It seems unlikely, however, that in
the near future health care will be transformed to adopt the
worst aspects of Western health care systems as feared by
some commentators. There simply is not enough money to do
that. While some 'showpiece' hospitals will certainly be developed
(and indeed always have been except between 1966 and 1976),
the basic day-to-day health care needs of both urban and rural
workers, and the level of demand which they exhibit due to
raised expectations, are unlikely to suffer dramatic change as
a result of increased interest in 'expert' medicine by sections
of the leadership. In terms of other areas of potential modernisation like agriculture, industry and weaponry, medical
advances are regarded as being of lesser importance and are
unlikely to attract a large share of resources.

What is important for China's health care is to consider how
those resources which are available will be used in the new
political climate, and how the balance between facilities for
urban and rural populations will be maintained.


CHANGING ORGANISATION AND FINANCIAL PERSPECTIVES -
'LAYING THE STRESS' ON URBAN AREAS?

In the first three years after Mao's death, 1976-9, official
reports where possible vilified the health policies of the Gang
of Four; praised much of the development in health care before
1965, and acknowledged the need to emphasise prevention,
concentrate research into common diseases (which by now
included cancer and heart disease), support mobile research
groups, and continue to stress the health needs of rural areas.
Since 1980 the financial and organisational aspects of health
care have received more attention. What is under scrutiny are
practical concerns about the viability of producing and maintaining an efficient, cost-effective service, for the spectre of
rising costs of health care, which the State might have increasingly to bear, looms over the existing system, let alone any
expansion that might be envisaged.

The social welfare fund for both urban and rural areas in
1978 was 19 per cent higher than in 1974.(79) The total budget
for culture, education and health (the three have always been
budgeted together) was 11.266 billion yuan in 1978, a 24 per
cent increase over 1977. In 1979 it was 12.08 billion yuan, a
less dramatic increase.(80)

In 1980 the Ministry of Finance issued a circular on a trial

measure to make the Ministry of Health responsible for its own
health budget, and to enable it to retain surpluses at the
year's end, rather than having them ploughed back into culture
or education. This is clearly a measure designed to encourage
economy.(81) Cuts have also been observed. In Xinjiang,
Lampton reports, the regional commune bureau made available
unauthorised health care benefits which had to be repaid by
the recipients.(82)

In 1981 it seems that medical expenditures were again
increased, and spent mainly to 'improve quality in the medical
service at the grass roots and strengthen existing networks
both in city and country.'(83)

The emphasis on 'strengthening' rather than expansion is
important. Whereas in 1977-9 a wide range of health care needs
was recognised, of late the emphasis has been on self-reliance
for the rural areas, stressing that health care and welfare
benefits must be derived from greater productivity and prosperity. In the cities, on the other hand, fiscal policies are being
constructed to provide better health and welfare benefits for
urban workers. Approximately 7.5 per cent of the total monthly
wage bill of neighbourhood co-operatives is to be set aside to
meet medical and welfare expenses.(84) Attention is also being
paid to those urban workers for whom benefits are not available.
A recent 'Beijing (Peking) Review' describes how a temporary
worker at a factory received a charitable donation from the
factory of three hundred yuan towards her son's medical
expenses. She said: 'I was overwhelmed, for I knew temporary
workers are not eligible for such assistance.'(85)

Urban services have somewhat improved. In Peking a city-
wide network of ambulance stations has supplemented the more
usual methods of transport to hospitals, like taxis, pedicabs,
bicycles and handcarts,(86) but there is a charge for transport,
first aid and medicine. Four of the biggest hospitals in Peking
have been expanded, adding 800 beds.(87)

Whether the service is improving fast enough to satisfy urban
demand is questionable. In 1979 the 'Peking Daily' commented
on

instances of patients and their families' beating and abus-
ing medical personnel and disturbing the normal working
order of hospitals... they sabotage the management of
hospitals and press unreasonable demands on medical personnel.(88)

The Public Security Bureau has now drawn up special regulations to 'safeguard order' in hospitals and doctors are being
instructed to 'prevent medical accidents... to use qualified
medical personnel and to abide by rules and regulations in their
practice of medicine'.(89)

These comments suggest problems in the availability of care,
as well as difficulties with standards of care too. Clearly

patients in the city have decided that their health care needs should be a priority on the agenda.

*'Developing the backbone' - supply and demand for care in rural areas*
(a) *County hospitals* The 'modernising current' of 1978-9 was demonstrated in the field of health care by the decision to bring one third of China's county hospitals up to standard by 1985.(90) Concentrating scarce state resources on county hospitals is a project dear to the heart of Qian Xinzhong who replaced Jiang Yizhen as Minister in April 1979.(91) This means that provincial funds which poured into the rural areas from 1976 to 1978 will be directed towards maintaining county hospitals rather than commune clinics, although they may also be used to help co-operative medical services in debt.(92)

Modernising hospitals is an expensive business; as experience in other parts of the world has shown, once established, even if building costs are controlled, hospitals tend to demand an increasing share of resources and dominate budget allocation. This is partly because staffing costs are high. This is not such a problem in China where salaries are strictly controlled and relatively low - nevertheless the use of more skilled staff will increase costs. A further reason is that increase and improvement in facilities increases demand which in turn produces either waiting and overcrowding, or forces more expansion.

By concentrating on modernising hospital care, the Ministry of Health is reverting to the policy of the 1950s and early 1960s; in short, its preferred style, in the latest pronouncements of the Minister, in gradualism:

> To set things right, both urban and rural areas must be taken into account under an overall plan.... Only in this way can health work in the rural areas be steadily elevated... thereby gradually narrowing the differences between rural and urban health work.(93)

A feature of this type of approach, as well as its barely perceptible forward movement, is the absence of any proper assessment of the role of hospitals in the rural system. At present it is claimed that 61 per cent of beds are in the rural areas. Although increases in X-ray appliances and hospital beds look good on paper, they do not in themselves guarantee, or provide, an index of good rural health care.

The setting of optimistic targets for 1985 has had no follow-up since. The cutback in capital building programmes in 1980 almost certainly affected hospital building, and the problems of rising costs in health care (which in the short run does not improve production levels, although it may in the long run) have probably led to a more circumspect view of hospital modernisation.

Another factor which could hinder modernisation is the lack

of skilled personnel. A visitor to one of China's hospitals reported: 'costly facilities such as brain scanners, but without technicians to operate them, or spare parts for repairs'.(94) Modernisation which is incomplete, therefore, as this example suggests, is wasteful. Complete modernisation however is expensive and will continue to be so. Probably in an attempt to forestall this, 'developing the backbone' is likely to be a parsimonious policy and is focused on county hospitals because the costs generated by them can be more readily controlled than if state funds were made available to lower-level units.

The 'backbone' policy founders on the problem of accessibility. County hospitals are frequently up to one hundred miles away from a commune. Lacking adequate transport, access will be difficult. Yet subsidised treatment will be available for those with a special note from their commune doctors.(95) Current economic policies, which stress the value of individuals' incomes to their households, rather than the team or brigade, make decisions on time spent going to hospital relevant to individuals and their families, for losses incurred will be borne by them.

The equation of rural health care which offsets State financing with what facilities can be achieved by local initiative is a difficult one to balance. That county hospitals cannot function without state support is certain. That they need improvement is also likely; but without adequate attention being paid to health care at commune and brigade level, county hospitals soon become overwhelmed by work, or peasants simply suffer declining standards of rural health. While local initiative and financing is the sine qua non of a basic-level service, any failure to achieve adequacy together with possible economic instability can only put at risk central government investment in county-level hospitals.

*(b) Barefoot doctors*   Ideally, provision of an adequate basic-level service removes problems of accessibility but the service provided may not necessarily be acceptable: it may be of too low a standard. Attempts to improve the training of barefoot doctors to ensure that they treated ailments correctly, and refrained, on the grounds of their insufficient skill, from referring large numbers of patients to the county hospital, have taken place. While these difficulties remained unsolved brigades were paying twice over for health care, once for the barefoot doctor's time, and once for county hospital treatment, an economic muddle that the barefoot doctor service was originally designed to remove.

It is important for the efficiency of county hospitals that barefoot doctors continue to treat the majority of ailments, and do not become a means whereby more work is generated. If, however, the barefoot doctors are uncovering serious unmet need, then such a development is inevitable. Their very accessibility increases the volume of patients. Paradoxically, their

improved training might do the same. It was suggested in 1981
that about one third had reached paramedical standard (this
also tells us something about the standards of the remaining
two thirds).(96)

New plans for 1980 have specified that there should be at
least two barefoot doctors, one of whom should be female, for
each production brigade. This number is actually less than
some brigades already have(97) but is an attempt to set a work-
able target, for there are great variations in the numbers and
distribution of barefoot doctors.

*'We don't have barefoot doctors any more'*
As 'socialist new things' the barefoot doctors carried with them
some of the stigma attached to the Cultural Revolution and
the discredited Gang of Four. Since 1980 their recommended
title has been 'paramedic'. Whatever they are called, there
has been a recent decline in their number from 1.8 million in
1977 to 1.6 million in 1978 and 1,396,000 in 1981.(98) The fall
in numbers could have serious consequences for the rural medical service, so serious in fact that some brigades are resorting
to measures previously condemned: fee for service payments as
salaries for barefoot doctors, and a reward system for excellence in prevention, treatment, use of Chinese herbal medicine
and fiscal management. Even more dramatic changes have
occurred. Private practice in individual enterprise type medical
service has reappeared. In these practices either barefoot
doctors or medical personnel with time to spare provide the
funds to run a clinic with all receipts for themselves.(99)
Licensing of private practitioners has already begun.(100) In
other cases barefoot doctors who have been trained for two
years and formally certified, 'will be under the direction of
the *county* authorities and generally brigades will have no
authority to transfer or replace them'.(101)

These two developments represent major changes in the
employment status of barefoot doctors. Both imply cutting the
links between the barefoot doctors and production brigades.
A degree of private practice means that the role of barefoot
doctors as a force in preventive environmental health will
diminish, and of necessity they will concentrate on individual
treatment on a fee-for-service basis. The change also suggests
that a degree of geographical mobility may be inevitable, as
barefoot doctors and others in fee-for-service clinics will establish their services where money is available to pay for them.

Converting doctors into state appointees responsible to
county authorities, rather than health workers chosen and
monitored by their brigades, might suggest a movement on to
the first rung of a semi-professional career ladder. The move
might be popular with those brigades who wish to perceive the
barefoot doctor as a full-time health worker, whose skills are
best used by treating sick peasants rather than marginally contributing to brigade productivity by their own participation in

agricultural labour.(102) It is probably also popular with barefoot doctors themselves, guaranteeing better pay, working
conditions, and job reliability.

Official Ministry policy is to encourage communes to support
barefoot doctors because 'they are what the people need *and
what we can afford* at this stage of development'.(103)

*(c) Co-operative medical service*  In China, still, the majority
of people receive health care that is paid for by a co-operative
medical service, but the proportion of brigades in the scheme
is at present declining. In 1978 approximately 85 per cent of
brigades had a co-operative medical service. In 1979 about 80
per cent, and in 1980 67.6 per cent. This is not the first time
that fluctuations have been observed in the numbers, but
nationally participation in the scheme is at its lowest since the
early(104) 1970s.

The co-operative medical service is a form of collective health
insurance, usually with a pre-set expenditure limit. If brigades
withdraw from the scheme, it can be for micro- or macroeconom
reasons. The former would include inefficient management of
funds, overuse and waste, and poor results from barefoot
doctors; Parish and Whyte(105) in their study of co-operative
medical services in Guangdong noted that small brigades, or
those with single-lineage systems were able to provide cheaper
and more extensive coverage, and that trust among members of
these smaller or related units was an important factor in keepin
the scheme going. Brigades which are composed of more heterogeneous populations might therefore be expected to be less
likely to maintain the service.

Macroeconomic factors are those economic policies which, sinc
1978, have tended to underplay the collective economy of brigade or commune, and promote the team or household economy.

Certainly some sections of opinion in China might say that the
present systems of work organisation on the communes lower
productivity and, because they are labour-intensive, hinder
mechanisation. Incentive schemes and the increased developmen
of private plots have brought into focus the inequalities that
exist between richer and poorer communes, teams and brigades
and it is inevitable that just as differentials may create incentives to 'catch up' and increase productivity and consumption,
they may also reduce the desire to support the co-operative
welfare and medical services where 'one or two get sick and
everybody has to pay'. A conflict may exist between incentives
to production and maintaining a co-operative medical service;
when the payment system of the co-operative medical service
consists of both payments from individuals and from the brigade's accumulation fund, a further difficulty occurs, for
brigade cadres might wish to change annually the amount of
surplus devoted to health and welfare. Observations(106) in
1978 suggested that 10 per cent of the fund was devoted to
health and welfare, but by 1981 this had reduced to 4 or 5 per

cent in some brigades.

For the service to function successfully, some degree of stability with regard to income is necessary. When hard times occur richer brigades and communes with better natural resources will have greater funds available to ride out the difficulties. The co-operative medical service is therefore vulnerable to two important external influences - the state of the weather and crops, and a changing political climate which at present may place it in an invidious position vis-à-vis other economic objectives.

While there is no doubt that a healthy workforce is an important factor of production, investment in health care by individuals and brigades has to be set against returns derived from - say - increased mechanisation. Explicit recognition of this has been made by central government. Although officially strongly committed to the co-operative medical service, a gradualist approach has been adopted towards financing health care 'in tune with local conditions' and the door has been opened to a variety of methods of payment including private practice. On the other hand government moves which restrict brigade freedom will also affect the service. Controls on the licensing of barefoot doctors, and the suggestion that their employment conditions be made more stable, will certainly lead brigades to be more cautious in their commitment. If they employ barefoot doctors, they will have to keep them on and not sack them when conditions change. If they decide to retain a co-operative service and utilise mainly county hospital treatment rather than paying for barefoot doctors they could be espousing an expensive solution. Controls on the manufacture and supply of pharmaceuticals, particularly traditional medicines, from which many brigades derive a proportion of income and supply their own needs, have also been instituted. Since 1980 such enterprises have been placed under a State Pharmaceutical Bureau.(107) These restrictions, by affecting overall brigade income and local pharmaceutical supply, could both increase the cost of and the income available for the service.

China cannot afford a National Health Service paid for from central government. The co-operative medical service is the most effective solution to financing much of rural health care. Locally based commune and brigade health care with skilled referral and technical back-up at county hospitals is the only viable prospect. China's rural areas are relatively poor however and the co-operative service is not cheap for families. Children and adults pay the same per capita fee. In Guangdong a family of five paying the going rate of 2.50Y - 3.00Y per person(108) into the service could be paying up to 10 per cent of the cash they would get from the collective, a not inconsiderable sum. Although in China about 760 million people pay for their health care not by insurance, or by state funding, but by money generated by and shared among themselves, the instability of the co-operative medical service, due to its dependence on local economic conditions, is its greatest problem. In Zhejiang province recently it was frankly admitted that 'at present no fundamental solution has been found for the lack of medicines and medical services in our rural villages'. (109)

If the system of co-operative medical care does not survive, the situation of the rural areas will be parlous indeed. The decline in co-operative services has not, given its new direction, aroused as much interest as it should have in Beijing, and the Minister of Health has refrained from passing any comment which might encourage the belief that the rural areas retain political priority in health care. Whereas before 1976 government 'rescue' of co-operative medical services in difficulties occurred, no promise of similar support is now forthcoming. The possible social divisiveness of self-reliance policies which exacerbate the difference between richer and poorer brigades is officially ignored. This coincides with economic policies which, while recognising the importance of agriculture, see modernisation as the key to increased production, stress the importance of oil resources and regard the urban industrial sector, particularly light industry, as the fastest means of achieving economic advancement.


## QUESTIONS AND CONCLUSIONS

China's attempts, as a poor country, to provide a decent health service for its enormous population provide a fascinating subject for study.

There is no doubt that China has provided a comprehensive cost-effective health care system for the majority of its citizens. The attempt to do this has been the subject of political debate as we have seen. These political struggles have foreshadowed or highlighted tensions in Chinese political life in general. While it could not be our aim to examine the wider problems in these closing remarks, it is necessary to mention them; they are political, ideological, economic and social problems.

Political problems include tensions over who should rule, what is the form of the political process, how are conflicts resolved, and the interests of all the sectors of society taken into consideration. What is the legitimate basis of political power?

Ideological problems include differences over the values attached to differing political objectives within an overall socialist framework. They are essentially normative conflicts about the nature of Chinese society.

Economic problems involve the amount and type of resources generated, the cost of various economic policies and the benefits achieved thereby.

Social problems include the divisiveness or cohesion of Chinese society, the relative value of different groups of people within the society and the problems and conflicts generated by economic, ideological or political tensions.

Fundamental to the changes which have been wrought in health care in China have been the guiding principles of socialism which maintain that a good state of health and the means to achieve it is a right to be enjoyed by the whole population. Health care is not, as in free market systems, a commodity to be bought and sold, and available only to those who can best afford it. This fundamental political commitment has been a necessary condition of China's achievements in health work.

These pages have shown, however, that political commitment alone is not enough. Problems of allocation of scarce resources, or the means of generating new ones, remain. While health care is a benefit available to China's citizens, the level of provision is not achieved without political and economic costs.

Looking at a number of evaluative dimensions, we can see how the system measures up.

In terms of efficiency, China has generated, at relatively low cost, large numbers of hospitals and health care personnel of varying levels of skill, and perhaps is the best example of the rule that with proper organisation decent levels of provision can be achieved without crippling expense. While not in themselves guarantees of improved health care, hospital beds, clinics and doctors are a necessary condition of it. Centralist initiatives and the direct use of political power to co-ordinate these have been crucial in obtaining the health care that is available in China. This provision has been achieved without (for the present at least) the spiralling costs experienced in many developed countries. One way of cost control has been to set relatively low salary levels. Whereas in the UK 72 per cent of hospital costs goes in salaries,(110) in China these account for only 25 per cent.(111) Also personnel are allocated to jobs, so a 'skills market' does not develop. Waste and overuse is limited by financing much of the care co-operatively (i.e. directly from people's incomes). Low levels of consumer spending have so far released funds for health care, although present policies to stimulate spending may in the future alter this. A relatively small proportion of the gross National Product is spent on health care (probably less than 4 per cent),(112) with generally sound results. Free market systems in the developed world suffer not only from rising costs, but insufficient returns on the investment. The richest country in the world, the USA,(113) spends more per capita on health care than almost any other country, yet its health profile is no better, and in some cases worse, than countries which pay less (see Table 5.6 at end of chapter).

We must remember, however, that the low expenditure of the Chinese system is related to the fact that there are many people as yet who do not enjoy benefits of free health care, or co-operatively financed care. This includes about 40 per cent of the rural peasantry at present and probably 20 per cent of urban workers.(114) Improving the lot of urban workers by increasing their access to health care benefits will undoubtedly

increase spending on health care, and will also increase demand
for care in the urban areas. The decentralisation which is a
feature of the system, with local units having a degree of
autonomy and control over financing and administration, has
ensured responsiveness to problems of waste, overuse, or gaps
in provision. There might be some disagreement over the degree
to which decentralist initiatives, as opposed to centralist ones,
have exerted a major influence on the health care system or
indeed that the power exerted locally is necessarily always
beneficial in terms of health care objectives. Nevertheless, there
exists a degree of structural tension in the distribution of power
between central and local decision makers which, over time,
cancels out the excesses or inadequacies of each in favour of
the other. It remains to be seen whether this creative tension
can be maintained, or whether the health care system will suffer
the inappropriateness and 'blanket' nature of over-central planning, and the patchiness and irregularity of provision which
results when local units are left to fend for themselves.

The medical profession in China is by no means a quiescent
group, as we shall see in chapter 11. Recently university
trained doctors have once again enjoyed the status and prestige
that they had been deprived of since the early 1960s. Yet in no
way does the medical profession represent a coherent self-
interested pressure group in the style of its Western counterparts. Political limitations on the power of any interest group
in China are provided by the existence of the Communist Party
as the supreme organising force and final legitimate authority.
Professional leaders in medicine, although having undoubted
influence, enjoy it on the basis of personal authority or prestige
rather than as representatives of an organised group. Financial
constraints in health care and education spending have proved
to be more potent influences on policy than the interests of
medical doctors. Allocation of work, rather than the freedom to
practise, also limits the economic base from which professionalism
might develop. Finally, medical educational policies have produced a group heterogeneous in training and skills, who do not
have an identity of interest, nor rely on professionally
controlled licensure as the basis of their practice.

Political and economic policies which are in general geared
towards low cost and the restriction of professionalism have
contributed towards a relatively efficient health care system
which compares well with that of other Asian countries. Maternal
and infant mortality has been almost reduced to Western
levels, and life expectancy has increased. Malnutrition still
occurs, especially as the results of recent vast crop failures
make themselves felt; but starvation has not been an unremit-
ting feature of Chinese life for thirty years. Parasitic and
infectious disease have been limited and in some cases eradicated
Much of the impact on China's disease profile has resulted from
the primary commitment to preventive health policies. Some of
these policies have espoused mass campaigns which have involved

the lay population in an attempt to undertake such work at low cost. The use of manpower in such a way, while no doubt raising the consciousness of the average Chinese in matters of sanitation and hygiene, may have proved ineffective in the long run; competing demands for manpower have occurred and political will to organise or participate in such campaigns has waxed and waned. New attempts at prevention face the health problems of an industrialising nation. In many cases these are too new to warrant evaluation, but projects to map cancer incidence nationwide, or the community coronary care programmes of cities and rural communes, show a willingness to tackle these difficult problems undaunted either by their enormous scale or the relative unavailability, world wide, of successful solutions. While China has not allocated massive proportions of her budget to buying expensive drugs and equipment, she has nevertheless managed a modest amount of expansion in this field. Shortages remain, and we cannot judge as yet whether in the field of medical care a climate more sympathetic towards curative medicine, which utilises surgical treatments and more modern diagnostic aids, is emerging. This is probably the case, but does not necessarily signal a turning away from the preventive medicine which has worked so well. The conflict between preventive and curative medicine characteristic of Western systems of medical care is largely an artificial one produced by historical circumstances, scientific advances and professional pressures which resulted in an inbuilt bias in favour of curative medicine.

Problems of accessibility bedevil all health care systems, but some more than others. A universal feature is the extent to which urban populations enjoy a relative advantage, a matter that is slowly being rectified in the newer Third World systems. In China accessibility to services is a problem which has been recognised for many years, and has been the focus of political struggle and conflict. The growth of a national network of primary clinics with secondary- and tertiary-level back-up has brought modern health care to the rural areas and improved that of the towns. The difficulties of access have by no means been solved, and current policies may well increase those difficulties. Systems of financing based on local income at best provide good coverage, at worst they are inadequate for those inhabitants of localities which are poorer than average. Advances in the availability of health care over the past thirty years need to be sustained.

By emphasising education and participation, and by retaining respect for traditional systems of medicine, the acceptability of the health care that is offered should be high. The Chinese, despite their needs for health care, have shown themselves unlikely to be 'passive accepters' of whatever is offered. Indeed, by requiring such a degree of direct payment for services, criticisms of levels and type of service are a continuing feature of a system which has by no means coped with all the unmet need in the Chinese population. Chinese traditional medical theory encourages a high degree of health consciousness, and makes people responsive targets for health education. Certainly in this matter, crucial to success in prevention, thoughtful and thorough attempts to understand patients' needs and resistances to certain kinds of treatment have been as evident as the rapid response to criticisms of skills and treatment. If services are not acceptable, means exist to voice difficulties and suggest remedies. In the past these remedies have sometimes been nega- tive - refusal and rejection of types of care - and sometimes positive, resulting in changes which are more acceptable.

The expansion of Chinese traditional medicine has also offered a new dimension of choice in health care to Chinese people.

D. Lampton, commenting on the historical changes in health care policies since 1949, has suggested that at present the bureaucracy which is responsible for policymaking, and faces the need to make choices in resource allocation, has gone for an 'optimising' policy. He says: 'Optimising does not mean "the best", but merely a process which can produce policy co- ordination and simultaneously take a decent range of inputs into account.'

Since this was written in 1977, we would suggest, the situ- ation has changed. The word 'optimising' no longer describes the style of health care delivery policy. This is for two reasons. First, optimising is essentially an unstable style of management, most unsuited to large-scale bureaucracies. Although capable of short-run survival, we would suggest that it cannot be sus- tained. Second, attention to the efficiency and effectiveness of health care over and above its accessibility and acceptability has been a feature of recent policy making, reflecting concerns in the Chinese leadership for a governmental system which is streamlined and managed more professionally.

The result has been a trend in health care policy we would call 'gradualism', which in real terms means that health care needs appear less of a political priority than at almost any time since 1949. In part this is because the system has generally performed well, and the stasis which can be observed at present - slowing down of development, 'gradual improvements' - may merely indicate that priorities are now being directed to other, needier areas like social welfare. Within health care itself we can observe a rearrangement of priorities towards the needs of the urban areas, and it appears that health care policy is being formed less in terms of needs than in terms of response to those capable of effective demand.

Those capable of making effective demands on the health care system are not only the urban industrial workers and cadres whose better insurance schemes have always put them in a more favourable position relative to their rural counterparts, but medical professionals who are now in a position to press for changes in the style of medical work; they want better equip- ment, more research opportunities, conferences and scientific exchanges with their counterparts in other countries. On the whole, professional demands are being met: resources are available for the latest medical technology in selected 'centres of excellence', trips abroad and study exchanges are being actively pursued.

One of the weaknesses of 'gradualist' policy is that it is not really a policy at all. It reduces those in charge of health care to the status of mere 'responders' to the strongest pressure, rather than 'initiators' or innovators. It is therefore essentially conservative, and some observers might justly argue that this is what is required now, that there have been enough experiments. This argument would be more convincing if we were not aware that the lack of development in health care at present stems less from thought-out policies than from an overriding concern with population control and economic development. We have also seen over the past thirty years how political intervention was necessary to make the health care needs of rural areas a fact of political life.

The weakness of the current position is that there is no 'built-in' method of ensuring that the needs of the disadvantaged appear on the health care planning agenda. While it would be impossible for the historical reasons cited above ever to ignore the health needs of rural areas, these areas are not homogeneous, containing variations of wealth and resources. To speak in broad terms of 'the urban areas' or 'the cities' is also often misleading, since we know that the cities also contain disadvantaged and unemployed persons. We wonder, therefore, how a 'gradualist' policy will be able to respond to the disadvantaged since, lacking power and direction, and constrained by national economic policy, it is more likely to move in response to pressures from the most economically valued (i.e. wealthier or more productive) groups. During 1982, economic reforms in agriculture have occurred, whose implications for rural health care are not yet clear. The 'Responsibility System' whereby each family in a production team assumes responsibility for growing a crop quota on a strip of communal land, from which they derive a personal income, may reduce collective funds available for commune health services, producing a decline which the upgrading of county hospitals will only partly offset.

Will new political directions emerge which seek to reaffirm commitment to disadvantaged sections of Chinese society, or will the stress on development be emphasised as a strategy for raising overall levels of health care by improving 'the best' as a model for everyone?
Will the consequent new interest in science and technology and policies of hospital modernisation prove an expensive and inappropriate attempt to solve China's health care problems?
Will inequalities in access and standards increase between urban and rural areas - and will steps be taken to prevent the development of intra-urban and intra-rural inequalities?

Will rising costs of medical care outstrip the benefits
accruing or lead to cutbacks both at national and local
levels?
Will the emphasis on improvement in county hospitals increase demand for curative services at the expense of
preventive health work?

In 1950 the stated objective of the Chinese health policy was
to make health care available to all sectors of society, to stress
preventive work and to utilise the treasure-house of Chinese
traditional medicine. In the 1980s these objectives still continue
to provide the broad guidelines of policy.

The health care system in China is not at present faced with
the crises that bedevil Western systems - increasingly low
returns in health set against investment; great inequality of
access, and inequalities between resources devoted to the
prevention and treatment of various conditions; over-reliance
on expensive quickly outdated technology. But as China increasingly faces the health problems of a developing industrialising
nation while still managing those of a relatively poor developing
country, health care policies have to be constructed which
enable China to continue to maximise its efforts to produce a
cheap, efficient and decent health service, which serves the
needs of all its people.

TABLES

Table 5.1  Organisation of rural health care in the 1980s

| | | |
|---|---|---|
| Provincial hospital | - | Teaching, research, specialist medicine (5-600 beds). State funded, university trained doctors. Large OPD. Serves population of 1 million. |
| County hospital | - | Training (barefoot doctors), internal medicine and surgery. State funded (40-100 beds), university and intermediate doctors and technicians. Large OPD. Serves population of 200,000. |
| Commune hospital/clinic | - | Some training (barefoot doctors), internal medicine, simple surgery, obstetrics, abortions, antenatal care. State/commune funded (10-50 beds, often more). Large OPD, intermediate and barefoot doctors. Serves population of 12-50,000. |
| Brigade clinic | - | Dentistry, out-patient treatment, preventive inoculations, antenatal care, family planning, brigade/commune funded. 2-5 barefoot doctors. 2-3 part-time health workers. Serves population of 2-4,000. |

| roduction team | - | Preventive work (organise mass campaigns), family planning, basic first aid treatments, antenatal care, brigade funded, 1 part-time barefoot doctor, 1-2 part-time health workers. Serves population of 200-500. |

Table 5.2  Organisation of the urban system of health care in the 1980s

| pecialist city hospital | - | Teaching research, specialist departments, medicine and surgery (100-700 beds). University trained doctors. State funded. Attached medical schools and research institutes. Serves national population. |
| Municipal/provincial hospital | - | Teaching, research, specialist departments, medicine and surgery, obstetrics (100-500 beds). University trained doctors. State funded. Attached medical schools, colleges. Large OPD. Serves population of 1 million and one sector of a city. |
| District hospital | - | Training (barefoot doctors, red medical workers, family planning workers), general medicine and surgery (100-200 beds). State/city funded. Large OPD. Serves population of 200,000 (one sector of a city). |
| actory/neighbourhood hospital | | General medicine and surgery (10-50 beds). Local/factory financed. Intermediate level (sometimes university trained) doctors, worker doctors, pharmacists, dentists. Large OPD. Preventive inoculations, obstetrics, family planning, abortion. Serves population of 10-20,000. |

Neighbourhood
clinics

Run by street doctors (red medical workers), 3-6 months training. Mainly family planning, preventive inoculations, care of chronic sick. Serve population of 2-3,000. Visits from local hospital personnel for antenatal, post-natal, and family planning. Municipal finance/local finance.

Lane clinics

Run by street doctors (part-time) and part-time sanitary worker. Organise preventive campaigns and family planning.

Table 5.3  Growth in medical and health care facilities, 1949-80

|  | 1949 | 1956[2] | 1960-3 | 1980[1] |
|---|---|---|---|---|
| Hospitals | 2,600 | n.a. | n.a. | 65,009 |
| Sanatoria | 65 | n.a. | n.a. | 440 |
| Out-patient departments | 775 | n.a. | n.a. | 99,643 |
| Epidemic prevention stations | 154 | 1,260 | n.a. | 1,066 |
| Maternity and child care units | 90 | 4,560 | n.a. | 2,559 |
| Pharmaceutical control units | n.a. | n.a. | n.a. | 1,159 |
| Research institutes | 3 | 6 | 100 | 295 |
| Public health stations | n.a. | 600 | n.a. | 3,049 |
| Hospital beds/1,000 population | 0.15 | 0.52 | 0.90 | 2.0 |
| Hospital beds | 80,503 | 328,000 | 724,827 | 1,982,000 |
| Higher medical colleges | 22 | 29 | 98 | 109 |

Source:  1  CMA, 'Medicine and Health Work in New China', 1981.
2  Ministry of Health Statistics (Health News), 'JPRS' 583, February/March 1957.

Table 5.4  Growth in medical personnel

|  | 1949[1] | 1965[2] | 1979[3] | 1980[3] |
|---|---|---|---|---|
| All medical staff | 540,000 | | 3,340,000 | 2,500,000 |
|  | 1.08 | | 3.4 | 2.53 |
| Medical technicians | n.a. | n.a. | 2,640,000 | 2,798,000 |
| Doctors of Western medicine/100,000 | 41,000 | 188,661[4] | 395,000 | 447,000 |
|  | 8 | 25 | 40 | 45 |
| Traditional doctors | 276,000 | 321,430 | 257,000 | 262,000 |
| Middle-level doctors | 53,000 | 170,000 | 435,000 | 444,000 |
| Nurses | 38,000 | 185,000 | 421,000 | 466,000 |
| Auxiliaries | n.a. | n.a. | 219,000 | n.a. |
| Pharmacists | n.a. | 20,000 | 96,000 | n.a. |
| Herbalists | n.a. | n.a. | 101,000 | n.a. |
| Midwives | 16,000 | 40,000 | 70,000 | n.a. |
| Barefoot doctors | n.a. | n.a. | 1,575,000 | 1,463,000 |
| Public health workers | n.a. | n.a. | 3,500,000 | 2,992,000 |

Sources:  1  Ministry of Health Statistics ('Health News'), 'JPRS', 583, February/March 1957. People's Republic of China, State Statistical Bureau, 'Ten Great Years', Peking, Foreign Language Press, 1960, p.2
2  V. Sidel, in J. Quinn (ed.), 'Medicine and Public Health in the People's Republic of China',

Sources:   Washington, John Fogarty Center, 1972, p. 156.
3 'Medicine and Health Work in New China', CMA, Beijing, 1981.
4 Dr Ma Wen Kan, Ministry of Public Health, Beijing, September 1981.

Table 5.5.  Rural health changes, 1962-80

|  | 1962 | 1980 |
|---|---|---|
| Hospitals and clinics | 28,656 | 55,413 |
| Hospital beds | 100,027 | 775,413 |
| Staff (qualified doctors, assistant doctors and paramedics) | 217,213 | 1,037,543 |

Source:  Ministry of Health, Beijing, September 1981.

Table 5.6   Per capita expenditure (pounds sterling) and infant mortality rates, 1979

|  | Per capita | % GNP | IMR/1,000 |
|---|---|---|---|
| Switzerland | 475 | 6.9 | 8.6 |
| Sweden | 437 | 8.6 | 7.8 |
| USA | 422 | 8.5 | 13.6 |
| FDR | 356 | 8.0 | 14.7 |
| Netherlands | 295 | 8.3 | 9.5 |
| Japan | 141 | 4.0 | 8.4 |
| United Kingdom | 123 | 5.5 | 13.1 |
| Greece | 43 | 2.4 | 20.4 |
| Cuba | 7 | n.k. | 25.0 |
| Thailand | 0.50 | n.k. | 26.5 |
| Philippines | 0.50 | n.k. | 56.9 |
| India | 0.50 | n.k. | 139.0 |
| China | 0.50* | 3.0[+] | 16.0 |
| World | - | - | 91.0 |

*Calculated from percentage of State expenditure on health, together with per capita expenditure on co-operative medical services.

[+]'Guesstimate' - no figures available.

Source:   International Comparison, 'Office of Health Economics', Compendium of Health Statistics, 3rd edn, London, 1979. Expenditure figures 'World Health Organisation', Vital Statistics and Causes of Death, Geneva, 1980, Infant mortality figures.

Table 5.7   Doctors and hospital beds per 10,000 population

|        | Doctors | Hospital beds | Life expectancy |
|--------|---------|---------------|-----------------|
| World  | 8.1     | 38.2          | 61              |
| Africa | 1.8     | 19.3          | 49              |
| Asia   | 3.5     | 18.7          | 58              |
| Europe | 18.1    | 95.0          | 72              |
| America| 11.6    | 45.4          | 68              |
| USSR   | 34.6    | 121.3         | 70              |
| China  | 4.0     | 22.0          | 68              |

Source:   All figures except China from 'WHO' Vital Statistics
and Causes of Death, Geneva, 1980. China figures are
my calculation based on Population figures of J.S. Aird
'Population growth in the People's Republic of China'
in 'Chinese Economy Post-Mao', US Government Print-
ing Office, Washington, 1978, pp. 465-7.

NOTES

1 Mao Tse-tung, Directive on Public Health Work, in Stuart
  Schram (ed.), 'Chairman Mao talks to the People', New
  York, Pantheon, 1964, pp. 232-3.
2 D. Lampton, 'The Politics of Medicine in China', Folkestone,
  Dawson, 1979, pp. 201-20. Lampton gives a most thorough
  and convincing analysis of relations between Mao and the
  Ministry of Health.
3 Chinese hospital praised for service to peasants, 'NCNA',
  Tsinan, 12 September 1965, 'SCMP', 3538, p. 14.
4 Gansu field conference on public health work, 'NCNA',
  7 April 1966 ('SWB'/FE/W362/A39).
5 Medicine and health work in Kwangtung Province is reso-
  lutely directed towards the countryside, Canton 'Yang-
  ch'eng Wan-pao', 15 September 1965, 'SCMP', 3550, p. 11.
6 Medicine for rural areas, 'NCNA', Peking, 12 October 1965,
  'SCMP', 3559, p. 18.
7 'SWB'/FE/W482/A/10, 14 August 1968.
8 'Ch'uan-wu-ti (Invincible)', 26 June 1967, Supp. 'SCMP',
  209, p. 31.
9 Shanghai medical team in rural area, 'NCNA', 1 November
  1968, ('SWB'/FE/W494/A/16).
10 Prelude to the Great March of orienting health work toward
   the rural areas, 'CMJ', 85, 4, April 1966, p. 212.
11 'SWB'/FE/W366/A20, 5 May 1966.
12 'NCNA', 11 November 1968 ('SWB'/FE/W495/A/16).
13 'Kunning, Yunnan Provincial Service', 22 May 1968,
   ('SWB'/FE/W470/A/20).
14 How do we implement the policy of prevention first?, Peking
   'People's Daily', 4 January 1969, 'Current Background'

872, p.27.

15 Production brigades to run their own medical services,
   Hofei 'Anhui Provincial Service, 7 December 1968
   ('SWB'/FE/W499/A14).
16 The Mao-Liu controversy over rural public health, Editorial,
   'Current Scene', vol. III, no. 12, 15 June 1969, pp. 14-17.
17 'Ch'uan-wu-ti (Invincible)', op. cit., p. 18.
18 S.M. Hillier, 'Interview files and travel notes', 1978, 1981.
19 The Mao-Liu controversy over rural public health, op. cit.,
   pp. 14-17.
20 Hu Teh-wei, 'An economic analysis of co-operative medical
   services in the People's Republic of China', John E. Fogarty
   Center, 1957, pp. 13-14.
21 Ibid., p. 14.
22 Ibid., p. 15.
23 Ibid., p. 29.
24 A great revolution on the health front, Peking, 'People's
   Daily', 13 December 1968, 'CB', 872, p. 13.
25 'Nanchang, Kiangsi, Provincial Service', 26 August 1971
   ('SWB'/FE/W658/A/12).
26 'SWB'/FE/W641/A/2, 13 September 1971.
27 S.M. Hillier, Travel Notes, Renho People's Commune,
   Guangdong province, 1978.
28 'Hung Ch'i (Red Flag)', no. 3, September 1968, in 'SCMM',
   628, p. 3.
29 Peking, 'People's Daily', 13 December 1968, 'CB', no. 872,
   p. 18, 'Hung Ch'i', no. 3, September 1968, in 'SCMM',
   628, p. 3.
30 Hu Teh-wei, op. cit., p. 20.
31 'SWB'/FE/W498/A/18, December 1968.
32 Struggle between two lines in Anhwei hospital, 'SWB'/FE/
   W499/A/15, 2 December 1968.
33 'SWB'/FE/W482/A/10, 14 August 1968.
34 'SWB'/FE/W601/A/17, 29 October 1970.
35 'SWB'/FE/W426/A/13, 9 July 1967.
36 Mao Tse-tung thought lights up the way for the advance of
   China's medical science, 'Hung Ch'i (Red Flag)', no. 3,
   28 February 1970, 'SCMM', 676, p. 49.
37 Ibid.
38 S.M. Hillier interview file no. 11.
39 'SWB'/FE/W366/A20, 5 May 1966.
40 Ibid., A21.
41 Ibid., A20-23.
42 Ibid.
43 Yuan Yung-ts'ai, Brilliant June 26th directive shows me the
   way forward, 'CMJ', 1, 4, July 1975, pp. 241-6.
44 'NCNA', Peking, 25 June 1976.
45 'SWB'/FE/W578/A1, 11 September 1971; FE/W574/A/8,
   29th May 1970; FE/W577/A/10, 24 June 1970; FE/702/A/1,
   6 December 1972; FE/W743/A/1, 28 February 1973.
46 Further grasp well health work in the countryside, 'Hung

Ch'i', no. 9, 25 August 1975, 'SCMM', 841, p. 41.
47 Ibid.
48 Hu Tei-wei, op. cit., pp. 11-12.
49 'SWB'/FE/W585/A/11, 6 August 1970.
50 Consolidate the dictatorship of the proletariat and run co-operative medical service well, 'CMJ', 1, 4, July 1975, pp. 233-6.
51 Ibid., p. 236.
52 Ibid.
53 J.A. Jewell, personal communication, September 1981.
54 Raise the level of medical techniques in the course of practice, 'Hung Ch'i (Red Flag)', no. 3, 2 March 1973.
55 Hu Teh-wei, op. cit., pp. 27-37.
56 Achievements in public health work must not be neglected - a criticism of the 'Gang of Four', 'Peking Review', no. 24, 10 June 1977.
57 Barefoot doctors are admirable in that they are barefooted, 'Kuangming Jih-pao (Bright Daily)', 26 June 1975, 'SCMP', 5893, 14 July 1975, p. 10.
58 'Peking Review', no. 24, 10 June 1977.
59 Further grasp well..., op. cit.
60 Conspiracy of the Gang of Four to usurp Party and State power in health departments, 'CMJ', 3, 4 July 1977, pp. 213-17.
61 'SWB'/FE/W731/A/1, 4 July 1973.
62 'SWB'/W749, 22 August 1973; W658, 2 February 1972; W660, 7 July 1972; W694, 11 October 1972.
63 Exercise the dictatorship of the proletariat on the health front, Peking, 'People's Daily', 27 June 1975, 'SCMP', 5893, p. 1.
64 D. Lampton, op. cit., p. 238.
65 'SWB'/FE/W701/A/1, 29 November 1972.
66 'SWB'/FE/W738, 22 August 1973; W683, 26 July 1972; W681, 23 August 1972; W668, 12 April 1972; W680, 5 July 1972.
67 'NCNA', 'SWB'/FE/W731/A/1, 4 July 1973.
68 Reversing verdicts for the Ministry of Health for urban overlords in a vain attempt at capitalist restoration, Peking, 'People's Daily', 15 May 1976, 'SCMP', 6136, p. 194.
69 'NCNA', Peking, 19 June 1977.
70 'SWB'/FE/W740/A/1, 5 September 1973; 'SWB'/FE/W885/A/3, 7 July 1976.
71 Ibid.
72 Exercise the dictatorship..., op. cit.
73 'Beijing Review', 25, 23 June 1980, p. 21.
74 Conspiracy of the Gang of Four to usurp Party and State power in Health Departments, 'CMJ', 3, 4th July 1977, pp. 213-17.
75 Ross Terrill, 'The Future of China', London, Andre Deutsch, 1978, p. 115.
76 Public Health Minister on modernisation, 'Beijing Review', 25, 23 June 1980, p. 18.

77 'SWB'/FE/W977/A/1, 26 April 1978.
78 'NCNA', English version, 5 June 1978, 'SWB'/FE/5837/BII/13, 8 June 1978.
79 'SWB'/FE/W1014/A/1, 17 January 1980.
80 Li Tai and Wang Chengyao, 'Zhonquo Baike Nianjian', August 1980; 'JPRS', 78774, 'China Report on Economic Affairs', no. 164.
81 'SWB'/FE/6313/B1/5, 8 January 1980.
82 D. Lampton, New revolution in China's social policy, 'Problems of Communism', vol. XXVIII, 5-6, September-December 1979, p. 1.
83 Health Minister on 1981 tasks, 'CMJ', 94, 4, April 1981, p. 240.
84 Wang Chengyao, Tax reduction and exemptions, 'China Report', no. 164, ('JPRS' no. 78774), op. cit.
85 Help came when I needed it most, 'Beijing Review', 11 January 1982, p. 27.
86 'SWB'/FE/W1102/A/1, 1 October 1980.
87 'SWB'/FE/W1118/A/1, 28 January 1981.
88 'SWB'/FE/6291/B11/4, 7 December 1979.
89 'SWB'/FE/6529/B11/4, 22 September 1980. Public Health Minister on modernisation, op. cit., p. 19.
90 'SWB'/FE/6320/B11/6, 15 January 1980.
91 'SWB'/FE/6084/B11/8, 4 April 1979.
92 In Kwangtung Province two thirds of drugs, equipment and staff go to county hospitals. 'SWB'/FE/W931/A/1, 1 June 1977.
93 Public Health Minister on modernisation, op. cit., p. 19.
94 S. Rifkin, Interview with Louise de Rosario, 1981, 'Hong Kong Practitioner', April 1982.
95 J.A. Jewell, personal communication, January 1982.
96 'CMJ', 95, 12, December 1981, p. 848.
97 'SWB'/FE/6313/B11/5, 8 January 1980.
98 'NCNA', 5 June 1978, 'SWB'/FE/W1053/A/1, 17 October 1979. Medicine and health work in New China, 'CMA', Beijing, 1981. Xinhua 26 August 1982.
99 Maintain the co-operative approach to medicine, institute measures in line with local conditions, Hangzhou 'Zhejiang Ribao', 14 July 1980, p. 3; 'China Report', Science and Technology, 10 September 1980; 'JPRS', 7640. 'SWB'/FE/6538/BII/9, 26 September 1980.
100 'SWB'/FE/6519/B11/2, 10 September 1980.
101 'Zhejiang Ribao', 'JPRS', 7401, 10 September 1980.
102 J.A. Jewell, personal communication, January 1982.
103 Public Health Minister on modernisation, op. cit., p. 19.
104 'SWB'/FE/5282/B11/10, 9 September 1976; 'NCNA', 5 June 1978, Medicine and Health Work on New China, 'CMA', Beijing, 1981.
105 W. Parish and M.T. Whyte, 'Village and family life in contemporary China', University of Chicago Press, 1978, pp. 90-1.

106 S.M. Hillier, Travel Notes, 1981.
107 'SWB'/FE/6442/B11/5, 11 June 1980.
108 Parish and Whyte, op. cit. p. 89.
109 'Zhejiang Ribao', 14 July 1980.
110 Costs of service: hospitals, 'Office of Health Economics, Compendium of Health Statistics', 3rd edn, London, 1979.
111 R. Blendon, Can China's health care be transplanted without China's economic policies, 'New Eng. J. Med.', 300, no. 26, p. 1457.
112 No recent figures are available. In 1973 about 1.7 per cent of budget was spent on health, and the amount has probabl' fallen.
113 International Comparisons, Office of Health Economics, op. cit. See Table 6.
114 Figures derived from co-operative medical services, and numbers covered by insurance, which accounts for between 70 and 80 per cent of urban workers.
115 D. Lampton, op. cit., p. 267.

# Part Two

# PREVENTIVE MEDICINE

# 6 PREVENTIVE HEALTH WORK IN THE PEOPLE'S REPUBLIC OF CHINA, 1949–82

## S.M. Hillier

Activities directed towards preventing ill health can be considered in a number of ways. At the simplest level prevention
can be concerned with those measures which stop disease or
injury from occurring. Examples of this are immunisation, good
maternal and infant care, adequate nutrition and environmental
hygiene. Preventive health work is also concerned with identifying and treating patients promptly, either to prevent more
serious injury or the spread of disease. To this end, finding
cases and screening people who are at risk are important activities. Finally, preventive work is also concerned with mitigat-
ing the effects of illness which has already occurred. Therefore
rehabilitation and the continuing care of the chronic or terminally ill are also important aspects.

Generally speaking, it is possible to identify all these activities in the preventive health work carried out in the People's
Republic of China. How this has developed since 1949 will be
the main focus of this chapter.

The definition of what constitutes prevention and the *direction*
of preventive health activities as well as the importance allotted
to them relative to other branches of medicine and health care
have changed over the last thirty years in China. These changes
will be described below. Preventive health activities are not
just a product of the post revolutionary period, however. Writings exist on the scope and practice of medicine in ancient times.

## PREVENTION IN ANCIENT TIMES

The philosophical background to writings on preventive medicine and public health go back as early as the sixth century
before Christ. Early Chinese natural philosophy employed the
concepts of Yin and Yang - to describe two fundamental and
universal forces whose balance and reciprocal nature should be
maintained. The basic cause of illness it was held was an
imbalance of Yin and Yang. The body must therefore be the
subject of constant vigilance. Some methods and techniques
known collectively as 'wei-sing' (the protection of life) were
practised, and included various forms of gymnastics, special
sexual practices, fasting and abstinence and even exposure
of the body to sunlight, moonlight and wind.(1)

The greatest Chinese medical classic which dates from the
early Han period, the 'Huangdi Neijing' stated 'The sage does

not cure the sick, but prevents the illness from arising', and there are numerous other references in medical books written during the first millennium AD to the high status attached to preventive medicine. Nutritional literature which saw correct diet as the basis of any therapeutic regimen flourished and was still being revised by the most famous Imperial dietitian Hu Suhui in about +1330. The Han also employed sanitary inspectors whose job it was to fumigate buildings and control insect pests, remove dead bodies, protect fisheries from pollution and control traffic.

Preventive medicine in Ancient China had two aspects - self-care and legislation for public health. Of the two it seems the former was accorded the greatest importance. The 'Huangdi Neijing' pays great attention to the achievement of good balance both in one's mental and physical states, believing that security and a calm mind were prerequisites of good physical health. The book says: 'When one feels naturally happy and free from self seeking and upsetting personal desires or greedy ambitions then the salutary "Chhi" of necessity guards and follows. Vitality thus guarding from within, how can diseases originate.' Personal hygiene was accorded great importance amongst the gentry. Frequent bathing and hair washing is recommended.(2)

However, communal measures to ensure public health were also important. Clean drinking water, for example, was a priority to be supplied, and extensive works were undertaken. Seasonal cleaning of wells was an important activity during the Han, and it was during this period that the oldest record of indoor drains can be found, but even in Qin times the 'Lu Shih Qun Qiu' (Master Lu's Spring and Autumn Annals) notes 'flowing water does not putrefy' and it was stated that 'if drains are unclogged and houses clean, there will be no foul odours and disease will not arise'.(3) The purity of the Six Wells which were the reservoirs of eleventh-century Hangzhou was jealously guarded and in the Sung capital of Kaifeng 'every spring people were told by the government to supervise the cleaning of the city's drains'.(4) Refuse removal and street cleaning were carried out either by people themselves under official supervision, or by a special group of refuse disposal workers who were individually paid.

Public lavatories in cities were set up as early as the Han as the result of public or private initiatives, partly for hygienic reasons and partly for the agricultural value of human faeces used as fertilizer. Lavatories were emptied daily by nightsoil collectors who then sold the contents to farmers or middlemen. The material was then transported to the countryside by barge.

The Chinese appear to have had clear knowledge of preventive medicine, and a concern for both public and individual health. Such an outlook originated in the theories of disease and the body which were fundamental to Chinese medicine, when it was necessary always to take measures to prevent the occurrence of physical or environmental imbalance. The imperial bureau-

cracy, and the extensive development of urban living made
public health activities necessary, together with the organisational means by which these could be carried out. Thus the
level of hygiene in Chinese cities up to the sixteenth century
far surpassed that of their European counterparts.

By the time of the Qing dynasty, however, the cleanliness of
cities had declined, and Mei quotes reports from the city of
Suzhou saying residents were obliged to hold their noses as
they walked the streets.(5)

However, the Chinese political system has always been geared
to the notion of prevention. It exists as basic to Chinese natural
philosophy, and a large-scale centralised structure has always
existed which allowed for preventive measures to be carried out.

## PREVENTION IN THE MODERN ERA

The early modern attempts at prevention are described in chapter 2; the Guomindang government, although making attempts
at prevention, lacked the organisational structure to tackle
problems over such a huge area. With the exception of a few
doctors, preventive health work was not the primary focus of
their 'professionalised' version of health care derived from the
medical schools of Europe and the USA. The Japanese invasion
and subsequent civil war produced a climate in which it was
impossible to carry through any reforms. However, in the
Communist-base areas of the Jiangxi soviet, a basic emphasis
on preventive measures was evident, and necessary to preserve
the health of Red Army soldiers. Even so, conditions left a
lot to be desired. If the army were not to be decimated more
by dysentery than the enemy, preventive measures had to be
put into action. 'Pay attention to sanitation' was one of the six
major disciplines of the Red Army General Ju De.(6) The Communist approach to preventive health measures derived much
from their guerilla experiences; these experiences set a style
of preventive health care which was particularly dependent
upon mass movements and the participation of ordinary people.

## PREVENTIVE HEALTH CARE IN THE EARLY POST-REVOLU-
TIONARY YEARS

The Communist Party's commitment to prevention was under-
lined at the first National Health Conference in Beijing on 7-9
August 1950. Li Dequan, the Minister of Health, wrote two
months later:

with China estimated as needing five million hospital beds,
five hundred thousand doctors and three to four million
auxiliary medical personnel of all kinds and with tens of
millions of people yearly suffering from preventable com-

municable diseases and epidemics it is obvious that a short
route must be found to the problem. And it has - keep people
from getting sick.(7)

EPIDEMIC DISEASES

Already in 1949 in those areas occupied by the Communists, a
three-level approach to the problems of sanitation and epidemic
disease had begun. A Central Plague Prevention Committee was
set up and was responsible for co-ordinating 'plague teams' of
medical staff who would be sent to deal with plague outbreaks
anywhere they occurred.(8) In October 1949 three teams amount
ing to 540 PLA (Peoples Liberation Army) and university staffs
were sent to Chahar. Soviet doctors were also called in to rende
assistance.(9) Other communicable diseases less immediately
urgent, and the organisation of health work in general, came
under the jurisdiction of the NE People's Government Department of Public Health. Their work also relied essentially on the
use of mobile teams; the method of organisation was to move to
rural areas where a particular disease was endemic, and to
attempt mass inoculations. Areas which had a rudimentary local
administration (and this applies to those parts of China which
had been longest under Communist control) had their own local
sanitary bureaux. By August 1949 the sanitary bureaux of
Dalien and its environs were beginning inspections of shops and
dwellings, and concentrating on local sanitation, 'including
attempts to eliminate mosquitoes and flies'.(10) Where possible
their job was also to organise the inoculation of townspeople.
In Shanghai that summer two and a half million people were
inoculated against epidemic disease.(11)

By early 1950 the Ministry of Public Health had announced its
immediate objectives - the eradication of plague and smallpox
within three to four years, and the regularisation and increase
in the numbers of drugs available for treatment and inoculation.(12) It also began to sponsor what was to be a constant
feature of preventive health work subsequently - public education by means of pamphlets and pictures. Success was claimed
for this 'shock team' and mass inoculation approach, giving as
an example the eradication of plague in Manchuria in the previous year.(13) Obviously the situation was well enough under
control by spring 1950 for a plague team bearing enough vaccine for a million people to be 'rushed from Manchuria to the
southern tip of Kwangtung province'.(14)

At that time the provision of pharmaceuticals was still a
serious problem. The Ministry demanded that 70 per cent of
supplies should be produced by local pharmaceutical departments.(15) A response appeared to be forthcoming. In the
north east smallpox vaccines for 40 million people were produced
but in Xinjiang, Sichuan, Henan and Shandong, external suppliers were still the main source of drugs.(16)

By summer of that year the New China News Agency announced the objectives of the fight against epidemic disease. In addition to the necessity of case notification and inoculation, increasing emphasis was placed on the need for a clean environment. China's cities began to 'clean up' and get rid of pests and vermin. In Beijing, 'gastrointestinal diseases that carry away thousands every summer and autumn [was due] to the network of underground sewers carrying sewage from the wealthier quarters of the city, which did not run into the grand canal, but surfaced in the city in the heart of a densely populated working-class quarter of the city'.(17) In north-east China 'the health service together with the mobilised people caught and killed 14,590,000 rats'.(18) By midsummer Shanghai had inoculated three million people, Guangzhou half a million, mainly against the 'summer disease' of cholera.(19) A modest programme of BCG inoculations for infants, children and young adults was also undertaken(20) in the major cities.

By the end of its first year's work, the Minister claimed:

in the first six months of this year, health workers gave 36,546,431 smallpox vaccinations, over 200,000 BCG inoculations, 6,842,949 injections against cholera, 4,701,063 against plague, 336,452 against typhoid.(21)

An evaluation of preventive work during these years can be seen as rapid and efficient responses to epidemics, but due to lack of resources only a preliminary attempt to tackle endemic disease occurred. Preventive work in the area of infant mortality too was recognised to be a difficult problem, awaiting the full training of midwives. Where these had been available, their success was obvious, reducing the infant mortality rate in one Shandong village from 37 per cent to 2 per cent.(22) In the western province of Xinjiang the infant mortality rate was lowered from 490:1,000 to 80:1,000.(23) Tuberculosis and venereal disease were difficult endemic diseases, whose treatment was relatively expensive, and they became the subject only of 'limited work on an experimental basis',(24) and in a major speech Vice-Minister of Health He Cheng warned against complacency saying that there were '6 million unnecessary deaths annually from infectious disease, and one in five of the population suffered some form of illness'.(25) However by 1952 the mobile anti-epidemic corps could claim success in the control of diphtheria, typhoid, kala-azar and, most notably, in smallpox, cholera and plague.

Preventive measures were given a considerable boost in 1952 with the use by the Americans of germ warfare in the Korean War. The Chinese Medical Association denounced the 'spreading of germs and poisonous substances over Korea and North East China'. It was proposed that mass supervision be organised 'to report every aircraft spreading poisonous insects or other matter'. Prevention classes were to be set up,(26) and swift

action by Chinese anti-epidemic units helped to obviate the
development of plague in Shandong and Manchuria,(27) but it
was claimed that the epidemic in Jiangsu was a consequence of
bacteriological warfare by the Americans.(28) An unexpected
side effect of bacteriological warfare was that impetus was given
to the setting up of epidemic centres and public health offices
in those areas far from the Korean border, which had been
somewhat tardy in their approach to prevention. In central
south China public health offices and health centres were set
up, and health departments created in all those areas where
land reform had taken place.(29) Two thousand midwives were
trained(30) with the aim of providing one to every settlement
of fifty thousand people. This period also saw the boost of the
first of the Patriotic Health Campaigns, those mass 'clean-ups'
which have characterised the Chinese approach to prevention
ever since. Using the People's fears about germ warfare as a
means of mobilisation 'shock attacks' lasting one to three days
were initiated. The population would clean and disinfect streets
and houses, destroy insects (later known as the 'four pests'),
clean wells and report possible instances of germ warfare.(31)

   The massive public response to these instructions resulted
in the acceleration of the cleaning-up campaign. Information on
infection and instructions on how to deal with animal and insect
pests was widely displayed and the first major assault on several
centuries of dirt and unsanitary living conditions was made.

PREVENTIVE MEASURES 1953-9

By the mid 1950s the first approach to prevention, control of
epidemics and mass inoculation was well under way. The second
aspect, environmental control, was basically established; the
third, training a corpus of medical and nursing staff to improve
preventive health, had made some modest beginnings (see
chapter 11 for a discussion of the training of medical personnel); and the fourth, the attack on endemic diseases, was
beginning. These difficult but linked areas of prevention will
be considered separately.

*Mass inoculation and the status of infectious diseases*
As we have seen, early attempts at prevention had used mobile
teams of medical and paramedical staff as a means of coping with
the disease burden and the shortage of locally available manpower. The teams were essentially 'on call' emergency measures,
but the hope was that with the inoculation programme, infectious
diseases would be brought under control. However, the teams
alone were not sufficient for the task and more stable local units
were obviously required. There were major successes in wiping
out smallpox and cholera.(32) A massive programme of 250 million inoculations had yet to be carried out as well as investigation into a whole variety of other diseases, notably malaria,

B-encephalitis, leprosy, Keshan disease, tuberculosis, bubonic
plague, cerebrospinal meningitis. The winter and spring of
1956-7 saw widespread epidemics. A Ministry of Health circular
stated:

> The prevalence of influenza, measles, epidemic meningitis
> and epidemic cerebrospinal meningitis may have been due to
> the increased contact resulting from the rapid development
> of communications, from the increased virulence of these
> diseases, and the increased susceptibility of sections of the
> population towards these diseases.(33)

In March 1957 Beijing had epidemics of communicable disease
in over two hundred units. Epidemic cerebrospinal meningitis
occurred in the winter months in Anhui, Hubei, and Shanxi.
The mortality rate was very high.(34) In November 1956 Beijing had a 14-fold increase in measles, Shanghai a 91-fold
increase.(35)

The official reasons given above only hinted at other sources
of strain in preventive inoculation work. The 'increased susceptibility of certain sections of the population' must surely refer
to the food shortages which immediately followed the decline in
agricultural production during the massive acceleration towards
collective agriculture which occurred in 1956-7. However, this
matter was quickly rectified when the 1957 harvest broke all
records.(36) A more fundamental reason was shortage of
financial resources; from the outset, Ministry policy had been
to decrease the financial demands on the central administration,
particularly in the matter of drugs and equipment. Provincial
health bureaux, faced with overstretched budgets, could not
cope. During the National Biologic Conference held in August
1956 the Ministry 'requested health departments and health
bureaux of fifteen provinces and municipalities to refrain from
large-scale reductions in the purchasing of biologic products'.(37)

By February the State Council notified the various provinces
and municipalities of available funds in order that plans could
continue.(38) It was clear that the central policy of 'putting
prevention first' was being undermined in a number of ways.
As the public health journal stated:

> Instruments and equipment, especially laboratory apparatus
> essential in the physical examination of the patient is lack-
> ing. For example there is no microscope in the Ting Hsien
> Prevention Station (no wonder there has been no further
> extension in the control of hookworm disease in Ting Hsien).
> Only 3 to 5 per cent of the medical treatment and epidemic
> prevention funds are set aside for epidemic prevention
> work.(39)

Not only finance, but organisational and medical skills were lacking. Paradoxically, the successes in 'clean-up work' organised by epidemic prevention stations took resources away from research into communicable diseases, and it was felt at this time amongst professionals that although the average cadre might be excellent at motivating people to exterminate rats and flies his theoretical knowledge and practical experience were insufficient to prepare him to face the complex health problems of growing industrial cities.(40)

The Ministry of Health and leading medical cadres felt that the amateur approach to prevention was no longer the best way to deal with many and widespread sources of disease - new sources in mines and factories, as well as the old familiar problems of diphtheria, measles and malaria and tuberculosis. Emphasis was given to strengthening the role of Epidemic Prevention Stations and professionalising their approach.(41) These stations were based in each city district and divided into five sections: food hygiene, industrial hygiene, environmental health communicable diseases of the intestinal tract, and parasitic diseases.(42) They also had a role in treating disease and it was clear that this would overstretch their slender resources. Despite Ministry demands that more professionalised work was required, in the medical schools

> the majority of high school graduates prefer the study of clinical medicine rather than that of public health. This results in a shortage of preventive medical personnel. Thus the quality of preventive health work from the provincial level down to the local public health units is low.(43)

While upholding the importance of expert opinion, health cadres failed to recognise opposition within the medical profession itself to undertaking preventive work.

It followed that expansion and upgrading of the basic preventive services were unlikely due to the shortage of resources. Further it was clear that these were policy differences between what medical professionals, the Ministry of Health and the Party wanted with respect to prevention. Where medical workers were placed under the lay control of Public Health bureaux friction occurred. During the 'Hundred Flowers' movement of 1957, when many aspects of Party policy were criticised, one leading doctor testily remarked that 'the Public Health Department was tyrannical and ostentatious and mess arose from the disregard of expert opinion by lay people'.(44)

Other doctors interested in prevention criticised the Ministry of Health. The public health expert Qin Baozhen said 'The Ministry has laid too much emphasis on medical treatment at the expense of preventive work.'(45)

*Environmental improvements and the patriotic health campaigns*
The massive health campaigns of the early 1950s which relied

on the participation of the population were still favoured by
the party as the major means of prevention. On 12 January 1956
the 'People's Daily' called for a nationwide movement to wipe out
mosquitoes, flies, rats and sparrows in order to protect public
health and guarantee increased production of grain. Provincial
health bureaux made plans for the campaign. In Heilongjiang
200,000 youths and children were organised into teams to catch
rats and sparrows.(46) The initial emphasis died out and by
1957 Li Dequan, the Minister of Health, was referring to 'the
occasional ineffectual Patriotic Health Movements which have
not successfully promoted a sustained health routine in a given
community'.(47) She emphasised that 'preventive health work
is a long-term target and cannot be accomplished within a short
time', and that reorganisation of basic-level health units, which
had prevention as their major priority, was a necessity as the
basis for the fulfilment of the Second Five-Year Plan.(48) The
main work of Epidemic Prevention Stations up to that time had
been

> the promotion of the Patriotic Health Movement and the era-
> dication of the 'Four Menaces' (rats, flies, mosquitoes and
> sparrows). These mass movements were responsible for
> reducing the occurrences of epidemics, lowering the death
> rate and improving the sanitation of cities.(49)

However, there were reservations as to the continuing effectiveness of such work, since 'there is no effective system to
popularize mass participation in health work'.(50)

*Achievements in public health work*
It was possible however to claim that there had been no cholera
for eight years, and that smallpox was basically eliminated.
Infant mortality rates in some places had been reduced from the
pre-liberation figure of 200:1,000 to 13:1,000.(51) In particular
mortality from measles had fallen from 8.6 to 1.5 per cent
between 1950 and 1957, while that from scarlet fever fell from
17.5 to 1.3 per cent.(52) Maternal mortality rates had fallen
from 35 per thousand to 0.5 per thousand.(53) Differences
emerged in the way these successes were evaluated. The Ministry was of the opinion that many improvements were related to
organisational changes in health care, especially in child health
and the midwifery training which had been sponsored by them.
In 1956 there were now some 4,560 maternal and child health
stations, compared with 349 in 1950,(54) and whereas before
1949 less than 0.9 per cent of births was attended by a trained
midwife, by 1957 the number had increased to a staggering
61 per cent.(55)
The dramatic fall in death rates from tuberculosis was attributed to the construction of sanatoria and the inoculation of
all newborn babies,(56) and the Ministry pointed out that it was
the mobilisation of medical treatment facilities which would make

the difference in any epidemic outbreak. Publications from the
Ministry of Health re-emphasised that although there had been
a fall in the mortality rate from tuberculosis in 1956 of 17.8 per
cent compared with the previous year and 72 per cent compared
with 1949,(57) and a dramatic growth in the numbers of patients
treated and numbers of beds available for TB treatment (there
were now over 40,000),(58) yet 'there are far too many tuberculosis cases in the nation to warrant establishing a definite
date for the final elimination of tuberculosis, but sooner or later
it will be eradicated'.(59) Furthermore, tuberculosis was still
the main cause of death.(60)

## The Great Leap Forward

By 1958 the Minister of Health was again speaking out enthusiastically in favour of the Party line on mass movements and
upholding the importance of the Patriotic Health Movement.
The change in her position can best be understood by remember-
ing that the Great Leap Forward represented a massive attempt
by the Party under Mao's leadership to speed up the industrialisation of China. The prominence of Mao was reflected in
the resurgence of those health policies most closely identified
with him – the mass movements. Renewed efforts in 1958 resulted
in the slaughter of 1.9 billion rats and 2.1 billion sparrows!(61)
The formation of People's Communes had made available an
organisational basis for these labour-intensive mass campaigns.
All the signs were that they would be pursued with renewed
vigour. In 1959 Li Dequan announced that 'more than a million
citizens in the capital, which is now one of the cleanest cities in
the world, have joined in the campaign in the past three days
to exterminate insects'.(62)

During the late 1950s, the mass campaigns were publicly
regarded as the major means of achieving the goal of prevention.
This was clearly the view of the Communist Party, and it was
apparently deferred to by the Ministry of Health. While much
had been achieved parasitic disease was still a major threat to
health. According to figures compiled in 1959, 280 million
people, or 1 in 3 of the Chinese population, suffered from some
form of parasitic disease.(63) The ratio could be slightly higher
since often diseases occurred in combination. It made political
and economic sense to concentrate on these diseases, but the
methods advocated to deal with them differed. While the Party
favoured mass action, particularly during the Great Leap Forward, health cadres in the civil apparatus, the Ministry, still
tended to trust an expert approach and were cautious as to the
impact of mass movements on the total health profile of the
Chinese people.

## Endemic diseases

The disagreement between the Ministry of Health and the Party
will be examined with particular reference to two troublesome
health problems, syphilis and schistosomiasis. In the first case,

one particular line of approach proved largely successful in the
eradication of disease. In the second, disagreements continue to
the present as to the most useful method of attack and the
disease, although under control in many areas, is far from
eradicated.

*The control of venereal disease*    The heritage of civil war and
foreign invasion prior to 1949, together with the poverty of
families forced to sell their girl children into prostitution, and
the absence of adequate health care, had produced a situation
where venereal disease was rife. Among minority people, about
10 per cent of the population were sufferers, in the cities and
urban areas 5 per cent and in the countryside between 1 and
3 per cent.(64)

When the Communist Party came to power, immediate measures
were taken to deal with prostitution. Brothels were closed and
prostitutes given free medical treatment. More importantly, a
number of large-scale reforms altered the social climate which
had produced prostitution. Land reform struck at the roots of
rural poverty. Increased industrialisation meant that jobs were
available for women. The economic and social transformation
of women's lives - as exemplified by the New Marriage Law of
1949 which gave women equal political and economic rights with
men - signified an important and irreversible change in the
status of women.

Alongside these social measures, the public health task of
case-finding and treating venereal disease had begun. In the
early 1950s Ministry of Health teams had organised medical
teams, which dealt with venereal diseases as part of their
general epidemic work. Mass campaigns against syphilis, urging
people to come for treatment, were combined with the Patriotic
Health Movement, and a specialised Central Research Institute
was given the massive task of co-ordinating case-finding,
research, treatment and training of specialised personnel.

First attempts were made with a survey of the Mongolian-
Tibetan minorities between 1950 and 1953, and by efforts to
treat active cases of syphilis in the cities. By 1956 the Beijing
Venereal Disease Conference noted that in eight major cities
only twenty-eight cases of infectious syphilis were reported
between 1952 and 1958.(65)

The incidence of active cases showed a steep decline during
the first ten years of antisyphilis work (1952-62) and, where
they could be identified, the incidence of latent cases also. For
example an examination of 1,262,403 pregnant women in Shanghai over an eight-year period (1954-62) revealed a drop in
seropositivity from 4.38 per cent in 1954 to 0.56 per cent in
1962.(66)

Finding latent cases is one of the major public health chal-
lenges in venereal disease. It seemed impossible to organise
serologic testing of all the population. By 1957 the slowness
of methods of case-finding, and the immensity and urgency of

the task, were already beginning to cause friction among those responsible for the eradication of venereal disease. By 1957 over two million members of national minorities had received serologic tests, and case-finding methods in the cities included examinations of pregnant women, army recruits and high school students.(67) The Great Leap Forward of 1957-58, however, would lead to a greater emphasis on case-finding and new methods and new personnel to deal with the task.

Professional doctors in the field of venereal disease had sought to increase efficiency by demanding more money and personnel to increase the numbers who could be screened by serological tests. This was not forthcoming. The cost of medical care had been rising in the mid 1950s, while the health budget itself was declining.(68)

The Great Leap Forward brought the establishment of health centres in many communes. Equally importantly, an ideology was espoused which stressed the importance of mass activity in overcoming problems. In the eradication of syphilis, the involvement of both the mass of people in 'at risk' rural areas and use of short-term trainees to undertake serologic testing and treatment, became the chief method of attack. Health propaganda work was given a boost. Meetings were held where activists would explain the causes of syphilis and urge people to come for treatment.

> Syphilis is a legacy of the old society. Our Party and people threw out the ruling classes... it is no fault of your own if you are afflicted. Cure is sure and free. If you have any of the clues come for an examination. Comrades, we cannot take syphilis with us into socialism.(69)

The 'clues' referred to in the quotation were a ten-point check-list of symptoms. The Institute of Venereology decided to use this method of case-finding in fifteen communes in Ningho county, Jiangxi, despite criticisms;

> some medical 'bourgeois experts' and conservatives who thought in the old way did not believe in the mass line. Some said that a lot of cases would be missed, others that the methods were too crude, and unscientific. Others said 'politics cannot eradicate syphilis'.(70)

This method of identifying latent and active cases by publicising symptoms uncovered over 90 per cent of venereal disease patients. The examination, diagnosis and treatment was carried out by specially trained lay workers and these trainees were successful in correctly diagnosing 89.7 per cent of cases(71) after a seven-day training.

Ma Haide, China's leading venereologist, writing at the beginning of the cultural revolution in 1966, claimed 'syphilis is now under full control through the country'. Surveys carried out in the early 1960s as a ten-year follow-up showed that no new cases had occurred, and in 1966 it was said that 'mass campaigns are over'.

The Chinese have always claimed that the campaign to eradicate syphilis has been successful, although no further information exists after 1966. It is also stated that other venereal diseases, e.g. gonorrhoea, were dealt with and eradicated at the same time. Presumably post-treatment 'mopping up' was required, and Ma Haide remarked that 'long-term post-treatment measures need to be further developed and strengthened... the measures used in the national minority areas need further study'.(72)

It is worth noting that while in 1949 10 per cent of cases in psychiatric hospitals were suffering from general paresis (late-stage syphilis), by 1970 no cases could be found.(73)

The control and eradication of syphilis was claimed at the time to be a victory for the 'mass line' and Mao's thought. The apparent speed-up of the campaign against syphilis during the Great Leap Forward was obviously an attempt to deal quickly with the rural areas where the disease had been neglected. It may be, however, that the bulk of the problem – which lay in the cities and national minority areas – had already been dealt with by 1957-8.

Urban groups had much more access to medical treatment. As Ma Haide said: 'in the cities measures are easier to carry out and have proved effective'. And even if eradication was not total in the national minority areas – 'they still need further study' – the problem was clearly defined and controllable. In any case, it would appear that large-scale social changes, which included raising the status of women, strengthening the position of the family and restricting internal travel and migration, were of equal, if not greater, importance than any particular treatment policy in the eradication of this disease.

*The battle against schistosomiasis* The comparison of different policies and approaches in the case of schistosomiasis is of considerable interest. Schistosomiasis continues to be a major threat to health at present. Like syphilis, the toll in terms of human suffering and disability is enormous. However, the scope of the problem was much greater, with approximately five times the number of people infected(74) than was the case with syphilis. During the 1950s mass surveys had been conducted. Approximately 10 million people living in the middle and lower Yangtze river valley were found to be infected and the health of a further 100 million was menaced in this, the major rice-growing area of China.(75) Essentially this was a rural disease. The most susceptible were the young, poor and lower middle peasants. Of the population in endemic areas 20 to 40 per cent were infected, and in some villages the rate was 70 per cent or more.(76) Injurious effects of schistosomiasis were obvious and devastating since it took a major toll of the agricultural

workforce. In 1955, in Qingbo county, Jiangsu province, the
paddy fields were uncultivated and more than half the 270,000
inhabitants of the county suffered from the disease.(77) In
many other villages the disease had been endemic for over one
hundred years. Many families died out, others fled from the
infected areas.

Schistosomiasis is caused by the fluke 'Schistoma japonicum',
which penetrates the skin and lodges in the large intestine. It
can spread to other parts of the body, especially the liver,
rectum and bladder. It causes an enlarged spleen, anaemia
and ascites and death occurs by liver failure or haemorrhage.
Eggs are carried in human or animal faeces and urine which is
discharged into water. The larvae hatch and parasitise water
snails, until full grown, when they enter their human host
through the skin from infected water. In order to control the
disease, a number of different measures are possible: the intermediate host the snail can be destroyed; the water supply can
be decontaminated; the faeces containing the ova can be regulated and rendered harmless; personal hygiene can be improved
and protective clothing worn, and treatment initiated to break
the cycle of disease. A combination of all these methods has
been used in the Chinese case but one problem has been the
close relationship between the life cycle of the fluke and that of
rice cultivation in paddy fields.

During the early 1950s overall responsibility for the control
of schistosomiasis had lain with the newly formed Ministry of
Health which, as we have seen, also carried responsibility for
preventive work in many other fields. The initial approach to
schistosomiasis followed that found effective in the treatment
of contagious diseases – case identification on a massive scale
and the setting up of a treatment network. By 1952 there were
17 anti-schistosomiasis stations, 61 sub-stations and 132 field
units.(78) However, this number was clearly inadequate to
cope with the enormous disease burden; although it was possible
to identify cases the disease proved extremely difficult to
treat; treatment alone, even if it could be effective, was clearly
insufficient to wipe out schistosomiasis. Problems of initial
infection and reinfection remained relatively untackled, largely
because the Ministry of Health had not had the organisational
resources available to mobilise the more complex preventive
work necessary to alter the life cycle of the fluke, and also
lacked the power to exact co-operation from other ministries,
like Agriculture or Water Conservancy, whose participation in
the project was necessary for success.(79)

The slow pace of anti-schistosomiasis work in the early 1950s
had decided the Party leadership, particularly Mao, to change
the organisational structure for dealing with the problem. In
November 1955 the Party Central Committee had created the
Nine-Man Anti-schistosomiasis Group which was given authority
to co-ordinate all agencies involved. This committee was essentially a lay organisation with a Chairman of Politburo level, and

the seeds of conflict between this group and the medical professionals in the Ministry of Health were present from the outset.(80) The Nine-Man Committee immediately undertook the
promotion of mass methods to control schistosomiasis. The main
method of attack was to alter the environment of the intermediate host, the snail, and thus break the infection cycle at
that point.

Peasants in the infected areas were mobilised to dig out the
earth inhabited by snails to a depth of a metre, and suffocate
the snails under a layer of earth. The work had got off to a
swift start, with a seven-year plan for eradication initiated in
1956:

> according to incomplete statistics more than seventy million
> square metres have been cleared of snails... extension of
> excreta control and water purification has been enforced and
> over forty thousand patients have been treated for schisto-
> somiasis.(81)

In Anhui province in 1956 1.5 million people had devoted 20
million man-days to the campaign.(82) Overall, over 2 million
farmers were mobilised to bury snails.(83) This was relatively
easy where ditches were small, but more difficult where there
were rivers and irrigation systems. The large-scale engineering
works involved in the production of irrigation systems were
monitored to control the water level, and so prevent an upsurge
in new schistosomiasis cases which often accompanies irrigation
construction.

By the second year of the seven-year plan some success in
snail clearing had been achieved. However, cases of reinfection
were noted, especially in Henan and Hubei provinces.(84) The
Ministry of Health involvement had diminished, since it no
longer controlled the programme, to research into appropriate
treatments for the disease and faeces control. Night-soil, as
human faeces is called in China, has been used for centuries as
a fertiliser. Left untreated on the land and containing parasitic
ova it provided a potent source of infection. Measures for storing night-soil in a compost to kill off ova were instituted, as
were stricter controls of faeces disposal. The night-soil was
collected in a 'cleanliness administration office', stored centrally
and treated to destroy parasitic eggs.(85) Washing night-soil
buckets in rivers and lakes was forbidden and to aid the orderly
collection of night-soil, many latrines were constructed.

Treatments were also being administered on a mass scale.
Between 1955 and 1956 the Party mobilised and trained 84,000
activists to undertake the work of administering sodium anti-
mony tartrate, and almost a million people were treated in
1956-7.(86) The period of treatment was shortened from twenty
to three days which enabled larger numbers to be treated.

The Seven-Year Programme received a boost during the
Great Leap Forward of 1958. The launching of People's Communes

and the collectivisation of all land created the opportunity for
the organisation of large-scale environmental attacks on schistosomiasis. The number of treatment stations was increased as
were the personnel working in the field. The first nine months
of 1958 saw the reported construction of 63 million public
latrines.(87) The disease had already been wiped out that year
in Yujiang county, Jiangxi province, and in eight counties and
cities and 116 districts and townships was 'basically under
control'. These achievements inspired Mao to write his famous
poem 'Farewell to the God of Plague'.(88) In 1958 over 3 million
patients were treated, including those with late-stage schistosomiasis, for whom combined treatment with traditional medicine
was found successful.(89) The mass movement to eradicate snails
was accompanied by a movement to educate the rural population
about the nature of schistosomiasis using films, slides, travelling shows and exhibitions and plays. According to Cheng Tien-
hsi, in Anhui province alone, a film depicting the life of 'Schistoma japonicum' had been seen by 440,000 peasants in 1,100
showings.(90)

> When the propaganda team called at Peiching production bri-
> gade of Yutai Commune in Hsiakau hsien, five or six young
> people on seeing a photo of a 'big belly' [late stage develop-
> ment of schistosomiasis] did not believe it and almost burst
> out laughing. An old commune member standing beside them
> said; 'What are you laughing at? I had a big belly before.
> Were it not for the arrival of the Communist Party I should
> have been dead long ago.'
> Hsiaossu Commune in Hangyang was situated in an area
> where schistosomiasis was prevalent. In the past some
> basic-level cadres said 'a red mark is left by a mosquito
> bite. Blood is shed as the result of a bite of ants and locusts.
> But the larvae discharged by snails is not even visible. How
> can they enter the human body?' Later a visit to the exhibi-
> tion convinced them. They said 'It is harmful not to believe
> in science.'(91)

Payment in terms of work points for taking part in snail clearing exercises, often done in connection with irrigation construction or during agricultural slack periods, was rationalised.(92) Throughout the campaign snail burying and burning
were the methods of choice and the use of expensive molluscicides played only a secondary role.(93) Research into the
disease was also intensified and the number of research institutes increased.(94)

*Achievements*
By the end of 1958 about 40 per cent of snail-infested areas
were cleared, about eight billion square metres.(95) In the
same year over 3 million people had received treatment and by
1960 the number had risen to 5.2 million, over half the number

of sufferers. In 1960 3,600,000 had been cured.(96) The work of the Nine-Man Committee speeded up the slow, cautious research-oriented approach which had been adopted by the Ministry of Health. The Committee's special status and single task made it an effective unit which could co-ordinate the variety of agencies and levels. Partly because of its lay composition and mass character, however, there was little attempt at professional evaluation of the movement's success. In general the impact of the massive snail eradication programme, patient treatment and cure of the overall disease burden remain difficult to assess, and achievement was often measured in terms of effort expended rather than the permanent halting of the spread of the disease. There was some impact, however. In villages where the disease was cleared, residents now enjoyed a higher standard of living,(97) and grain production increased 33 per cent,(98) but the problem of this endemic disease, tied to the rural way of life, was unsolved and the committee's activities were severely curtailed by economic failures following the Great Leap Forward. The collapse of rural health structures made mass campaigns increasingly difficult to organise, and preventive activity during the next phase, prior to the Cultural Revolution, was played down.

## PREVENTIVE WORK PRIOR TO THE CULTURAL REVOLUTION, 1960-4

### Mass health movements

One prominent feature of this period was the growth in the status accorded to professionals and a relaxation of the intellectual climate. In preventive work, officials now stressed the importance of combining the role of professionals with the efforts of the masses. Mass movements declined in popularity. Indeed the Minister of Health, Qian Xinzhong, appeared directly opposed to 'health movements of the masses', saying 'when the dust of the east is fanned up, that gives people more chance of inhaling viruses and spreads tuberculosis'.(99)

When sanitation campaigns did take place they were largely directed towards urban rather than rural conditions and involved the major cities: Beijing, Guangzhou, Tianjin. The Great Leap Forward had produced a decline in urban sanitation standards. In Beijing in 1961 '13 shock sanitation movements have been carried out, during the course of which 1.7 million tons of garbage, night-soil and other waste were cleaned up'.(100) Rather than relying on the 'broad masses' to undertake the work, street cleaners were appointed. In Guangzhou a major clean-up was put under the control of the army.(101) In fact the army played an important role in sanitation work at this time, working mainly in the major cities and border regions. In Xinjiang 'red banners' were awarded to 'the headquarters and political department of the Sinkiang military region for their

meticulous sanitary work during the recent mass movement for
public health'.(102) Appeals rather than directives were issued
and although sanitation campaigns continued, they lost their
mass character; responsibility for organisation devolved to the
public health bureaux, who tended to carry out long-term plans
rather than engage in shock campaigns.

*Epidemic and endemic disease control*
Despite the floods, famine and drought of the early 1960s epidemic prevention measures were well organised enough to prevent any major disease outbreak. In a sense the Ministry of
Health continued working in the style of the early 1950s relatively uninterrupted by the need to organise mass campaigns.
They stressed organisational growth wherever possible given
limited resources, professional control of health care and the
development of research. This inevitably meant a move away
from the emphasis on preventive health care and one towards
curative health measures. The basic preventive infrastructure
based on local public health bureaux was not geared for any new
developments. In contrast, a new emphasis on the role of count
hospitals was more responsible to centralised direction from the
Ministry of Public Health.(103) Preventive work sponsored by
the Ministry tended to take the form of generalised directives on
inoculations, on occupational disease, the health of schoolchildren, and students' eyesight.(104) The diseases which
caused concern were mainly those attendant on unhygienic sanitation in cities, for example dysentery, or those related to
malnutrition (there had been widespread famine in the early
1960s). There were some notable achievements, however, the
result of ten years of persistent work. By 1961 it was claimed
that over 70 million cases of all types of parasitic disease had
been treated.(105) By 1962 preventive measures against kala-
azar had reduced the incidence of this disease from 3,500 per
million to 6 per million.(106) Infant mortality in Beijing, which
had been 86.6 per thousand in 1951 was now 29.9 per thousand.
Neonatal mortality over the same period fell from 44.4 per
thousand to 11.3 per thousand. In Shanghai, neonatal mortality
fell from 19.5 per thousand in 1957 to 7.5 per thousand in
1964.(107) By 1964 90 per cent of children had received BCG
vaccination.(108)

*Anti-schistosomiasis work*
The fall in agricultural production which was the aftermath of
economic experimentation, flood and drought at the end of the
1950s produced a situation where peasants were unwilling or
unable to expend time and energy in large-scale campaigns of
snail clearing. By 1962 molluscicides were being used(109) in
Hunan, and specialised prevention and control groups at the
behest of the county health bureaux were undertaking clearing
work, but on a much smaller scale than previously envisaged.(110)

By 1964, however, emphasis on schistosomiasis prevention again became prominent, with model villages which had rid themselves of the disease being cited as examples(111) and Yujiang county the subject of Mao's poem was once again in the news.(112)

## THE INFLUENCE OF THE CULTURAL REVOLUTION ON PRE-VENTIVE HEALTH WORK 1965-70.

Changes in the emphasis on schistosomiasis work towards the end of 1964 were among the early signs of a change in the political system in China.

Mao had always favoured the mass campaigns, and other policies in health which the Ministry of Health had pursued less than vigorously. Ministry emphasis on professional control of health, full professional training of doctors, on research, on urban development of health care and a professional management of preventive work were not the sorts of policies which, he felt, served the peasant and disadvantaged base from which Mao sought to draw his support. For economic reasons basic-level rural health care had remained relatively underdeveloped in the early 1960s, and this lack of development proved a valuable political weapon with which to attack official health policy, as well as giving voice to peasant demands for better health care. The 26 June directive of 1965 was a major speech by Mao, in which he maintained that the Ministry of Health in directing resources for health care was biased towards the privileged sectors of urban society:

> Tell the Ministry of Public Health that it only works for 15 per cent of the total population and that this 15 per cent is mainly composed of gentlemen, while the broad masses of the peasants do not get any medical treatment.(113)

Of course, his views did not go unchallenged, as those in charge of health policy sought to forestall criticism by discussing the means by which better health care for peasants could be obtained. This meant new efforts to eradicate schistosomiasis and the swift mobilisation of propaganda teams to revitalise the flagging or defunct mass movements. These teams - later to be regularised as mobile medical teams - trained the local peasantry in methods of preventive health.(114)

*Schistosomiasis prevention and rural sanitation*
Late in 1965 a major conference in one of the provinces where schistosomiasis was prevalent was held, and optimistic targets involving mass movements again proposed. Those areas which had progressed in anti-schistosomiasis work, it was said, should seek to eliminate the disease in one or two years. 'In other areas effort should be made to eliminate schistosomiasis in the shortest

possible period of time... the most important question... was to overcome hardship-dodging feelings and lethargic ideas....'(115)

By 1966 Mao's importance as a moving force in the new anti-schistosomiasis campaign was clear.

Revolutionary fervour must be combined with a scientific attitude. Areas which had or were about to eliminate the disease must prevent arrogance and lethargy and persist in the struggle to consolidate and increase victory. The Party Committees in areas where the disease was common must strengthen leadership.(116)

The revolutionary treatment mode which emphasised attempts to cure even the most advanced stages of the disease was encouraged. The number of splenectomies performed increased. (117) Research foci altered dramatically. A leading professor speaking on the state of medical research in China emphasised that 'the focus of attention for some time would be on common diseases. Many people were engaged in research on drinking water which held the key to preventing intestinal diseases, typhoid and dysentery'.(118)

'Slackness and lethargy in the work must be shaken off' stated a stern directive from the Shaanxi Public Health Bureau, warning of the dangers of epidemics of influenza and cerebrospinal meningitis.(119)

'Public health work has only started to face the countryside' declared speakers at a Hunan Public Health Conference,(120) and throughout the year provincial public health departments echoed the triple themes of sanitation, rural health, and the battle against schistosomiasis, underscored with the idea that all 'should seriously implement the Party's mass line'.(121) Throughout the next three years preventive health work became less of a matter for centralised direction and, increasingly, the success of prevention depended on local initiatives to carry it through. The Ministry of Health itself was occupied by Red Guards, and effectively closed between 1967 and 1969.

Three important developments in the organisation of health care, all of which affected preventive health, took place during the Cultural Revolution. These were: (a) mobile medical teams, together with the transfer of about one third of staff of the major city hospitals to work in the rural areas: (b) the large-scale training and deployment of paramedical health workers – the famous 'barefoot doctors'; (c) the co-operative medical service, a new method of payment for health care.

These developments represent a major shift in the balance of health work, in response to Mao's suggestion that the rural areas receive priority over urban areas.

*Mobile medical teams*  It was initially hoped that the transfer of large numbers of trained doctors to the countryside either permanently or for periods of time in small teams of twenty or thirty with specific tasks to perform would be potent force in raising the general level of health in the countryside. Early in 1964 the Ministry had sent a number of high-ranking prominent doctors as teams to selected rural areas,(122) but by 1965 the pressure to increase the scope of the operation was increasing. In Hebei province 10,000 health workers were transferred from urban hospitals.(123) In Guangdong province the initial response was much less and the persons sent were by no means all qualified doctors:

> In recent days... comparatively experienced medical staff of the Chungshan Medical College... [will] stay for long periods in the countryside. The staff, who include professors, lecturers, nurses and technicians will set out for 22 counties... at the beginning of May. A few of them are being sent to special district and county hospitals, but most will work at commune health centres.(124)

On their transfer to the countryside, the jobs of urban medical workers varied. They often found very unsanitary conditions, and a population in poor health. Their tasks therefore included curative measures and training the population (and later the barefoot doctors) in preventive measures and hygienic practices.

As a result of mingling with the poor and lower middle peasants the staff have gained understanding of how and whom to serve. They say that while they are curing the peasants' physical illness, the peasants are curing their ideological illness.(125)

The teams however were too sporadic and small in number to make much impact on the backward nature of rural health services. Although some of the city-trained doctors were in favour of the teams, many complained of the lack of facilities for modern medical treatment. There were few drugs, and often not even the simplest piece of equipment which might help in preventive work. As one ophthalmologist said:

> For urban medical workers, going down to the countryside is a deep-going ideological revolution... some medical workers face two ideological obstacles. First, they fear filthy, difficult and fatiguing work. Second, they fear that they may not learn anything in the countryside and will lose their skills.(126)

In the end the number of medical workers on mobile teams were fewer than had originally been intended. Instead of half the staff of urban hospitals, the figure that Mao had demanded, only about one third went down.(127) Those who went often included very new graduates, doctors with 'ideological problems' and old or handicapped doctors.(128) Nevertheless the teams appear to have tried earnestly to carry out the tasks required of them – the curing of disease, the supply of medicines, the training of medical personnel, sanitary measures for fertiliser accumulation and water storage and the launching of mass movements, within the resources available and the constraints of political upheaval. Interviews with hospital staff who had worked on mobile teams during this period indicate that those who were not medically qualified took charge of organising 'clean-ups' in the villages, educating the peasants in the basics of prevention which had worked well in the cities during the 1950s. In general they found this a difficult task.(129) Medically qualified personnel were more likely to work in the local hospitals and commune clinics, performing surgery,(130) while the non-medically qualified dealt with health education:

> We tried to persuade them to put chlorine in the water but they said 'Oh it's a bad smell, we don't like to use that'.... Then we would take a microscope and show them.... 'Take a look at that. That is what happens if you don't put chlorine in'... actually it was not the schistosome they saw, but they had plenty of worms in the water anyway, and it helped to convince them.(131)

> I volunteered to go to a very backward part of China. I was a teacher in the medical school. I went there for a year. I wanted to go and see what the situation was and I was influenced by Chairman Mao's teaching. I couldn't have imagined such a poor and backward situation. Where I went was the poorest commune. The first thing I saw was a woman giving birth. They don't think that birth should be in a clean place – it should be out of the house and very dark – in the pigsty, very dark and wet. That woman was just sitting there – there was not even clean paper let alone a blanket.... They had some water boiling I was relieved to see... but they said – 'That's to boil the eggs to give the woman after birth.'(132)

The Minister of Health was less than enthusiastic about the whole policy, in 1965 he wrote:

> Due to the lack of systematic investigation... and also the lack of experiences methodically summed up, we know very little about the characteristics of the outbreak and spread of various common diseases in the countryside, and the most effective methods for their treatment and prevention, the way to carry out effectively most of the elimination of the four pests, for publicising hygiene and for the prevention and control of diseases in the countryside.(133)

By 1966, according to his Red Guard accusers, he was saying: 'If everybody goes down to the countryside and does not
make a success of his work, he increases the burden on the
countryside.'(134)

Although it is difficult to evaluate the work of the teams,
they clearly helped to get preventive work in the communes
'off the ground': even if their own work was more in the direction of curative medicine, their presence gave impetus to a
growing view of public health as 'a revolutionary task'. Those
who complained about the arrival of the mobile teams in the
villages, and the new emphasis on sanitation and health measures, were condemned as 'bad elements' and medical workers
were reminded that they should have 'implacable hatred for
these class enemies'. Attempts were made to integrate mass
campaigns with spring farming to avoid the disruptive nature
of earlier campaigns.

This early period of the Cultural Revolution, 1966-7, demonstrated the confusion which confronted those responsible for
organising public health and preventive work. The new emphasis on rural health work (clearly an attempt to correct the
neglect of previous years) presented local health bureaux
with very large problems. First, with political changes they
received only the vaguest of central direction, and calls for
action. Second, they often did not have the powers of persuasion, money, or personnel to do what was required, even if the
task itself had been clear, but nevertheless in the prevailing
political climate felt impelled to make some attempt to follow
the general line, fearing criticism themselves. However, among
students in medical colleges and some of the younger staff
there was a genuine belief that to volunteer for a mobile medical
team was a revolutionary act. Many believed at this early stage
that this was a short-term measure; indeed it was only towards
the end of the decade that temporary 'going down' to the
countryside became 'permanent settlement'.

By the end of 1967 mobile teams could no longer be seen as
the solution to the problems of rural health. By 1968, two other
important developments occurred.

*Barefoot doctors*   Barefoot doctors were conceived as a force of
rural health workers, part peasant and part paramedic. Financed
by the commune, their medical work credited with work points,
and with brief periods of training ranging from three to six
months at county hospitals, their job was to cope with the basic,
common diseases and act as part of a referral chain to the county
hospital. One of their major tasks was prevention in all its
aspects: environmental sanitation, particularly of pig-pens and
water supplies; 'clean-up' campaigns; maternal and child health;
antenatal care and preventive inoculations:

At ordinary times the barefoot doctors went deep into the
fields and reservoir sites to give medical treatment to the

sick and make propaganda, *thus bringing preventive work
to the first line of production.* In winter we launched manure
accumulation movements on a large scale... exterminating
insect pests at the same time. In day-to-day preventive work
we laid emphasis on the control of water and manure and
improvements in cooking facilities and environmental hygiene.(135)

Despite the specialised personnel, the emphasis was once
again on the efforts of 'the masses' to achieve a higher level of
rural sanitation:

After one year of effort the poor and lower middle peasants
in their spare time converted 786 latrines which were for-
merly 'the paradise of pigs and dogs' into hygienic latrines
... at present there has arisen a movement among the masses
to regard the promotion of hygiene as glory.(136)

Their desire to be involved in such movements depended
upon the propaganda efforts of health workers to convince them
that prevention and a cheap and effective medical service went
hand in hand. The incentives, as we shall see below, were
economic.

*The co-operative medical service*   The co-operative medical
service is a means of financing rural health care at commune
level and below. Commune members pay a small fee and this is
subsidised by sums from the commune to provide a co-operative
medical fund. In addition commune members in some schemes
pay a registration fee and fees for medicines. Although there
are variations, the basic principle is much the same throughout
China.
Prevention was emphasised as a sine qua non of the co-
operative medical service. Clearly, preventing disease reduced
the burden on the co-operative service to which the peasants
all contributed. It also released funds for health personnel and
equipment, which in turn meant that more cases could be dealt
with on the commune without referral upwards to the county
hospital.

Some people have misgivings that after the establishment of
the co-operative medical service, and since medical treatments cost nothing, people would lay emphasis on medical
treatment and disregard prevention thus incurring waste...
such misgivings are superfluous [they] will pay even greater
attention to prevention and economy.(137)

However, as exponents of preventive health are often now
aware, prevention had to go hand in hand with curative activities. As the Vice-Minister of public health Zhang Kai drily
remarked when speaking of mobile medical teams in 1966: 'it

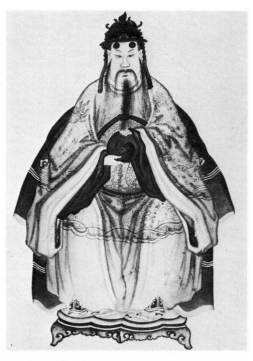

1(a) Fu Xi, a legendary deity and founder of medicine
In this painting he is holding the symbol for Yin and Yang and is believed to have divided nature into these aspects. He is also 'god' of hunting and animal husbandry.

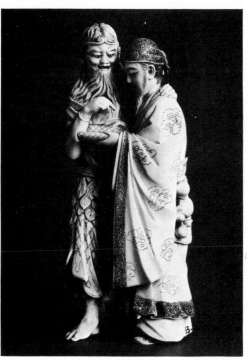

1(b) Shen Nong and Huang Di, ivory figures of the Yellow Emperor
Huang Di legendary author of the 'Nei Jing' (Canon of Medicine) discussing the book with Shen Nong a 'god' of Medicine, Pharmacy and Agriculture. He was supposed to have written the original 'Ben Cao Jing' (The Herbal).

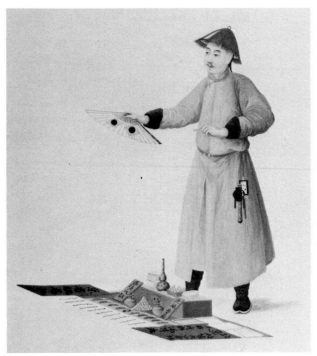

2(a) A nineteenth-century watercolour of a Chinese doctor
He has his wares laid out on the pavement and the symbols on his fan
represent medicinal plasters.

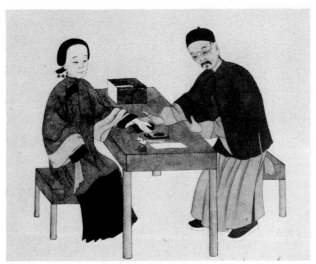

2(b) A nineteenth-century watercolour of a traditional doctor feeling a
patient's pulse
He is wearing glasses and the pen and paper is for writing the
prescription.

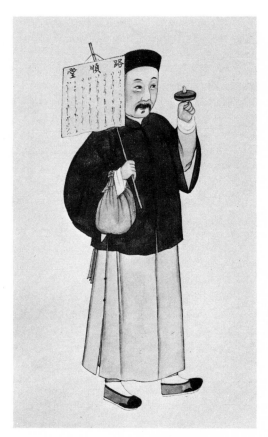

3(a) A nineteenth-century print of a 'medicine seller' He would wander around advertising his special prescriptions and is holding a bell on his finger.

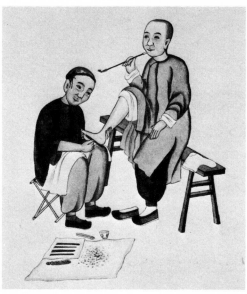

3(b) A nineteenth-century print of a chiropodist at work with his instruments laid out.

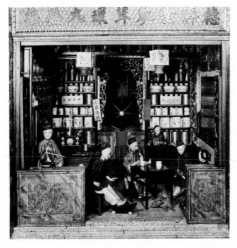

4(a) Model of a nineteenth-century pharmacy
At the rear of the shop is an altar to the god of medicine where incense was commonly burnt. The proprietor is serving two customers with tea. The assistant in the foreground is using a 'boat-shaped' mortar operated with his feet.

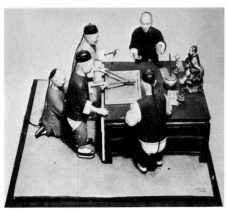

4(b) Model of a scene in a Medicine Temple
The worshipper is kneeling in front of the altar to the god of medicine. Two assistants are holding a planchette above a tray of sand on which the prescription is to be written. The prescription will be transcribed for the supplicant to take to the pharmacy.

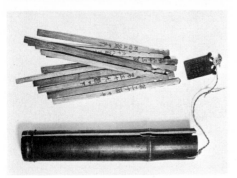

4(c) Bamboo container with sticks marked individually
The container is shaken while praying until one stick falls out and this indicates the appropriate prescription.

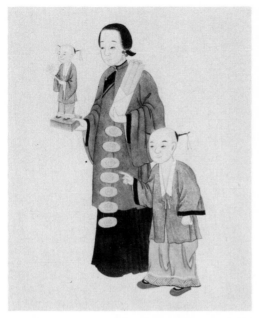

5(a) A nineteenth-century watercolour of a mother taking her child and effigy to the temple
The model, incense and paper money would be burnt for the gods in an appeal for the child's recovery.

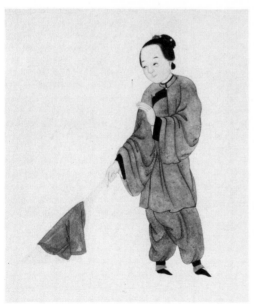

5(b) A nineteenth-century watercolour of 'Calling for the return of the soul'
If a child had convulsions, fainted or became comatose the relative would place a piece of clothing on a broom and wave this about calling the child's name in order to attract the soul back into his body.

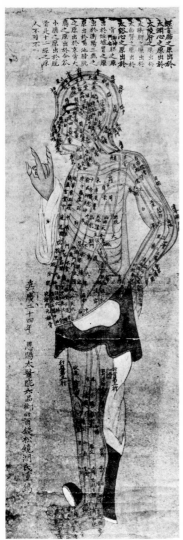

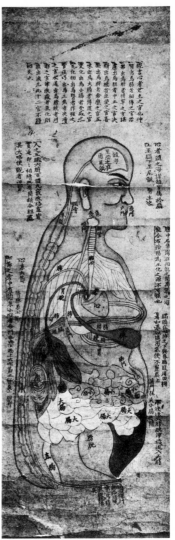

6(a) Anatomical chart of the Ming period illustrating the course of the acupuncture channels on the body.

6(b) Anatomical chart of the Ming period showing the internal Zang-fu organs.

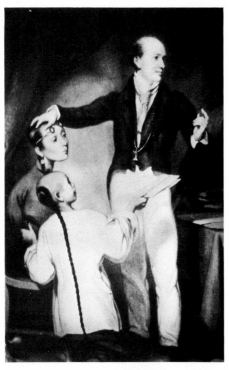

7(a) Thomas R. Colledge, surgeon of the East India Company
He established the Opthalmic hospital in Aomen (Macao) in 1827.
Taken from W. Daniell's engraving of George Chinnery's portrait.
(photo by Dr S. S. Brooks)

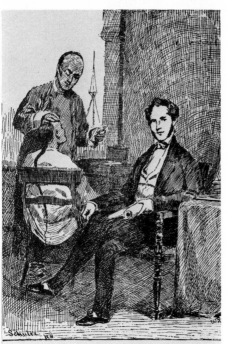

Rev. PETER PARKER, M.D.,

7(b) The Rev. Peter Parker, the first medical missionary in China
He opened the Canton Missionary Hospital in 1835.
In the background is the Chinese assistant Guan Yadu (Kwan Ato) who he trained to be an expert surgeon. He was the first Chinese trained in Western surgery and was surgeon to the Imperial forces during the 'Taiping rebellion'.
(photo by Dr S. S. Brooks)

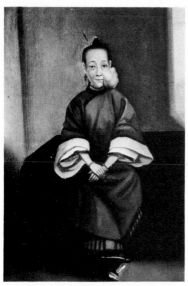

8(a) This case was a 41-year-old-woman 'one of the First Society of a native village' (Parker's notes), possibly with a parotid tumour.

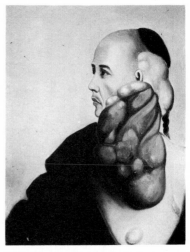

8(b) A 45-year-old man who had other small tumours on his body
The main mass arose from behind his ear with a 2-inch pedicle. After incision it weighed 4 lbs and may have been a case of multiple neurofibromatosis.

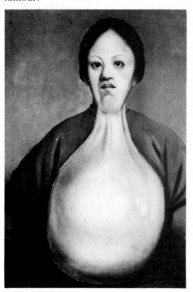

8(c) A 20-year-old woman with a mass arising from her chin
This had grown slowly over ten years but at the time she was also some 5 months' pregnant. It was excised in 12 seconds, was probably a lipoma and she had a son.

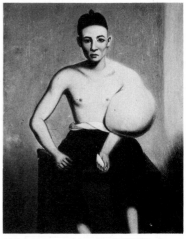

8(d) A 23-year-old male who had broken his arm six years before
It had fractured again six months prior to the operation. A cystic swelling had developed and amputation was recommended. This was probably the first amputation by a Western surgeon in China.

(These photographs by courtesy of the Gordon Museum, Guy's Hospital Medical School, London. They have a collection of paintings of some of Peter Parker's patients by 'Lamqua'. He was the uncle of Guan Yadu, Parker's assistant and was a student of the artist George Chinnery.)

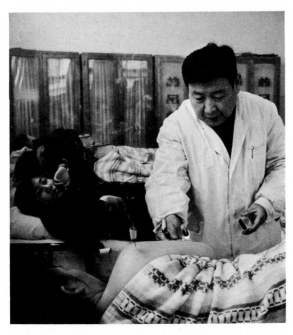

9(a) A modern acupuncturist treating a patient with 'warming needle', i.e. moxa burning on an inserted acupuncture needle
The patient may be suffering from a painful shoulder that in the West is sometimes referred to as a 'frozen shoulder'!

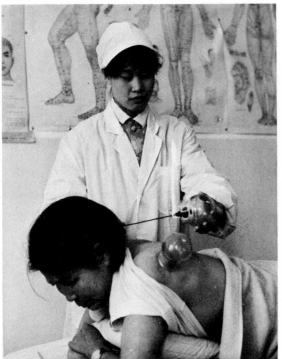

9(b) Cupping method
The practitioner is flaming the glass cup with a lighted, alcohol-soaked cotton-wool ball. The skin is sucked up into the cup when the hot expanded air cools.

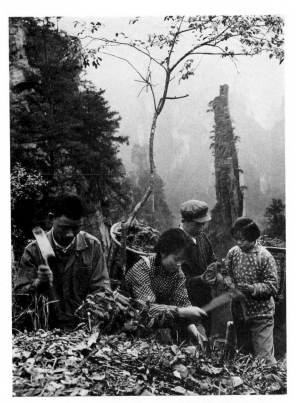

10(a) and 10(b)
Collecting and
processing medicinal
plants at a local level.

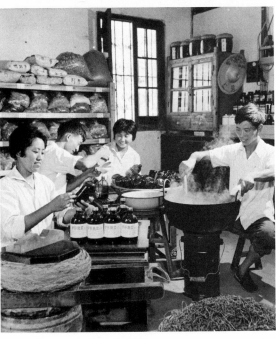

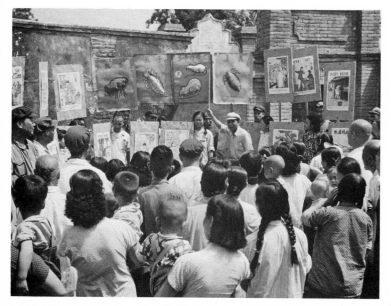

11(a) Public street campaign against the 'four pests' and to promote hygiene.

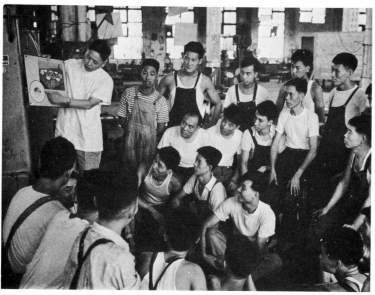

11(b) Health campaign in a factory workshop about contamination of food by flies.

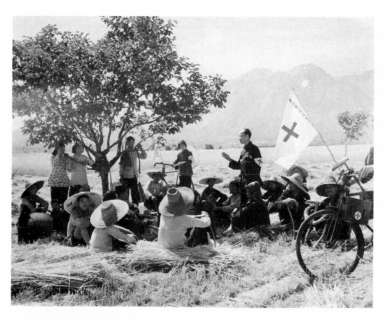

12(a) A rural health t[...]
campaigns amongst t[...]
peasants.

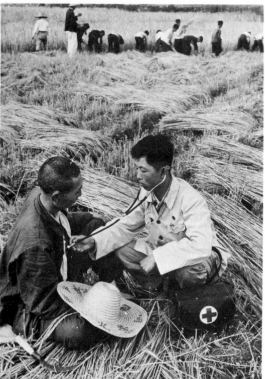

12(b) A 'barefoot' do[...]
consults in the fields.

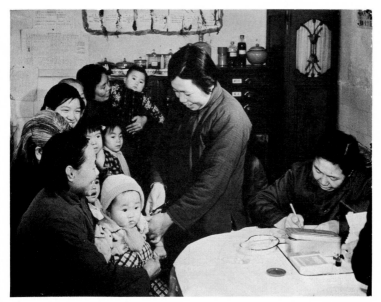

13(a) Childhood inoculation in a Neighbourhood clinic.

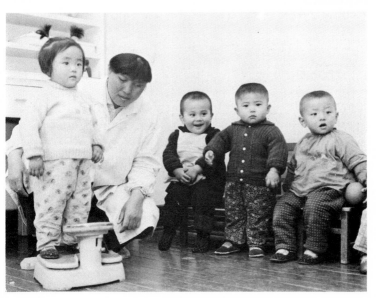

13(b) Children in a factory kindergarten have a 'check-up'.

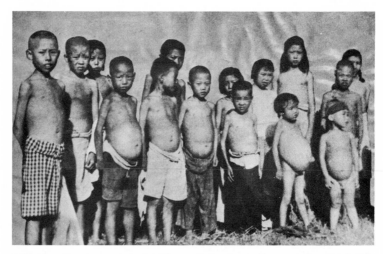

14(a) An earlier picture taken of children suffering from schistosomiasis or 'big belly' disease.

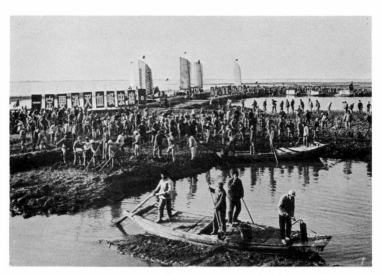

14(b) Mass preventive campaigns were necessary to bring this disease under control. The snail vector was one of the targets and they were buried during major irrigation works.

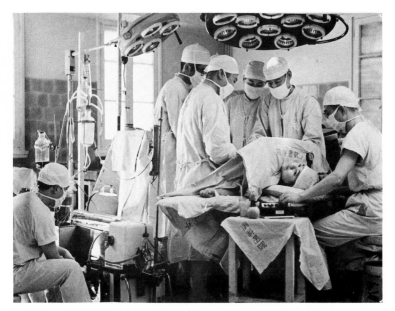

15(a) Open-heart surgery with a 'heart-lung' machine done under acupuncture analgesia

The acupuncturist's electrical stimulator is connected to the needles.

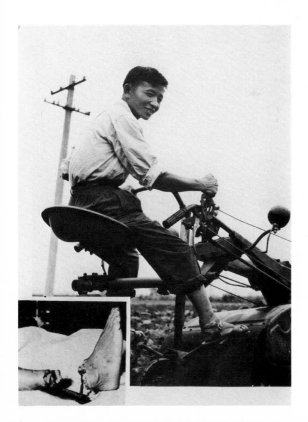

15(b) A 'pinnacle' for Chinese surgeons is their success at reattachment of severed limbs with good functional recovery.

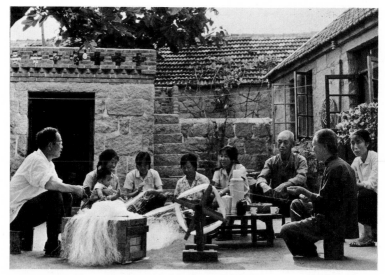

16(a) A family-planning representative explaining the government's policies to a peasant family encouraging them to have one child only.

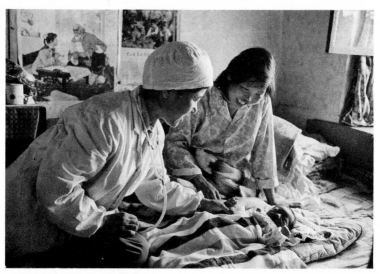

16(b) Good maternal and child-care services are recognised to be an important adjunct to the 'one child policy'.

is difficult for the masses to accept medical teams who talk only of prevention without giving medical treatment'.(138)


## POST-CULTURAL REVOLUTION PERIOD 1970-6

During the various phases of the Cultural Revolution it appears that, as with other services like education, there were varying amounts of disruptions in the field of health, as well as various innovations. Political developments emerging at the end of the Cultural Revolution - the introduction of the army to restore order, the dissolution of mass organisations and the restoration of party authority - can be seen to have had an effect in the field of health.

*Environmental health*
The first development was the revival of the Patriotic Health Campaign, led, this time, by the army. PLA units organised their own medical teams to rural areas and also mobilised city dwellers:

> PLA commanders and fighters throughout China are taking the lead in improving environmental hygiene as part of the Patriotic Health Campaign. In mid July a campaign to exterminate mosquitoes, flies, rats and bedbugs has taken place. The medical workers of the PLA units in the Peking area have organised large numbers of health workers and propaganda teams to go to the factories and rural areas to disseminate Mao's instructions on health work... in Kunming [the Army] dispatched more than ten thousand propaganda teams to go among the masses.(139)

Cleaning up the cities and communes and routine collections of night-soil were organised. The urgent nature of exhortations at the time give some idea of the scope of the problem: neglect of mass campaigns during the Cultural Revolution, it was felt, had led to a decline in the level of public sanitation. Faced with problems of reorganisation the government was understandably reluctant to countenance the prospect of new epidemics.

The new form of political organisation - the Revolutionary Committees, which operated at provincial, local and unit levels - issued urgent calls to the population to join in the clean-ups, but there were already signs that public, and certainly professional, confidence in this form of preventive activity was waning.

> There are those who do not believe that mass campaigns are very effective. We must persuade them that this is not so by publicising the needs performed by advanced units... the patriotic health movement should not be opposed to the struggle criticism transformation movement.... Stress must

be laid on practicality and effectiveness together with
frugality and industriousness.(140)

Provincial Health Departments appeared to be responding to
a number of different pressures. In order to carry out their
work, public health cadres, with very little detailed central
direction, tended to rely on the cheap, tried and tested methods
of mass campaigns. However, to public unwillingness or inability
to take part could be added other sources of strain. One was
from professionals who doubted the effectiveness of effort in
this area; the other from new political cadres who feared that
undertaking organised medical work on a large scale was a
diversion from the political objective of the Cultural Revolution.
Such work would see all people, irrespective of their political
stance, as important sources of labour. In addition, the skills
of discredited medical cadres and doctors would be required in
the campaigns, and skills might be regarded as more important
than political attitude.

The urban emphasis of patriotic health campaigns was clear.
Major cities like Wuhan, Beijing, and Shanghai were always
leaders in the field. Reports of the time also illustrate the
scope and variety of these activities with more advanced areas
beginning to concentrate on environmental pollution as well as
the more routine and by now familiar 'Four pests'. In Beijing
in 1973-4 two campaigns were launched to reduce smog and protect water, although some aspects of the campaign might cause
even an uncommitted ecologist to pause for thought:

> Coal mines near the Yungtung River, one of Peking's water
> sources, are discharging treated waste water into nearby
> fields instead of into the river itself.... It is stipulated that
> factories with intense pollution discharges shall not be situ-
> ated on the windward side of the city.(141)

*Schistosomiasis campaigns*
Political struggles surfaced again during campaigns against
schistosomiasis. Their novel feature was that while at one time
mass campaigns had been boosted with 'left' rhetoric these
same campaigns now suffered from ultra-'left' criticism. During
the Cultural Revolution reports of anti-schistosomiasis activities
had been confined mainly to reviews of achievements in the
most affected provinces. By 1970 it seemed that the seven-year
target had fallen behind schedule. Indeed in 1971 the Nine-Man
Committee which oversaw schistosomiasis work in south China
was dissolved.(142) In spring of that year, the officials of
eleven provinces, one autonomous region and one municipality
(Shanghai) again called for all-out war on the schistosome(143)
and the 'People's Daily' remarked: 'some people have set the
control of schistosomiasis against struggle-criticism-transformation. This attitude is wrong. Schistosomiasis prevention is a
major part of the Cultural Revolution.'(144)

In Hunan 'vigorous measures to control snail fever' were undertaken: 'At first the barefoot doctors were reluctant to take part in this work fearing the difficulties and troubles which might arise... and even certain cadres were afraid to join in this work.'(145)

In Yunnan those who worked in snail clearing campaigns were made aware of the importance attached to local responsibility and initiative.

The campaign would fail if reliance were placed on a small number of persons and doctors posted specially for the work; if drugs had to be requisitioned from the State and if the elimination of snails were to depend solely on those drugs.(146)

The work of provincial health departments in the elimination of schistosomiasis was probably aided considerably by the setting up of a better organised programme of rural health during the Cultural Revolution. By 1970 all of China's 50,000 communes had access to some form of medical care and more health personnel could be mobilised to lead anti-schistosomiasis campaigns than was the case in the early 1960s. Mass stool surveys, one of the major diagnostic techniques, were carried out by the new 'barefoot doctors'. New techniques enabled more samples to be tested in five minutes with a 73 per cent success rate.(147) However the task was still enormous - and there were competing demands for resources, as well as the need to co-ordinate with other ministries: 'departments of agriculture, electricity and water supply, light industry, material supply, trade, culture, education and public health should take the elimination of schistosomiasis as a political task'.(148)

Provincial health departments might have found the burden of total responsibility for schistosomiasis eradication in their area too great, and sought to share the load. The signs are, however, that there was considerable variation in the methods of organisation, with some areas attempting to develop research, others to co-ordinate efforts across departments, and others to devolve the responsibility on to brigade cadres and pay lip-service to 'wiping out' objectives.

By 1972 all the major infested provinces were listed as having made some improvements in schistosomiasis work: 'Since the Cultural Revolution 3,600,000 people have been treated and cured, and 4,000 million square miles of snail infested land cleaned.'(149)

It is important to remember that this figure *fails* to include the 3,600,000 who, it was claimed, were cured by 1964. This is in keeping with a political climate which could not admit to any achievements in health work before 1966. Political pressure must have been strong indeed for health cadres to actually underestimate the total achievement. An alternative explanation is that this figure is the total figure cured since the programme began in 1955, which suggests little progress since the early

1960s, or that major reinfection had occurred.

Difficulties continued: 'some places set anti-schistosomiasis work against running agriculture *in a big way* holding that they are so busy with revolution and production they have no time for prevention of disease'.(150) Later Zhang Chunqiao, one of the presently discredited 'Gang of Four', was said to have remarked that the Party Committees in charge of anti-schisto-somiasis work were 'busying themselves about tiny flukes while neglecting major affairs'.(151) By 1973 some provinces were setting targets for total elimination of the disease. Hubei, Zhe-jiang and Fujian claimed total or partial success. By 1976 it was claimed that

> roughly two thirds of all identified patients in China suffer-ing from schistosomiasis have been cured and restored to health... 5,000 million square miles of contaminated land have been cleaned and 3,500,000 patients cured.(152)

The results achieved seem impressive, but the figures are confusing. The number of those claimed to be cured - 3,500,000 - is 100,000 less than in 1972 yet the figure covers the period from 1971 to 1976.(153)

Perhaps we should not be too scrupulous when dealing with such an enormous number of patients on whom figures have to be collected from many different sources. It does sound some-what odd however that on three separate occasions, 1960, 1972 and 1976, the figure of 3 million plus cures had been quoted. If all the cures are added together, they amount to more than the total number of patients originally identified, but we must remember that of that total, some would have died, or new ones have been added. What is lacking is data on reinfection rates. That there must have been some is suggested by nil growth in the number of cures in the period 1970-6.

These figures, although impressive and difficult to interpret, remind us of some important points. The first was commented on by the American Schistosomiasis Delegation who visited China in 1975. They noted that 'little attention was paid to ecological immunological and sociological factors determining transmission, infection and disease... or careful measurement of incidence'.(154) It was therefore difficult to judge progress, although the delegation agreed that sanitary measures had halted transmis-sion, resulting in decreased incidence. It is likely, although not proven, that measures to control the spread of parasitic ova by proper night-soil management have been more effective than attempts at snail clearing.

The organisation of mass efforts requires a stable political climate, and a degree of authority which rural cadres have not always enjoyed. Doubtless, mass campaigns were impossible to organise during the years 1967-70, and in this period snails could breed and reinfect land previously cleaned. The dis-solution of the schistosomiasis group in 1970, probably on political rather than organisational grounds, removed the only effective co-ordinating unit.

The disease is woven into the fabric of rural life in South China. As one peasant put it: 'You try walking along those little dykes, between channels, without coming in contact with the water.'(155)

In order to deal with the disease, cadres in the schistosomiasis-ridden areas had adopted three basic strategies:

The first of these was to attempt to change the agricultural pattern which promoted the spread of the disease. Thus peasants were encouraged to grow dry rather than wet crops - i.e. to change from rice production. 'People in the affected areas should cultivate green manure crops instead of going into the lakes to collect weed. They should also grow some dry land crops.'(156)

The second is the attempt which had met with success in the past - the combination of snail clearing work with irrigation construction. In other countries in the world irrigation construction is a particularly high risk activity with regard to the disease, since the expansion of ditches and canals increases the availability of marsh for snails to breed.(157)

The third was a tentative suggestion that people ought to be credited with work points during hospital treatment in order to encourage people to come forward for treatment. 'The question of work points for sufferers should be solved reasonably during their treatment.'(158)

These measures were suggested in addition to the Central Government funds that were made available to provide free treatment, to ensure that the cost burden did not fall on the communes. At the same time, in an attempt to make costly treatment more effective, there was a resurgence of research into methods of treatment. As far back as 1965 the Chinese worried at the side effects of antimonial therapy, especially the five-day short courses which had been developed, had begun to focus research on non-antimonial compounds. In 1965 a nitro-fural compound F-30066, which possessed both curative and prophylactic powers, had been discovered. Extensive testing and further development of the drug showed that it could be best used in acute cases, but was less effective for chronic schistosomiasis.(159) By 1973 research into the role of traditional Chinese medicines was intensified and some discontent was being expressed as to the adequacy of diagnostic tests carried out by barefoot doctors as a method of tracing all cases of the disease:

The diagnosis of the disease used to be based solely on the results of night-soil culture. Now a comprehensive diagnostic method is widely in use which bases the diagnosis on a combination of reading from night-soil culture immunity reaction, ultrasonic detection and a check of rectal tissues.(160)

There are signs during this period of the tentative emergence of the professional 'expert' in the treatment of schistosomiasis. Although officially the line was to support mass campaigns and the courageous work of barefoot doctors at the front line of the disease, examination of new laboratory diagnostic techniques was beginning.(161)

*Other infectious and parasitic diseases*
In addition to the upsurge of campaigns to eradicate the snail vector for schistosomiasis, the first half of the decade sought to emulate the activities of the late 1950s in its attempt to 'work through' a series of diseases and deal with them. If the problems of malaria, hookworm disease, schistosomiasis, fili-ariasis, leptospirosis, tuberculosis, trachoma, not to mention the diseases of advanced urban civilisation like cancer or heart disease were not enough, fresh attacks would be made on hitherto untackled diseases like chronic bronchitis, chronic tracheitis and dacryocystitis.(162)

In 1973 Zhou En-lai gave instructions to find the cause of Keshan disease, and a composite research group was formed under the Academy of Medical Sciences. Research into lepto-spirosis (disease carried by rats) was also revived.

As well as encouraging consideration of new problems, or continuing to attack diseases systematically, some successes were being claimed in tuberculosis control. Tuberculosis pre-valence rates in Chongqing and Guangzhou suburban areas dropped 43 and 53 per cent respectively between 1964 and 1974.(163) In Beijing's eastern district prevalence rates of TB were only 20 per cent of the 1952 figure. In Beijing as a whole, in 1973, the tuberculosis rate was 14.8 per 100,000, compared with 230 per 100,000 in 1949.(164)

In general, however, success was somewhat patchy. A report of the work of the epidemic prevention station in Jishan county, Shaanxi province, told of their inability in dealing with a serious epidemic of encephalitis in 1967, bacillary dysentery in 1972, and outbreaks of measles between 1969 and 1970.(165) Between 1968 and 1969 there were malaria epidemics through Jiangsu, Shandong, Henan, Anhui and Hubei.(166) Records of 156 cases of epidemic haemorrhagic fever in the rural and suburban counties surrounding Shanghai indicate failures to control the farm rat.(167) Even the model Dazhai brigade had its problems:

> When we mobilised the masses to carry out the revolution, they said 'Life and death is pre-ordained. It makes no dif-ference whether one is hygienic or unhygienic'. Cadres took the lead in popularising scientific knowledge and repudiating superstitious ideas.(168)

The problem in organising major epidemic prevention work was not dissimilar to the problems of combating schistosomiasis. While small-scale local political and administrative structures were capable of flexibility, spontaneity and political sensitivity, they lacked the centralised direction necessary to co-ordinate large-scale public health measures, and often, even if the will was there, the authority to carry such measures through.

Where centralised policy and direction did occur, it was largely in specialised fields like cancer. This type of research, while superficially retaining a 'mass' approach, was more appealing to professionals. During 1972-3 some of the previously discredited cadres, including Vice-Minister Qian Xinzhong, were back at the Ministry of Health; the 'Chinese Medical Journal' resumed publication in 1975 after seven years, and a gradual, barely perceptible change came over public health work. If success in the fight against disease was not to be gained by mass movements at the local level, perhaps specialised research could be held to provide the answer.

## MATERNAL AND CHILD CARE

During the Cultural Revolution, a network of rural health care, which extended and developed to the brigade and production team level, was built on the commune health infrastructure of the 1950s. In the towns, where extensive coverage of populations had always been a feature of health care, neighbourhood provision of clinics and health workers, as well as that afforded by industrial enterprises, was strengthened. The outcome of these changes made improvements in accessibility to medical care. It also meant that the task of preventive health work was carried out down to the basic level. Control of epidemic disease, either by the Patriotic Health Campaign, or by programmes of inoculation, was thus made easier although, as we have seen, the enthusiasm for mass health programmes and belief in their effectiveness was diminished.

Most importantly, however, the availability of maternal and child health care was improved. Undoubtedly the recognition of the central importance of maternal and child health was linked to new attempts at population control, for the growth rate in 1971 was 2.1 per cent, adding over 20 million people a year to the population. Writers who visited China during this period were enthusiastic about the care given to mothers and babies. Maternal and infant mortality figures which would give some real indication of the benefits for the period are hard to come by, although it is claimed that by this time vaccination and immunisation reached over 90 per cent of children. Sidel, in her account of maternal and child health written after a visit to China in 1971, noted that babies under one year were immunised for TB (using BCG), diphtheria, pertussis, tetanus, polio and measles, and vaccinated against smallpox. At one year, and thereafter annually up to the age of 14, encephalitis B and meningitis immunisations were available,(169) and the take-up in most cases was over 95 per cent. The exception was smallpox, where the side effects were greater, with a still impressive take-up of 80 per cent being reported. The TB prevalence rate for children in Shanghai in 1972 had been reduced by 96.8 per cent since 1957.(170) Antenatal care was stated as being available to 95 per cent of women in some of the suburban counties of Shanghai.(171) Most communes employed a number of trained midwives or barefoot doctors to carry out antenatal care, hospital delivery and post-natal care.(172)

The availability of health care from trained paramedical workers, constant surveillance of health records and systems of checking vaccination and immunisation clearly had effects on the mortality rates of infants and children.

The bureau of public health in Shanghai made available figures to Lamm and Sidel which suggested a very low crude birth rate of 6.1 per thousand (a reflection of the intensity of the family planning campaign) for 1972, a crude death rate of 5.6 per thousand, an infant mortality rate of 12.6 per thousand and neonatal mortality rate of 3.2 per thousand. The mortality rates for children are remarkably low and compare favourably with the 1972 rate for New York City of white babies, 18.8 per thousand.(173) The rate for China as a whole in 1972 was given as 18.7 per thousand. This is a dramatic fall from the 150 per thousand in 1948, and the 39 per thousand in 1959.(174

However, differences between the life chances of children in the town and countryside were seen to exist. In Shanghai in 1975 the city's infant mortality rate was 11.85 per thousand, compared with that of the surrounding Jiangsu province which was 33.9 per thousand live births.(175)

Studies of physical development in children and adolescents carried out in August 1975 in urban and rural areas throughout China showed slightly better infant physical development in urban babies, and earlier age of puberty for urban adolescents Comparison with earlier samples taken between 1937 and 1940 in Beijing's eastern district and urban Beijing children in 1975 showed significant increments in weight and height. Comparison of rural children in 1975, with urban children measured in 1952-5, showed that average weights and heights of their rural children surpassed those achieved earlier by urban children.(17 Overall heights and weights were rising, but there is no evidence as to whether or not the rural-urban gap was increasing or decreasing. The authors attributed the changes to immunisation, physical exercise and training in the kindergarten and school, and the facilitation of breast feeding. An American paediatrician who visited China in 1973 compared the mean heights and weights of a sample of Shanghai children of 6 months to 7 years with those of children in Hong Kong and Singapore, and found the Shanghai children had better height and weight gains.(177)

The Cultural Revolution developments in health care brought new impetus to the level of care available to factory workers. A study of neonatal and infant mortality among the children of textile workers born between 1954 and 1965, and 1964 and 1975, showed the latter group had an infant mortality rate of 12.2 per thousand compared with the former 27.1 per thousand. There were fewer deaths from infectious diseases, including respiratory infection, in the latter group.(178)

Maternity care was also better organised, specified periods of time were laid down for paid maternity leave, continuing the practice of the 1950s. In rural areas the situation was somewhat different - no paid maternity leave for example - but the model Dazhai brigade claimed that:

> women's health has been given appropriate attention. In arranging farm work, we emphasise that her physiological characteristics be taken into consideration. During menstruation, pregnancy, puerperium and lactation the women are assigned light work on dry land near the village. It is further stipulated that no work points are detracted when women go home early to cook [sic].(179)

In the countryside, ending traditional practices like only allowing women to eat gruel after childbirth were seen as important. We do not know whether the proportion of rural births attended by a trained midwife had increased from the 61 per cent quoted in 1957.(180) It is possible that since the absolute number of midwives had increased, the proportion of deliveries attended by trained staff had also slightly increased. However, a study of urinary fistulas among peasant women in Jiangxi from 1961 to 1971 found that 95 per cent were due to poor obstetric management.(181)

Although there had been improvements in rural health, the lot of the rural woman as compared to her urban sister was probably relatively poor.

*Cancer surveys*
The early 1970s were characterised by the redirection of mass surveys away from infectious and parasitic disease towards the screening of populations for cancer. This was because much surveying work had been done on such diseases in the late 1950s and early 1960s and it seemed that, even if they were not fully controlled or eradicated, the extent of the problem was recognised. Cancer surveys, which had begun in 1958 as part of a general attempt to tackle carcinoma of the cervix among female textile workers (see below), began to be extended to a number of other cancers. In 1972-3 it appears that decisions were taken to establish cancer registers in the major cities, and establish registers devoted to single cancers in those areas which had particularly high rates. A National Office of Cancer Control with headquarters in Beijing was instituted to organise cancer-co-ordinating groups in Zhengzhou (oesophageal cancer), Shanghai (liver cancer) and Guangzhou (nasopharyngeal cancer).(182) The objectives were to use

screening methods to record the incidence and prevalence of th
major cancers, and to carry out mass surveys of the population
in high risk areas. The methods resembled those used with
parasitic and infectious disease. Prevention of cancer was unde
taken in two ways: early detection so that early treatment was
possible; environmental modification, for example diet, as in th
case of oesophageal cancer. In cancer of the cervix, clear bene
fits were obtained (see below), but as far as oesophageal cance
is concerned insufficient time has elapsed to allow a proper
judgment to be made.

The restructuring of the health care system following the
Cultural Revolution provided an infrastructure for the execu-
tion of mass surveys. Generally, these were carried out by
barefoot doctors, backed by more specialist staff, and clearly
such large population studies over vast areas need to have an
infrastructure able to obtain the data and co-ordinate properly

*Cervical cancer*   In 1972 mass screenings for carcinoma of the
cervix were carried out in ten urban and ten suburban countie
of Shanghai. In the following three years 1.4 million women
were examined,(183) while screenings which had begun among
Shanghai textile workers in 1958-72 were already revealing
promising results. The prevalence rates for carcinoma in situ,
the earliest stage when cancer cells are observed, had fallen
from 53 per hundred thousand in 1963-7 to 22.9 per hundred
thousand by 1972 and 8.7 per hundred thousand by 1974.(184)
The incidence had decreased from 66.1 per hundred thousand
in 1958 to 23.8 per hundred thousand in 1972. Survival rates
with early detection were excellent - over 90 per cent of Stage
I patients survived up to twenty years,(185) which compared
favourably with quoted rates of 70 per cent in the West.(186)

*Other cancers*   During 1970-2 600 barefoot doctors in Southern
China screened 436,786 people for nasopharyngeal cancer. The
proportion of Stage I and II cancers thus identified rose from
24 per cent to 87 per cent.(187) Screening of 417,644 workers
for liver cancer uncovered 57 with raised alphafetoprotein
values. In Shanghai, in 1973, an analysis of those patients
with early stage cancer was made; patients in the mass survey
group were compared with 1,200 patients seeking medical advic
at various hospitals in Shanghai. The proportion of early cases
in the mass survey group was 44.7 per cent, and in the hospital group 0.4 per cent. The three-year survival rate for these
patients in whom an early cancer was detected and treated was
57.1 per cent.(188) In Linxian, Henan province, an area with
a rate of oesophageal cancer fifty times that of anywhere else
in the world, over 100,000 persons have so far been screened
for the disease since 1971. The early detection method by mass
screening has reaped benefits. Of the 170 patients with early-
stage cancer of the oesophagus operated on at Linxian hospital
93 per cent have survived for five years.(189) In addition to

screening health education was also emphasised. Firstly, education was aimed at aiding the recognition of the symptoms of
oesophageal cancer. Travelling shows visited all areas in Linxian,
and with the aid of songs and dance illustrated the symptoms
and emphasised the message of: 'early detection, early diagnosis and early treatment. Surgery, drugs and radiation combined is most effective.' The song went on to list the 'seven
clues':

> Feeling obstruction when swallowing food
> Sharp pain behind the breastbone
> Feeling of something stuck in the throat
> Stomach ache, dry throat
> Belching when taking food and soreness at the back
> These are the seven symptoms.(190)

An attempt was also made to change the eating habits of
peasants and measures undertaken to prevent fungal contamination of food. Research carried out had revealed the likelihood
of carcinogenic agents in pickled or mouldy food. This view was
supported by the occurrence of gullet cancer in chickens who
had been fed table scraps by the peasants.(191) Further preventive work includes the use of ammonium and molybdenum in
fertiliser and the treatment of patients with epithelial
hyperplasia.(192= There had been some local resistance to the
'balloon test' used for screening, which is painful. Doctors
who worked on the project reported the peasants as saying
'The only way we'll be able to stop having this balloon test is
if we develop cancer'. They noted that the procedure was very
unpopular, and peasants required much persuasion.
   It was also difficult to persuade economically active peasants
who were asymptomatic to undergo a major operation which,
among other things, betrayed the fact that they had the disease
and ruined their own or their children's marriage chances.(193)

*Conclusion*
Summing up preventive work in the period 1970-6 is very difficult, partly because subsequent political events led to a very
negative evaluation of most of the public health activities of
the period. The fall of the 'Gang of Four' after Mao's death in
1976 was rapidly followed by accusations that, among other
things, the Gang had inhibited or neglected public health work.
It seems clear from what evidence is available that public health
work in the 1970s exemplified some of the major problems of
the forms of organisation extolled in and immediately after the
Cultural Revolution. The devolutionist perspective of those
who attained leading positions of power in the early 1970s,
vaunted as one of its successes the large-scale coverage of
rural health systems, which readjusted the balance between
town and country. However, it seems clear that the success or
failure of the rural system depended, like the mass movements

to eradicate schistosomiasis, on local initiatives, resources and motivation. Prevention, even if undertaken without mass campaigns, required direction and organisation, as well as some form of evaluation of the success or failure of activities. In those areas of preventive medicine where an infrastructure had long existed, like maternal and child health, gains were made. Areas which aroused professional interest, like cancer research, also showed progress. Least effective were those areas of prevention which required mass support or basic-level efficiency It is for this reason that we observe patchiness, and apathy in public health campaigns. It is also the reason for the greater need to involve the army as a labour force when public support for mass campaigns was lacking.

We also observe that the life chances of those in urban areas, who experience a higher standard of living, better health care resources and the means to buy them, continued to improve, and urban/rural gaps, although lessened, still remained. The medical profession, especially medical research, began to enjoy a cautious revival, and although publicly the exploits of barefoot doctors continued to be praised, privately the mass approach to research was modified and, in addition to preventive work, circumspect attempts to investigate the etiology of many diseases, began.

## PREVENTIVE HEALTH WORK IN THE POST-MAO PERIOD

*The Patriotic Health Movement and environmental health*
In the early 1970s the re-establishment of a measure of centralised control had been marked by an upsurge in the Patriotic Health Movement. After the fall of the Gang of Four a similar resurgence of the Patriotic Health Campaign was observed. Criticism of the Gang's interference in public health was widespread:

> their vicious interferences reached every corner of the country and caused widespread havoc. Not only was the Patriotic Health Campaign interrupted or entirely neglected, but worse still, most of the organisations for preventive medicine and their field services were either disrupted or disbanded.(194)

Concrete evidence of their disruptive effect is difficult to come by except in the case of schistosomiasis, where progress was halted, although it does seem that the particular political style of the leadership of the 1970s was not very conducive to the development of public health.

By Spring 1978 the Central Committee of the Communist Party approved revival of the Central Patriotic Movement Health Committee which was to be headed by Party Vice-Chairman Li Xiannian. A three-point programme which stressed environ-

mental protection, health education and rural sanitation was
adopted.(195) The appointment of such an important member of
the Central Committee to head the movement can be taken as
some indication of the stress that was being laid on the problem
of preventive public health work, and the fears that political
disruption had caused the disintegration of much of the preventive health infrastructure.

The State Council called on all provinces, municipalities and
autonomous regions to:

> reinstitute their Patriotic Public Health Campaign commit-
> tees.... The re-establishment and reinforcement of the
> sanitary and anti-epidemic centres, anti-tuberculosis centres,
> centres for the control of various specific endemic diseases
> and maternal and child health centres.(196)

The State Council directive on rural health prevention was
still tentatively linked to the now defunct campaign to 'learn
from Dazhai' (the model brigade which had amongst many other
achievements rehoused its members, resited pigpens, correctly
composted night-soil and provided the brigade members with
clean tap water),(197) but the real emphasis was upon a unify-
ing spirit and the re-establishment of centralised Party author-
ty espoused by the new regime, with its practical goal of 'the
four modernisations' (industry, science, agriculture and national
defence).

Although mass participation in the campaigns was emphasised
the tone was more restrained than when the mass line was in its
heyday:

> the need for mass participation in the campaign - the mass
> line - hardly requires further emphasis... for it directly
> benefits the people and they contribute their creative talents
> to the campaign... aiding the building of a powerful socialist
> country.(198)

The problem which campaigns had run into before were hinted
at. Health campaigns were not to be: 'an isolated and useless
extra chore unrelated to production'. Furthermore, they

> cannot be expected to produce lasting effects if carried out
> only once in a blue moon... in every season of every year
> an all-round assault [must] be made under the auspices of
> the campaign and in every organisation a once-a-week clean-
> up must be practised regularly.(199)

The low-technology nature of the campaign was re-emphasised,
underscoring the point that these campaigns were to provide
valuable economic results (a healthy population), by the
cheapest means, even if these were less effective:

general environmental sanitation can be improved by the
use of... simple... implements such as picks, spades,
brooms etc.... the important elements are strong leadership and firm determination... this does not of course deny
the greater efficiency and advantages of more modern equipment and newer techniques employed by the economically
more developed countries.(200)

In the cities of Shanghai and Beijing, Harbin and earthquake-
stricken Tianjin, the campaign took the by now familiar style:

millions in Shanghai have participated... tunnels, basements
and other breeding grounds for flies and mosquitoes have
been checked and disinfected.(201)

approximately 3,400,000 throughout Tangshen Prefecture
have... removed 3,950,000 tons of rubbish and dredged
191,000 metres of ditches.(202)

In Peking 1,200,000 people, cadres, workers, student
neighbourhood residents and medical workers turned out
to clear streets and yards.(203)

By spring 1978 public health rallies had been called in only
five of the provinces. This was a set-back which suggested
that, as before, the campaign's greatest effectiveness was
confined to the major cities.

Following the initial impetus, relatively little attention has
been paid to the sanitation aspect of the Patriotic Health Movement, suggesting that the uneasy balance struck by 1977-8
between motivation, political respectability and effectiveness
of action had gone out of kilter. By 1980 only Beijing and
Shanghai were in the news, their residents faithfully fulfilling
their tasks.(204)

By now three features characterised the state of the Patriotic
Health Movement. The first was its lack of success in motivating
mass health campaigns along the lines of the 1950s. There often
appeared a need to call on the extra manpower afforded by
the army and workers in the non-productive centres of the
economy (cadres, teachers and students).

The second was the recognition of the need to employ paid
workers, not just volunteers, for sanitary duties. 'Normally in
Peking more than 7,000 of the sanitary workers work from 9
o'clock in the evening until daybreak. They remove two to three
thousand tons of garbage each night.'(205) The lot of sanitary
workers was not a happy one. In Jiangsu, one complained:
'Sanitation workers are poorly paid, their welfare is poor and
they are despised. We have more than twenty young men who
have great difficulty in finding a wife.'(206)

The third was the urban emphasis in campaigns. A definite
change of direction could be observed away from the mass

eradication of four pests to the more complex environment problems of urban life. The only 'pests' mentioned were dogs. A health circular in Sichuan stated: 'All dogs must be destroyed in April before the rabies season.'(207)

Throughout there were only a few references to the sanitary standards of rural areas, and the impression is that they were to be left to their own devices:

> At a meeting to promote 'two controls and five transformations' (control of drinking water and night-soil, and transformation of wells, stores, toilets, livestock rings and the environment) in Haiken county, it was proposed that every effort be made to carry out this work over large areas of the province by taking advantage of leisure time now hoeing was finished.(208)

The new urban emphasis in preventive work now took several forms: (a) the emphasis in health and safety in industrial enterprises, (b) the concern with environmental pollution in the cities resulting from the activities of factories, or traffic.

The current trend towards concern with new problems seems to represent a move away from the 'laying the stress on the rural areas', a doctrine so strongly espoused by Mao during the Cultural Revolution. It also appears to be a valiant effort at prevention of some of the major health hazards of an industrial society. Essentially the change in direction seems to represent a degree of sophistication in the approach to problems of prevention, which integrate well with the new government's commitment to modernisation. We shall examine each aspect in detail below.

*Health and safety in industrial enterprises*

*1 Accidents*  A number of disasters in industrial enterprises were publicly reported and factories criticised for their poor safety records. In November 1979 an explosion in a Jilin coalmine 'killed and injured dozens of people'.(209) 'Serious action is being taken against those responsible,' New China News Agency reported. The basic cause of the explosion was reputed to be the management's desire to step up production - workers had been offered very substantial bonuses. However, excessive excavation had led to concentrations of gas in the tunnels which lacked suitable ventilation, and the fatal explosion occurred.

After the explosion other mine managements were quick to set up rules and regulations governing extraction(210) and the 'People's Daily' carried an editorial in May headed 'production must be safe and civilised', and attributed the major responsibility for the decline in standards of industrial safety to the interference and sabotage of the 'gang of four'.

under the pretext of abolishing the 'control, check and
suppression of workers', the gang of four abolished many
rules and regulations. Some people lack a sense of discipline
and wilfully violate operational procedures... some leading
cadres do not pay attention to labour protection adopting a
devil-may-care bureaucratic attitude towards workers' safety
in production.(211)

The editorial went on to suggest that better legislation was
necessary to 'overcome the erroneous thinking of concentrating
on production disregarding safety, and of regarding safety
as non-essential'.

The Vice-Premier Kang Shien remarked that although some
improvements in industrial safety had been made, 'major accidents continued to occur... for which he blamed lack of discipline and technical training, and poor management.'(212)

A second 'People's Daily' editorial of September, commenting
upon the Bohai oil rig disaster, which cost seventy-two lives,
remarked angrily: 'What is disgusting is that some leaders consider funerals joyous events, and they regarded as heroic
deeds in laying down one's life for the revolution what were in
fact accidents resulting from negligence'.(213)

Those responsible for a gas explosion in Shandong in which
eight people died were arrested and sent for trial.(214)

*2 Occupational Disease*   The immediate and dramatic hazards to
life and limb which are highlighted above do not directly con-
front other problems of industrial safety - the long-term 'invi-
sible hazards' in the work environment. The annual medical
check of workers in all industries in China, itself a major contribution to prevention, is not always detailed enough to provide
data on industrial hazards. For example, blood lead levels were
not checked at a factory producing lead and mercury batteries
nor were blood tests given to family members who lived in
adjacent factory housing.(215)

Some developments have occurred, however. In the chemical
industry, where it is admitted that 'many workers contract
occupational diseases', air filters and purifiers have been
recently installed at plants.(216) Research into occupational
risks is now being encouraged, rewards presented to those who
undertake prevention,(217) and ministerial regulations on
occupational health have been issued.(218) Noise hazards are
being cautiously investigated as are problems of aplastic anaemia caused by industrial toxins. However, measures to protect
workers from occupational disease, especially from newer
hazards like those produced by the development of nuclear
power, remain inadequate. A distinguished radiobiologist who
visited China in 1980 noted an excess of hepatitis amongst
uranium miners, a lack of long-term monitoring for chromosomal
abnormalities; problems of the disposal of nuclear waste, and
radiation hazards for those working in nuclear power plants.(219

Workers at the Capital Iron and Steel Company in Beijing suffer a very high incidence of lung cancer, 18.5 per hundred thousand. Most cases have occurred in workers in the coke ovens. The American cancer delegation noted that the concentrations of hydrocarbons were not measured at the plant, nor was there rotation of workers to minimise exposure.(220) The 'Cancer Atlas' confirms a definite high prevalence of lung cancer in the major industrial cities, e.g. Changchun, Harbin, Shenyang, Beijing, Tianjin,(221) Shanghai, Taiyuan, Nanjing, Hangzhou, Zhengzhou.

In contrast in Tianjin, doctors from city hospitals monitored the toxic levels of lead, benzine, mercury and chromium in 600 factories,(222) and it was reported in 1978 that over 80 million workers in factories and mines had been checked for chronic bronchitis.(223)

The approach to occupational disease seems to lack co-ordination at present, and it is likely that prevention of occupational disease will require yet another special planning group, such as those in cancer, schistosomiasis, pharmaceuticals, and family planning which will be expected to oversee and control developments in occupational health from Beijing.

3 *Pollution*   The control of environmental pollution is a relatively new development with which industrialising China is faced. The declaration of the 'four modernisations' meant that accompanying industrialisation are the health hazards of environmental pollution. At a battery factory in Anyang visited in 1978, waste products were discharged straight into the town's main drainage system.(224) The Beijing Iron and Steel factory, however, monitors surrounding air and water and has 'taken measures to reduce the discharge of liquid pollutants'. The new blast furnace is equipped with dust absorbers. Recovery of valuable chemicals from the factories' waste products is part of the pollution control programme.(225) In Guangzhou local factories are being fined for discharging pollutants above permitted levels.

A factory will be fined 20 yuan a day if it discharges fifty to one hundred tons of waste water containing more pollutants than the permitted amount. Penalties will rise 50 per cent until the factory brings the problem under control.(226)

In Wuhan twenty-five factories were fined for discharging waste into the Yangzi River, and one, a pharmaceutical plant, was ordered to move out of town because the people around complained of the 'bad smell in the making of furan drugs'.(227)

The wastefulness of environmental pollution has also been emphasised recently:

Some comrades still cannot see the importance of environmental protection, but simply treat it as an economic burden. As a matter of fact, due to the backwardness of

industrial techniques and equipment in some enterprises a
lot of energy and materials become waste in the course of
production and pollute the environment.(228)

An 'environmentalist lobby' appears to be emerging in China.
In August 1980 there was a major row in Beijing over the siting
of a cotton mill in the Evergreen suburban commune, and letters
to the 'People's Daily' stressed that the mill would 'pollute the
source of drinking water for two million residents of the city'.
A visit to the mill by experts of the National People's Congress
confirmed this. They stated that 'industrial waste water, even
if it is treated, can never be entirely free of pollutants'.(229)
The siting of this mill exemplified urban planning problems
which have emerged in other parts of China, due to lack of
co-ordination between public health officials and those responsible for economic and urban planning.

They have built wherever there is space. Waste water discharged from the Xixiashan refinery has polluted the source
of water nearby... even the fish in the ponds have died...
staff living in Nanjing have to bring their own drinking
water from home. Ninety per cent of the industrial liquid
waste discharged into rivers is untreated.(230)

Air pollution is also regarded as a hazard, and a serious cause
of bronchitis and lung cancer. Beijing in particular has a
dusty atmosphere, which compounded with the effects of wood-
and coal-burning stoves, creates smog. In China at present
respiratory diseases are the major cause of death in males and
females,(231) and are also one of the major causes of neonatal
death in the cities.(232) The amount of soot released annually
by industry and households in China is estimated at over 10
million tons, in addition to the 15 million tons of sulphur dio-
xide.(233) The drive to control pollution is clearly being treated
very seriously. It is seen as a problem for the whole of China.
In a country committed to rapid industrialisation, it is a major
decision for officials to state the following:

Production *must* be subordinate to environmental protection,
when contradictions occur between the two. Decisive action
must be taken to clear up the problem. Where it is currently
impossible to find ways of halting pollution, factories causing pollution must cease production or be closed. We must be
resolute in dealing with the problems.(234)

*Schistosomiasis control*
The American schistosomiasis delegation which visited China in
1975 was cautious in its evaluation of the success of what had
been achieved in schistosomiasis control. After the fall of the
Gang of Four criticism of the inadequacy of co-ordination of
programmes was made, but it was less virulent than that which

was made of the Gang's activities in other areas of Chinese
life. The measures that had been taken after 1970 – attempts
to change agriculture production – were no longer in fashion.
The emphasis on curing the disease as an attempt to break the
cycle of infection, on research into the better method of diagnosis
(but not into evaluation of anti-schistosomiasis programmes
was maintained and increased, and there was a resurgence
of mass activity of snail clearing often in combination with
irrigation work, with targets set for the elimination of the
disease by 1985.(235)

A major conference on the treatment of schistosomiasis was
held in 1977 in Shanghai,(236) and the schistosomiasis research
committee which had been suspended for twelve years became
operative again.(237) It was claimed that schistosomiasis had
increased under the Gang of Four, due to the policy of closing
research institutes: 'Even today there are still 3,000 million
square miles of terrain where snails are multiplying unchecked.
Some two and a half million people still suffer from snail fever'
[schistosomiasis].(238) Evidence from Guangxi province, which
claimed to have 'basically eliminated snails in 1972' suggested
new outbreaks with seventeen new anti-schistosomiasis stations
being set up.(239)

Almost a year later successes were claimed for the anti-
schistosomiasis work. These were attributed less to the efforts
of the masses than to the leadership of local Communist Party
committees, and scientific research on prevention and cure.
Summing up the two years since the fall of the Gang, it was
claimed that schistosomiasis was basically eradicated in 200
counties and that the number of patients had been reduced by
two thirds, a proportion previously quoted in 1976.(240) An
editorial in the 'People's Daily' was sober in its assessment of
progress:

> We... must be ready to fight over a long period... the
> intermediate host of this disease spreads wide, breeds fast
> and is difficult to wipe out... we must adopt scientific
> methods and advanced technology... under the leadership
> of the party... we must organise the concerned departments
> of sanitation, agriculture, water conservancy, light industry
> and so forth.(241)

The editorial clearly identified some of the major problems
concerned with schistosomiasis control and eradication, chiefly
the need for persistent well co-ordinated work. There was no
mention of attempts to alter the cycle of agricultural production,
but the need for good night-soil management was stressed. Subsequent scientific research into schistosomiasis has not been
greatly in evidence; what has been done has drawn attention to
the possible role of the immune system of the body in treatment
of schistosomiasis and the development of a vaccine against the
disease. This latest approach, which has been the subject of

research for twenty years outside the People's Republic, is now being considered, if not as an alternative, as another valuable weapon in the armoury to be used against the disease.(242) Technological advances are also being utilised: for the first time in China, the tegumental surface of the adult 'Schistoma japonicum' has been scanned by the electron microscope.(243)

*Other infectious, endemic and parasitic disease*
The present period of Chinese history is one where shortcomings in the health care system and in the attitudes towards prevention can be more freely stated. This is because deficiencies are seen to be pointers for development, and there exists a set of political scapegoats to take the blame. Therefore assessment of the status of many diseases is more sober than it might have been several years previously. Despite an increase in the volume of pure laboratory research, and some use of Western advanced techniques, it would be a mistake to say that there has been a decline in the commitment to prevention in China. What does appear to be the case is that the old concepts and methods of prevention are regarded as no longer sufficient to cope with the changing pattern of disease, or the alterations in the environment due to industrialisation, and that there is a new emphasis on the more complex problems of urban areas. However, there are enough of the 'old' problems of environmental hygiene, infectious and endemic disease (particularly in the rural areas) for a gap to have emerged in their management. Mass effort has declined: basic inoculation of children and adults against infectious disease remains undoubtedly the most efficacious aspect of preventive work, but infectious and parasitic diseases still pose big problems as do the endemic diseases. The case of schistosomiasis is but one example of this. However, in terms of prevention, the trend with infectious disease is towards better diagnostic techniques which are seen as an adjunct to attempts to wipe out the source of the infection. In malaria control in Guizhou, for example, 'The use of insecticide has been cut down and stress is placed on making blood tests to trace infection.'(244)

The networks of epidemic control, based on the anti-epidemic stations, are now of vital importance, both in administering inoculations and keeping up basic health work. The emphasis appears to be not only on maintaining basic sanitary measures and inoculation, but on the early discovery and prompt notification of disease.(245)

Responsibility for epidemic disease control is now located at county level, where new attempts are being made to understand epidemiology. In Jishan county anti-epidemic disease station: 'we have conducted comprehensive analyses of bacillary dysentery, epidemic encephalitis, influenza and smallpox'.(246)

This trend towards more centralised control, under expert direction, accompanies the movement towards making county-

level units the linchpin of the system of health care delivery.
The work of the station also gives some indication of the still
important presence of infectious diseases in the countryside.

In the cities anti-epidemic stations are now engaged in more
rigorous attempts at epidemiology. In one Shanghai anti-
epidemic station collection and analysis of 'flu epidemics are
used in attempts to forecast impending risks. The data showed
peak incidence as being usually two weeks earlier than case
reportage, and it was concluded that there was a need to
tighten up reporting procedures, as well as using seasonal
forecasting.(247)

The tuberculosis prevention and treatment networks set up
in the cities have kept records which show a steady decline
in the incidence and prevalence of TB, and TB mortality.(248)

In Shanghai, the young age-group 15-29 and those of over
50 showed the greatest morbidity. This might be due to present
conditions in Shanghai, or to the difficulties in ensuring adequate vaccination due to political disturbances when the young
adults were babies or adolescents.(249) The regular X-ray at
two-year intervals at factories, and the 96.3 per cent take-up
of BCG vaccines has doubtless had an excellent preventive
effect. In Beijing the 1970s have witnessed the absence of
deaths in the 0-4 age-group from TB, due to the high inoculation rate.(250)

New problems are admitted to exist however. A meeting of
health officials from Kiangsu, Shantung, Anhwei and Hebei
reported that the incidence of malaria had increased 43 per cent
in all the provinces except Jiangsu.(251) Trachoma also appears
to be increasing in incidence. Visits to a very well equipped
children's kindergarten in the heart of Beijing revealed that
very special precautions were being taken to avoid it - strict
rules about washing and the use of flannels and towels.(252)
Figures from mass surveys of peasant populations presented at
the 1979 Convention of the Chinese Ophthalmological Society
showed an incidence of trachoma of 64.93 per cent among
northern peasants in Inner Mongolia, Heilonjiang, Shaanxi and
Henan, and 32.95 per cent among southern peasants of Guangdong, Hunan, Anhui.(253) The incidence of trachoma is
reported as higher in rural communities than in urban areas,
and is plainly a problem to be dealt with.

In 1978 a conference was held at which a 1985 target was set
for the eradication of endemic diseases like goitre, Keshan
disease and Kashin-beck.

The following year a meeting in Shenyang reported the results
of research: 'goitre caused by lack of iodine, flourine disease
by too much flourine in drinking water, undulent fever by
Brucella abortus... and Keshan disease which may cause heart
disease and death'.(254) However, since 1977 3 million goitre
patients had been cured and 20 million provided with iodised
salt. By 1980 it was claimed that 10 million had been cured and
130 million given iodised salt.(255)

Water supplies were treated to reduce the incidence of Keshan disease, and mineral supplements added to the diet.(256) The disease remains of unknown etiology, and a medical controversy is emerging in China as to whether in fact Keshan disease is a variety of viral myocarditis, or a distinct disease entity, whose etiology depends upon specific geographical factors such as selenium deficiency. Whichever hypothesis is adopted has important preventive implications. If the latter, then attempts to find the cause by modifying the diet, mainly by prophylactic administration of sodium selenite,(257) might have to be altered Proponents of the thesis that Keshan is a variety of viral myocarditis have made somewhat different observations and come to different conclusions:

since high incidence of Keshan disease is often observed in large and not well-to-do families and at present there are no specific prophylactic measures, improved living standard and cultural level through increased agricultural and industrial production and family planning are of fundamental importance.... It is worth mentioning that in Jilin province where the people's living standard has risen, and some of the non-specific sanitary and medical measures for mass prevention have been carried out since 1949, the incidence of KSD (Keshan disease) has steadily declined... many diseases cannot be effectively controlled by mere medical measures without attention to standard of living.(258)

These remarks suggest a trend towards consideration of the role of the general standard of living in producing change in the disease pattern. It marks a shift away from the idea that adequate hygienic measures and medical services are sufficient or major aspects of prevention, and points to the resilience of the host as being equally if not more important in the prevention of disease. In a study of pellagra prevention (a disease due to niacin deficiency) found in populations with a high maize and low animal protein diet (e.g. Uygurs in Xinjiang), the researchers recommended that the best results could be obtained if animal husbandry or soya bean diet was encouraged in areas where pellagra is endemic. However, they recognised that such a change in habit could not be immediately obtained and suggested instead that maize with higher protein and niacin content should be planted.(259) This was actually an American strain of maize, and the recommended change is an example of co-operation between the Ministries of Agriculture and Health.

The important influence of life-style on disease patterns occurs again in the latest work on diabetes. In 1978 a mass survey of 100,000 people carried out in Shanghai discovered an overall diabetes prevalence of 10.12 per 100,000. It was found to be closely associated with age, female sex, and being overweight: 'The highest prevalence occurs in retired workers, housewives, workers in heavy industry and then cadres. The

lowest prevalence is in the peasant group, students excluded.'
The study noted the difference in prevalence between those
engaged in heavy physical labour and those in sedentary occu-
pations.(260)

Noting occupational difference in disease patterns has never
been a major aspect of Chinese epidemiology. The discipline is
itself relatively new in China, the first national epidemiology
conference being held in Harbin in 1980. These studies on
endemic disease point to new directions and considerations in
preventive work. Other areas now emerging, with the impetus
being given to research, are studies of the preventive and
curative action of vaccines and medicines themselves.(261)
Studies of measles vaccine, sulphonamides, drugs used in the
treatment of leptospirosis, polio, rice growers' dermatitis and
hookworm have all been published recently. Such changes
underline the present political view that modern scientific research is most likely to provide the answer to the large-scale
problem of endemic disease in China.

*Maternal and child health*
The improvement of maternal and child health, in conjunction
with birth-control work, has been one of the major themes of
the 1980s in China. Government policy is to reduce the natural
growth-rate of population to zero by the year 2000.(262) In
order to persuade couples to accede to these targets, it is felt
necessary that measures to ensure the healthy survival of
children should be pursued with even greater intensity, particularly in the rural areas. The improved training of barefoot
doctors which is now under way, and the specification that
each production brigade should have two certified barefoot
doctors, at least one of whom should be a woman, emphasises
the importance of raising basic-level child health care and
midwifery standards.(263)

The production of a healthy child begins even before conception. Since recent research has suggested that a staggering
ten million people in China suffer from various congenital
defects, the question of 'the quality of the population' has
arisen.

In recent years the birth rate of various congenital deformed
babies has increased, congenital diseased patients who would
otherwise die young now live and get married... prohibiting
the mentally retarded from procreating will greatly decrease
the births of congenital mentally retarded children.(264)

The marriage of cousins up to the third degree is now forbidden in the new Marriage Law, and several cases have recently
been reported in the Chinese medical press of the consequences
of marriage within too close a degree of kindred. Amniocentesis
and early abortion is recommended where the possibility of
abnormal offspring exists.(265)

China's children, especially in the major cities, are among the healthiest in the Third World. Neonatal mortality rates for Beijing were 10.1 per thousand in 1979 compared with 12.21 per thousand in 1978 (compare UK 11.1 per thousand in 1973), the infant mortality rates for 1979 were 17 per thousand, and 17.1 in 1978 (cf. UK 16 per thousand).(266) These of course represent an amazing drop from the pre-revolutionary figure of 147 per thousand.

British obstetricians visiting Shanghai in 1978 noted the low reported incidence of low birth-weight births which is at least partly attributable to the lower parity of Shanghai women due to population control policies. Only 4.7 per cent of Shanghai babies weighed less than 2,501 grams at birth, compared with 8.7 per cent of babies in Cardiff, Wales.(267)

Maternity care has always been provided free, and maternity leave is fifty-six days which may be taken at any time before and after the birth. Planning of future pregnancies involves the work unit. Many women work up to the end of pregnancy although it is suggested that they should be given 'light work'.(268) However, recently a letter of complaint appeared in a Liaoning newspaper claiming that 'maternity leave is counted as absence from duty and 0.1 mark is deducted for every absent day during women workers' maternity leave'.(269) If maternity leave is not so easily available, this could affect both maternal and perinatal mortality rates.

An interesting trend may be observed in China which occurs in other developing countries: that is a movement away from breastfeeding of infants. One advantage of the existence of factory and brigade crèches has been that they enable mothers to continue breastfeeding after they return to work. In general, two nursing periods of half an hour per day are allowed and no deduction of wages takes place. Similarly in the rural areas up to one hour per day can be allowed for breast feeding.(270) While the proportion of mothers breastfeeding one month after birth – even in a sophisticated city like Shanghai it is some 44 per cent according to one study(271) – is high by our standards, yet artificial feeding of infants appears to be on the increase. In one neighbourhood committee in Beijing, two thirds of the infants were artificially fed.(272) This of course has its consequences: an examination of infants with acute infantile gastro-enteritis admitted to the paediatric ward at the Sichuan Medical College hospital showed that only 10 per cent were breast fed.(273) Major reasons for these findings are the difficulties in sterilising bottles and keeping feeds hygienic. Full breast feeding usually continues for six months, after which it may be supplemented with other foods or milk substitutes until weaning finally takes place between twelve to eighteen months. As in other countries, the association of breast feeding with poverty has led more prosperous urban workers to turn to formula feeding. This is often also more convenient if crèches are not provided at the mother's place of work, or if babies are

cared for by other relations at home, but the milk itself is
sometimes difficult to buy.

One study of physical development of children and adolescents
actually attributed the difference in the length and weights
of rural and urban infants partly to the tendency of rural
mothers to delay weaning.(274) Artificial feeding has problems
attached, however. The Shanghai newspaper Wenhui Bao condemned the substitute milk powder for infants as 'not suitable
for babies - but there is hardly any choice'.(275) In Shanghai,
where a regular system of health checks for the children in
the city has been instituted, trained staff in crèches and
kindergartens supervise children.(276) In the first three months
after a baby is born medical workers visit the home three times,
keep records of the child's health and give advice to new
mothers on infant feeding.(277)

Disturbing news came however from a national conference on
rickets prevention which recently reported results of a mass
survey held throughout China. The incidence of rickets in
children under three was about 33 per cent in Xinjiang, Shandong, Gansu, Hupei, Jilin and Heilongjiang. In a few provinces
(unstated) the incidence exceeded 80 per cent.(278)

If the welfare of infants and mothers is closely linked to need
to promote the one-child family, the restoration of formal examinations and tightening up of the educational system are behind
the new stress on the health of schoolchildren and students:

> As China's students are studying harder more attention
> must be paid to their health... among students there is a
> growing incidence of such diseases as myopia, trachoma,
> caries, roundworm, liver trouble, neurasthenia, tubercu-
> losis and bronchitis.(279)

In the 1980s infant and child welfare is being seen as in need
of greater improvement. Seasonal bouts of gastroenteritis still
occur, and in 1978 a million and a half cases of measles resulted
in 6,162 deaths.(280) Improvement in maternity care also seems
to be indicated but this has received less emphasis. In both
cases, more importance appears to be given to the provision of
medical care and basic medical measures than to nutritional
status; yet both good and poor nutritional status seems to be
implicated in the developments of the diseases described above.

*Cancer prevention*
As we have seen above, in the early 1970s a number of mass
surveys of cancer were undertaken. Some of these took a few
years - as many as eight - but an impressive retrospective
(1973-5) nationwide survey was done which culminated in the
publication of the 'National Atlas of Cancer Mortality' in
1979.(281) In fact the mass surveys for cancer in areas of high
incidence often did not have a closure date set, but continued
to steadily screen and treat as many patients as possible. The

combination of mass screening and early treatment seems to have had an impressive effect upon survival rates. Figures for survival from oesophageal cancer and cervical cancer have been quoted above. An evaluation of screening for hepatocellular carcinoma has recently been carried out. Comparing cases found by mass AFP (alphafeto protein) screening, and those with pathologically proved liver cancer, the authors showed that they were able to identify very early stage cancers in the mass survey group. Resection was successfully performed in 56.1 per cent of the mass survey group compared with only 17.7 per cent in the clinically treated group.(282) Less satisfactory has been the attempt to discover the etiology of cancer. The clear geographical distribution of some cancers in China, e.g. oesophagus and nasopharynx, seemed to suggest that environmental factors might be implicated and research into these was undertaken. So far researchers appear to have come up with a number of etiologic pointers in the case of particular cancers, none of which on their own are sufficient to explain the incidence, but which, taken in combination, gives some clues for prevention. In the case of oesophageal cancer in Linxian, Honan province, methods of food preparation, abrasive or mouldy diet, and molybdenum deficiency are all suspect. For nasopharyngeal cancer, infection with Epstein Barr virus and food with a high nickel content, are implicated,(283) and in the case of liver cancer, liver damage from hepatitis B infection interacting with an environmental chemical agent perhaps concentrated in stagnant drinking water.(284) However no clear clues have emerged as to the cause of gastric cancer which is the major killing cancer in China.(285)

The cancer prevention networks which have been set up function by organising local health workers to aid in surveys of the population. The Cancer Institute under the Chinese Academy of Medical Sciences revealed that cancer was the second leading cause of death in males and third leading cause of death in females. One million people contract cancer a year and the fatality rate is 70 per cent. Cancer of the stomach (gastric cancer) is commonest in both sexes, followed by cancer of the oesophagus in males and cervix in females.(286) In one people's commune investigated over five years the mortality rate from cancer has risen 36 per cent from 75.33 per hundred thousand in 1975 to 111.5 per hundred thousand in 1979.(287)

Recently preventive activities have taken a new turn. Lung cancer mortality is higher in cities than in the countryside, and in big cities rather than small towns (the highest lung cancer fatality is in Shanghai, Tianjin and Beijing) and the three north-eastern provinces. These being northern industrial towns suggested that atmospheric pollution was involved. Until recently, despite a consistent public denial of the effects of smoking on lung cancer (it is said not to explain the rates of lung cancer in Chinese women, who smoke little), epidemiologists privately agreed that lung cancer and cigarette smoking are linked. In 1979 the government began a propaganda campaign against smoking which apart from cancer was implicated in bronchitis and heart disease. The statement said that growing numbers of people in both towns and cities were taking up smoking and that the number of women and youthful smokers was increasing: 159 per cent more cigarettes were sold in 1978 than in 1965.(288)

The Minister of Health said that 'cigarette smoking is harmful to the people's health, and cigarette smokers should voluntarily stop smoking or control it'. He remarked: 'the incidence of cancer has increased year after year in Peking, Shanghai, Nanking and other cities in the country... the incidence of cancer in Shanghai has increased fivefold(289) in the past fifteen years'.

In October 1979 the Chinese Medical Society held a meeting in Beijing on the dangers of smoking. 'Medical and health experts pointed out that excessive smoking over a long period could lead to lung cancer and cardiovascular disease.'(290)

By 1980 a well-worked-out anti-smoking drive was under way in Shanghai. It stated 'Smoking is prohibited in hospitals, conference halls, theatres, kindergartens, schools, buses and other public places. Students may not smoke, cigarette packets and match boxes must carry anti-smoking warnings.'(291) However, at almost the same time, three Chinese cigarette factories signed agreements with British and American tobacco companies to produce cigarettes 'to be sold in China and abroad'. While aimed primarily at tourists, the move definitely provides an inroad to markets in China for those tobacco companies.(292) The Chinese Tobacco industry is the largest tobacco monopoly in the world and their exports are an important source of state revenue. It will be interesting to see the resolution of this contradiction which was made worse by Mao's chain-smoking and longevity.

This approach to the prevention of smoking is a change in attitudes, but action remains at a fairly rudimentary level as yet. An almost contradictory trend could be seen at the beginning of 1979 when, moving away from attempts to identify etiology, curative measures are being stressed. For example, the oesophageal cancer project in Linxian has recently been criticised for concentrating upon attempts to find the cause of cancer at the expense of treating the disease:

Work at our centre is at a low ebb and some people even think that this work is dispensable. At present, other countries are studying the treatment of cancer in its early stages, but we have not really given it proper attention.(293)

Research into cancer is one of the 'key areas' of the 1980s. The mass surveys may have resulted in the early detection and treatment of many different types of cancer but it seems they, too, are out of fashion. Attempts to find the causes of cancers are being rapidly superseded by developments in medical and surgical treatments for the disease, and in this, we must conclude, professional pressure, as well as the need to provide results to the peasants who pay for medical services, must have played a part.

*Heart disease*
Chinese people suffer more strokes, but less heart disease and myocardial infarctions, than the people of Europe and the United States. This was the conclusion reached at a conference held in 1980.(294) In Beijing the first cause of death at present is heart attack, followed by cerebrovascular disease and cancer; about 66 per cent of the deaths in greater Beijing in 1979 were accounted for by one of these three. In the urban areas cerebrovascular disease was the main cause of death(295) and in eight out of twelve major Chinese cities surveyed in 1976, cerebrovascular diseases were the main cause of death.(296)

In the early 1970s some large-scale mass surveys of hypertension were carried out. These surveys, which included all people above fifteen years of age, showed a prevalence rate ranging from 2 per cent to 10 per cent, with higher rates in urban (7.52) than rural populations (3.94), and northern (9.68) than southern (3.52) Chinese. Reports from factory hospitals suggested that hypertension is often the first or second most frequent cause of medical visits or sick leave.(297) Hypertension is therefore a major public health problem and its prevalence, in industrial areas at least, appears to be increasing. In 1958 a study on Beijing showed a prevalence rate of 7.4 per cent. In 1970 the rate of a group surveyed was 10.9. In Shanghai, in 1958, the prevalence rate was 6.7 per cent and in 1973 had increased to 8.3.(298)

As a result of surveys which have been carried out, community control measures to monitor and treat hypertension were started in 1969 among factory workers. By 1974 programmes had been set up by research teams in a number of cities. Under local health authorities specialised teams worked with local health workers to survey, register and treat hypertension and coronary heart disease. The work included primary emergency care. By 1976 these control programmes had been united to form regional networks covering 50-100,000 people. An example of such a programme, in one health district of Beijing (Peking), is illustrated in Figure 5.

Special training is given to medical personnel in the treatment of cardiovascular diseases.(299) The demand for such networks, as indicated by the prevalence of hypertension in the population, is enormous. The existing CCCP network 'merely constitutes a small fragment of the total need, but it is hoped to extend the network to major cities, factories and communes by 1985.'(300)

The existence of cardiovascular community control programmes has clearly had benefits. In practice the programme has

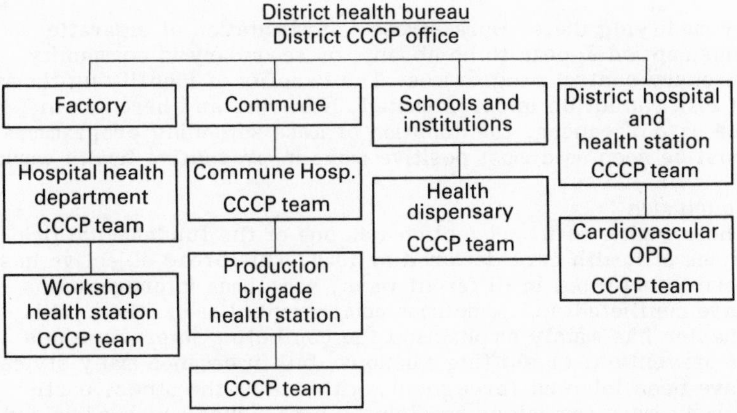

District health bureau
District CCCP office

Figure 5   Organisation scheme of CCCP of Shijingshan district, Beijing

wo aspects: hypertension control, and coronary heart disease control. At Shijingshan commune all the population over fifteen years have been screened (10,810 people). Blood pressure BP) levels of 140/90 or a diastolic pressure of 90 were taken as indications of hypertension in the first round of screening. Later the WHO criteria of hypertension 160/95 or 95 diastolic was applied. In the control of hypertension drugs were taken daily, with BP levels being checked at three to four weeks. Hypertension was satisfactorily controlled in 65 per cent of those identified. Stroke management includes control of hypertension coupled with herbal medicine and acupuncture. The methods of management are reported to have produced a 23 per cent reduction in stroke mortality over five years. Persons identified as suffering from coronary heart disease are followed up and treated with both Western and herbal preparations. A 13 per cent drop in cardiovascular mortality was noted over the five-year period.(301)

The methods of monitoring, screening, treatment and follow-up described above clearly demand a degree of co-ordination and utilise the skills of all levels of workers; however, little attention is paid to the 'self-management' of hypertension, although people are encouraged to take their medicines. The model of prevention appears to be that of 'guidance-co-operation', where patients accept the medical regime, but where as yet little attention is paid to the modification of personal habits; nor are more general factors like stress or the level and type of nutrition within the population considered. Education is seen as one aspect of the preventive programme, and this seems to centre around displaying to the public, via posters, pamphlets and media, the causes, manifestations, prevention and management of hypertension, stroke and acute myocardial infarction. However, more far-reaching attempts to control hypertension, by modifying diets, work stress, and limitation of cigarette consumption appear to be absent, or secondary in community coronary control programmes. The benefits of identifying those at risk cannot be underestimated, however, and here, as in the case of cancer, the adoption of mass screening programmes must be seen as a most positive move in preventive health work

## Conclusion

The commitment to prevention was one of the fundamental principles of health care declared in 1950. This broad objective has been interpreted in different ways; sometimes interpretations have conflicted and sometimes complemented each other. This chapter has mainly emphasised the conflicting interpretations of prevention, or shifting fashions, but in essence many styles have been followed throughout, with one or the other, particularly mass campaigns receiving a prominence which coincided with the political ascendancy of the group which backed them, and the temporary eclipse of those who opposed them.

We are not in a position to fully assess the impact that strains in preventive work may have imposed on its overall effectiveness. For few countries as yet have been faced with the massive problems which beset the Chinese in 1949, and attempted some form of solution to them. In this the Chinese must be seen as pioneers, and it is almost impossible to answer the question 'how might it have been done differently?' Mistakes in policy were made: over-reliance on mass campaigns is probably one example, failure to formulate an adequate policy for rural preventive health in the 1950s was another.

The efficiency of some mass campaigns, especially in the control of schistosomiasis, is questionable; but this disease is extremely intractable as it is entwined with the form of rural agriculture. The modernisation of agriculture and increased mechanisation may provide a better basis for controlling the disease, simply by removing the numbers of persons at risk. The campaigns against schistosomiasis often served objectives other than health – the utilisation of underemployed agricultural labour, for one. Other examples of the mass approach, involving large numbers of people and semi-trained medical personnel, as in the case of venereal disease and environmental improvement, have shown better results, and were low-cost measures which ensured a moderate degree of success for a small economic investment. Experience has shown that when mass campaigns dealt with those diseases or environmental conditions where the opportunity costs of improvement – i.e. time and effort expended, costs of seeking treatment, set against other activities – were less than the benefits – a cleaner or healthier or more beautiful environment, relief from a disabling condition – some success was achieved. Where the costs were greater, for example in the case of schistosomiasis where the disease in its chronic stages can be tolerated by peasants with only a marginal effect on agricultural output, success was considerably less. Time spent on snail clearing had to be set against time spent on other activities: when campaigns took up the slack in rural unemployment or were combined with irrigation work, participation was high; when they interfered with private plot cultivation enthusiasm was muted. The 'commandism' characteristic of some cadres urged to motivate those peasants who looked upon snail clearing as a type of corvée labour, suggests that resistance to the mass campaigns lay not only with officials of the Ministry of Health who resented the diversion of resources towards what they regarded as ineffective action, but with the peasantry too. It is probably a calculation of what can be achieved successfully by mass campaigns that has made environmental improvement in the urban areas the focus of current concerns, while mass campaigns in the rural areas have been dropped. A city population is probably more accessible to mass campaigns, and to the influence of example. Thus in March 1982 we see the chairman of the Chinese Communist Party taking a broom and sweeping the streets of Beijing. Motivating the population in this low-cost exercise of environmental and moral improvement is easier in cities; results are quickly seen and communicated; for the eradication of chronic, endemic diseases in the countryside, where immediate large-scale benefits may not be apparent, motivation is much more difficult.

Attempts to increase the effectiveness of rural preventive work still utilise a 'mass' approach, if not whole-scale mass movements. Efforts continue to be made, for example, in the treatment of oesophageal cancer to saturate the rural population with information, and exhortations to come forward for treatment. To rely on the mass approach alone, without any proper organisation of treatment and primary prevention (i.e. removal of those conditions which cause the disease), has been a waste of time. Signs suggest that for the rural areas, those mass campaigns which are combined with some form of effective treatment, even if primary prevention is absent, stand a better chance of success. It is for this reason, for example, that the basic etiological work at Linxian into the causes of oesophageal cancer is being redirected in favour of research into more effective treatment, with the mass campaigns being used as means of motivating early detection.

Other more formal attempts at building up a basic adequately staffed preventive health structure with the continuing and routine tasks of secondary prevention such as screening, vaccination, immunisation and referral for treatment, which was largely the job of the Ministry of Health, have proceeded moderately well: much progress was made in the cities in the 1950s. However, there was neglect of preventive work in rural areas which was only partly solved by the imaginative use of mobile medical teams from the mid-1950s onwards. The current organisation of rural and urban public health networks, some of which dates from the late 1960s, extends all forms of preventive health

work down to the basic level and, while occasionally providing
duplication of effort and wastefulness, also ensures accessibility
The organisational form of health care detailed in other
chapters has strengths and weaknesses, which are reflected in
the style of preventive work. When overcentralised, local
problems were not dealth with; when devolved there was often a
lack of co-ordination and resources to deal with all but the
most pressing health care problems.

Central initiatives towards prevention (which are not necessarily the same as centralised organisation) have undoubtedly
been of great benefit in the identification of major health problems. Vestiges of the 'mass approach' can be seen in the large-
scale screening of populations at risk for cancer, and in registers of cancer and hypertension. This 'totalising' approach to
health care problems, which is an attempt to get a broad picture
of the scope of the problem and then develop an overall strategy
for dealing with it, is typical of current attempts to come to
terms with the disease profile of an industrialising nation. It is
probably the most efficient fusion of 'mass' and 'routine structural' approaches that has been made in China. Political changes
have sometimes supported and sometimes neglected or undermined the role of expert knowledge. Current strategies of
prevention have sought to combine the role of the expert in
research and treatment, with 'mass' dissemination of knowledge
and basic-level organisation of health propaganda and surveillance. This is a fruitful collaboration, best exemplified in the
work on cancer and hypertension, and if successful will present
the world with the first co-ordinated attack on the 'diseases
of civilisation' - heart disease and cancer.

Table 6.1  Some vital rates for all China, 1949-80

|  | 1949 | 1980 |
|---|---|---|
| Life expectancy | 35 | 68 |
| Mortality rate | 25/1000 | 6.2/1000 |
| Infant mortality | 200/1000 |  |
| rural |  | 20-30/1000 |
| urban |  | 12/1000 |

Source:  Ministry of Health, Beijing, 'SWB'/FE/W1154/A/3,
         7 October 1981.

The effectiveness of Chinese approaches to prevention is
perhaps best shown in the simple measures of life-expectancy
and infant mortality, and the control and sometimes eradication
of many types of infections and parasitic disease (see tables
6.1 and 6.2). In general, best results have been achieved when
organisational structures of prevention (e.g. TB networks,
epidemic prevention stations, maternal and child health stations)
have been linked with movements for environmental sanitation

(e.g. night-soil management, domestic cleanliness, clean drinking water), whether or not these latter changes were produced
by mass campaigns. Given the poverty of both rural and urban
China, the mass campaigns were the easiest and cheapest method
of improving environmental health, but of course they were by
no means the only way in which this was achieved. The combination of primary prevention with secondary prevention has
proved most effective, but in the absence of the former, the
latter has proved its value. A more tangible benefit of mass
campaigns may have been raising the health consciousness of
the population to a new awareness of the importance not only of
individual health, but of public health, and the relationship
between one and the other.

Table 6.2  Present disease profile of China (selected cases)

| | | |
|---|---|---|
| Eradication of: | * smallpox | |
| | *. venereal disease | |
| | * opium addiction | |
| | * kala-azar | (some cases |
| | * haemorrhagic fever | identified |
| | * leptosirosis | 1978) |
| Control of: | * maternal and infant | |
| | ....mortality | |
| | * diphtheria | |
| | * measles | |
| | poliomyelitis | (cases still occur) |
| | * whooping cough | |
| | + tuberculosis | |
| | scarlet fever | |
| Problems with: | Japanese B encephalitis | |
| | * malaria | (rising incidence) |
| | * hookworm | |
| | * schistosomiasis | |
| | * typhoid fever | |
| | * meningococcal | |
| | meningitis | |
| | * trachoma | (rising incidence) |
| | * rickets | (rising incidence) |
| | + hypertension | (rising incidence) |
| | + stroke | (rising incidence) |
| | *+ cancer | |

* mainly rural
+ mainly urban
Source:  WHO Health Statistics, All China, 1980.

China is now having to fight new health problems (see Table
6.2), while still attempting to defeat the old ones. The weapons
which may prove most effective in the long term, those of
primary prevention, which concentrate upon the causes of

disease whether they be patterns of agriculture, impure water, environmental pollution or malnutrition, are precisely those which are hardest to utilise and which cause most political difficulty either by interfering with production in the short term, or making demands which the system cannot or will not afford. Yet it is in these, combined with effective methods of secondary prevention, the major achievement of preventive medicine in China, that the greatest successes may be achieved.

NOTES

1 J. Needham and Lu Gwei-djen, Hygiene and preventive medicine in Ancient China, in 'Clerks and Craftsmen in China and the West', Cambridge University Press, 1970, p. 344.
2 Ibid., p. 360.
3 Ibid., p. 356.
4 J. Gernet, 'Daily Life in China on the Eve of the Mongol Invasion 1250-1276', London, George Allen & Unwin, 1960, p. 45.
5 J.Y. Mei (1971), Public works and community health in pre-industrial China, 'Papers on China', vol. 24, Cambridge Mass., East Asian Research Centre, Harvard University, 1971, p. 15.
6 A. Smedley, 'The Great Road', New York, Monthly Review Press, 1956, p. 257.
7 Li Teh-ch'uan (Li Dequan), Health work in New China, 'People's China', vol. II, no. 7, 1 October 1950, p. 10.
8 'New China News Agency', 29 October 1949.
9 'NCNA', 4 November 1949.
10 'NCNA', 24 July 1949.
11 'NCNA', 24 July 1949.
12 'Shenyang Provincial Service', 2 February 1950.
13 'NCNA', 29 January 1950.
14 'NCNA', 5 March 1950, 'SWB', 47, 14 March 1950.
15 'NCNA', 29 January 1950.
16 'SWB', 47, 14 March 1950.
17 'NCNA', 15 May 1950.
18 Li Teh-ch'uan, op. cit., p. 11.
19 'NCNA', 28 May 1950.
20 'NCNA', 31 March 1950.
21 Li Teh-ch'uan, op. cit., p. 11.
22 'NCNA', 13 January 1952.
23 'NCNA', 21 March 1952.
24 Li Teh-ch'uan, op. cit., p. 31.
25 'NCNA', 3 August 1950.
26 'NCNA', 17 March 1952.
27 'NCNA', 14 March 1952.
28 'Nanchang Provincial Service', 10 March 1952.
29 'Wuhan Provincial Service', 23 March 1952.

30 'NCNA', 22 March 1952.
31 P. Wilenski, 'The delivery of health services in the People's Republic of China', Ottawa, International Research Development Centre, 1976, p. 18.
32 'Chien K'ang Pao (Health News)', 19 March 1957, 'JPRS', 583, p. 8.
33 'Ta chung I-hsueh', nos 4-8, 1957; 'JPRS', 583, p. 15.
34 Ibid.
35 'China: Diseases of Man', in 'Health and Sanitation in Communist China', 'JPRS', 583, p. 15.
36 J. Domes, 'The Internal Politics of China 1949-72', London, Hurst, 1973, p. 70.
37 'Chien-K'ang Pao (Health News)', 29 March 1953, 'JPRS', 583, p. 13.
38 Ibid.
39 'CKP', 12 February 1957, 'JPRS', 583, p. 14.
40 Ibid.
41 'CKP', 18 January 1957, 'JPRS', 583, p. 30.
42 'CKP', 1 February 1957, 'JPRS', 583, p. 30.
43 Yin Fu-ching, Some problems in the expansion of public health work, in 'Health and Sanitation in Communist China', August 1957, 'JPRS', 583.
44 R. MacFarquhar, 'The Hundred Flowers', London, Stevens, 1960, p. 127.
45 Ibid., pp. 127-8.
46 'People's Daily', 12 January 1956, 'SWB', part V, Far East, p. 18.
47 'Chung-chi I-K'an', August 1957, pp. 1-3.
48 Ibid.
49 'CKP', 12 February 1957, 'JPRS', 582, 1 July 1958.
50 Yin Fu-ching, op. cit.
51 'Kuang-ming Jih-pao (Bright Daily)', article by Ministry of Public Health, 'NCNA', 5 September 1957.
52 Ibid.
53 'NCNA', 5 September 1957.
54 Li Teh-ch'uan speech at 4th session of the First National People's Congress, CCIK August 1957, in Section I Public Health Work, 'JPRS', 583.
55 'NCNA', 24 December 1958.
56 'NCNA', 5 February 1957.
57 'Jen-min Jih-pao (People's Daily)', 20 February 1957.
58 Summary of article by Tuberculosis Association of China in 'Chung-chi I-K'an', April 1957, pp. 3-5, 'JPRS', 583, p. 29.
59 'JPRS'.
60 Huang Kun-yen, Infectious and parasitic diseases, in Joseph P. Quinn (ed.), 'Medicine and Public Health in the People's Republic of China', Washington, Fogarty Center, 1972, p. 240.
61 Speech by Li Teh-ch'uan, Minister of Health, 'NCNA', 27, April 1959.

62 'NCNA', 11 August 1959.
63 T.C. Hou, H.L. Ching, L.Y. Ho and H.C. Weng, Achievements in the fight against parasitic disease in China, 'CMJ', 79, December 1959, pp. 493-520.
64 Ma Hai-teh (Ma Haide) (George Hatem), With Mao Tse-tung's Thought as the compass for action in the control of venereal disease in China, 'China's Medicine' (1), October 1966, p. 52.
65 Ibid., p. 55.
66 Ibid.
67 Ibid., p. 62.
68 Nai-ruenn Chen, 'Chinese Economic Statistics', Chicago, Aldine, 1967. Quoted in D. Lampton, 'The Politics of Medicine in China', Folkestone, Dawson, 1979, p. 59.
69 Ma Hai-teh, op. cit., p. 61.
70 Ibid.
71 Ibid.
72 Ibid., p. 64.
73 Paul Lowinger, 'The Solution and Treatment of Narcotic Addiction in the People's Republic of China' (mimeo), Departments of Psychiatry and Community Medicine, University of California, San Francisco, 1976.
74 Calculation based on comparison of figures given by Ministry of Health and Ma Hai-teh.
75 National Schistosomiasis Research Committee, Studies on schistosomiasis japonicum in New China, 'CMJ', 78, 1959, pp. 368-79.
76 Cheng Tien-hsi, Schistosomiasis in mainland China: a review of research and control programmes since 1949, 'Am. J. Trop. Med. & Hyg.', 20 (1), January 1971, p. 35.
77 Pan Yueh, Ending the scourge of schistosomiasis, 'China Reconstructs', 6, 8, 1957, pp. 9-10.
78 Cheng Tien-hsi, Some aspects of research in the prevention and treatment of s. japonicum in New China, 'CMJ', 73, 1955.
79 D. Lampton, Policy change and China's anti-schistosomiasis programme: an evaluation, 'Am. J. Trop. Med. and Hyg.', 26, 3, 1979, p. 458.
80 D. Lampton, Health policy during the Great Leap Forward, 'China Quarterly', no. 60, 1974, pp. 668-98.
81 'Ta chung I-hsueh', nos 4-8, 18 July 1958, 'JPRS', 528, p. 14.
82 Li Teh-ch'uan, New tasks for the protection of public health, 'NCNA', 18 June 1956.
83 'CKP', 15 February 1957, in 'JPRS', 83, p. 5.
84 'CKP', 22 March 1957, in ibid., p. 7.
85 'People's Daily', 5 February 1957.
86 Report of the American Schistosomiasis Delegation to the People's Republic of China, 'Am. J. Trop. Med. & Hyg.', (1977), 26, 3, p. 460.
87 Hou Tsung-chang *et al.*, Achievements in the fight against

parasitic diseases in China, 'CMJ', 79, 6, December 1959, pp. 493-520.

88 'NCNA', 30 June 1958.

89 'NCNA', Shanghai, October 1958.

90 Cheng Tien-hsi, op. cit., p. 45.

91 Canton 'Yancheng Wanpao', 5 September 1965, 'SCMP', 3545, p. 13.

92 F.R. Sandbach, Farewell to the god of plague - the control of schistosomiasis in China, 'Social Science & Medicine', vol. 4, 1977, pp. 27-33.

93 Report of the American Schistosomiasis Delegation, op. cit., p. 441.

94 D. Lampton, Policy change, op. cit.

95 Ch'ien Hsin-chung (Qian Xinzhong), Summing up of mass technical experiences with a view to expediting eradication of the five major parasitic diseases, 'CMJ', 77, 1958, pp. 521-32.

96 Shen Ch'i-chen, Report on the prevention of schistosomiasis, Speech given at 2nd session of 2nd National People's Congress, April 1980, 'JPRS', 6256, p. 1.

97 Jen Shih-yen, Jenkun village after the wiping out of Schistosomiasis, 'China Pictorial', 15, 1960, pp. 20-1.

98 Wei Wen-po, Battle against schistosomiasis, 'CMJ', 80, 1960, pp. 229-301.

99 Ch'ien Hsin-chung quoted in Chairman Mao's June 26th directive, 1967, Supp. 'SCMP', 198, p. 34.

100 'NCNA', 19 December 1961.

101 Canton municipality mobilised to tidy up its general appearance, 'Nanfang Jih-pao', 16 December 1963, 'SCMP', 3144, p. 15.

102 Sinkiang symposium on Public Health and Sanitation, 10 June 1964, 'SWB'/FE/W262/B/21.

103 D. Lampton, 'The Politics of Medicine in China', 1979, op. cit., pp. 159 *et seq.*

104 'NCNA', 11 October 1966, 'SWB'/FE/W288/B33.

105 Li Teh-ch'uan, speech at 2nd session of 2nd National People's Congress, April 1960, 'SCMP', 2237, p. 21.

106 'SCMP', 2 September 1964, 3291.

107 A. Minkowski, Care of the mother and child. Data from 1st Maternity Institute of Shanghai, in M. Wegman *et al.*, 'Public Health in the People's Republic of China', New York, Josiah Macy Jr Foundation, 1976.

108 Huang Kun-yen, Infectious and parasitic diseases, op. cit., p. 242.

109 'NCNA', 20 October 1962, 'SWB'/FE/W189/B15.

110 'Nanchang Provincial Service', 16 March 1963.

111 Village of happiness, in East China Schistosomiasis Area, 'NCNA', 22 September 1964, 'SWB'/FE/W285/B18.

112 'NCNA', 26 July 1965, 'SCMP', 3508.

113 Chairman Mao's June 26th directive, 'Survey of Mainland Press Supplement', no. 198, in D. Lampton, op. cit., p. 34.

114 Medical education, 'NCNA', 11 August 1965, 'SCMP', 3538.
115 Kwangtung holds conference on prevention and care of schistosomiasis, Canton 'Nanfang Jih-pao', December 1965, 'SCMP', 3607.
116 Kiangsu Provincial Conference, 'NCNA', 12 January 1966.
117 'SWB'/FE/W349/A/53, 12 January 1966.
118 'NCNA', Peking, 29 March 1966, 'SCMP', 3671.
119 'Taiynan Provincial Service', 12 March 1966, 'SWB'/FE/W356/A25.
120 'Changsha Regional Service', 2 April 1966, 'SWB'/FE/W361/A/31.
121 National Schistosomiasis Conference held in Chengtu, 'NCNA', 8 September 1966, 'SWB'/FE/W383/A8.
122 'Jen-min Jih-pao (People's Daily)', editorial After stepping out from the hospital and going to the countryside, 10 May 1965, 'SCMP', 3468, p. 8.
123 Directing focus of health work on the countryside, 'Kuang-ming Jih-pao', 5 August 1965, in 'SCMP', 3527.
124 Canton Medical Staff for Countryside, 'SWB'/W364/A/30, 23 April 1966.
125 Report of Hunan Provincial Public Health Conference, 'Changsha Regional Service', 2 April 1966, 'SWB'/FE/W362/A.
126 Chin. Wei, Continue to make a success of the revolution in public health work in the countryside, 'Red Flag', 12, 1 December 1963, 'SCMM', 765.
127 Mayflies lightly plot to topple a giant tree, 'Ch'uan-wu-ti (Invincible)', 26 June 1967, 'SCMP Supplement', 209, p. 18.
128 Ibid.
129 S.M. Hillier, interview file no. 4 (1980).
130 S.M. Hillier, interview file no. 3 (1980).
131 S.M. Hillier, interview file no. 4 (1980).
132 Ibid.
133 Ch'ien Hsing-chung quoted in Mao's revolution in public health, 'Current Scene', vol. VI, no. 7, 1 May 1968, p. 5.
134 Ibid., p. 4.
135 'People's Daily', 4 January 1969, 'CB', 872, p. 27.
136 'People's Daily', 19 December 1968, 'CB' 872, p. 20.
137 Ibid., p. 18.
138 'Current Scene', vol. VII, no. 12, 15 June 1969, pp. 1-18.
139 'SWB'/FE/W595/A/9, 22 October 1970.
140 Nanking 'Kiangsu Provincial Service', 29 January 1970, 'SWB'/FE/W557/A17.
141 Peking protects environment, 'CMJ', vol. 1, no. 4, July 1975, p. 301.
142 Schistosomiasis research committee becomes active, 'SWB'/FE/W998/B, 20 September 1978.
143 Cheng Tien-hsi, Schistosomiasis in mainland China, op. cit. p. 49.
144 'Peking Home Service', 27 January 1970, 'Jen-min Jih-pao',

commentary, 'SWB'/FE/W557/A/16.

145 'Peking Home Service', 27 January 1970, 'SWB'/FE/W558/A/11.

146 Kunming, 'Yunnan Provincial Service', 'SWB'/FE/W559/A/11, 13 February 1970.

147 Report of the American Schistosomiasis Delegation, op. cit., p. 435.

148 Nanking, 'Kiangsu Provincial Service', 'SWB'/FE/W577/A/11, 12 June 1970.

149 'SWB'/FE/W662/A/1, 1 March 1972.

150 'SWB'/FE/W678/A/1, 21 June 1972.

151 Southern China launches anti-schistosomiasis campaign, 'CMJ', 3, 4 July 1977, p. 286.

152 'NCNA', 3 February 1976, 'SWB'/FE/W870/A/1.

153 'SWB'/FE/W863/A/1, 4 February 1976.

154 Report of the American Schistosomiasis Delegation, op. cit., p. 442.

155 J.A. Jewell, personal communication.

156 'Hupeh Provincial Service', 'SWB'/FE/W678/A1, 21 July 1972.

157 P. Rosenfeld, R. Smith and M. Gordon Wilman, Development and verification of a schistosomiasis transmission model, 'Am. J. Trop. Med. Hyg.', vol. 26, no. 3, 1977, pp. 505-15.

158 'Hupeh Provincial Service', 'SWB'/FE/W701/A/2, 29 November 1972.

159 H.C. Chow, F.M. Chuang, H.L. Chow and M.H. Wei, Clinical evaluation of F-30066 in long course treatment of schistosomiasis japonica, 'CMJ', 84, September 1965, pp. 591-8.

160 'NCNA', 2 October 1973, 'SWB'/FE/W749/A/1.

161 Book reviews in 'CMJ', 1, 3, May 1975, p. 226.

162 'Peking Home Service', 30 August 1971, 'SWB'/FE/W639/A/1.

163 'NCNA', 'SWB'/FE/W958/A1, 7 December 1975.

164 Peking Tuberculosis Research Institute, TB control in New China, 'CMJ', 3, 4, July 1977, pp. 218-33.

165 Anti epidemic station of Chisan County, Shansi Province, Communicable disease control in Chishan county, 'CMJ', 3, 6, November 1977, pp. 358-60.

166 News and notes, Malaria control, 'CMJ', 94, 3, March 1981, p. 156.

167 News and notes, Epidemiological and clinical studies of epidemic haemorrhagic fever, 'CMJ', 94, 3, March 1981, p. 143.

168 Tachai Production Brigade Party Branch of Hsiyang County, Shansi Province, Upholding the dictatorship of the proletariat and deepening the revolution in health work, 'CMJ', 2, 2, March 1976, p. 80.

169 Ruth Sidel, 'Women and Child Care in China', Baltimore Md, Penguin, 1973, p. 64.

170 Peking Tuberculosis Research Institute, TB control in New China, 'CMJ', 3, 4, July 1977, pp. 218-23.

171 Shanghai improves maternity and child care, 'CMJ', 2, 1,

January 1976, p. 77.
172 Sidel, op. cit., p. 61.
173 S.H. Lamm and V.W. Sidel, Public Health in Shanghai: an analysis of preliminary data: 1972, in J. Quinn (ed.), 1974, 'China Medicine as we saw it', Washington, John Fogarty Center, 1974, p. 139.
174 Ibid., p. 119.
175 Medical Activities, Child health care in New China, 'CMJ', 1, 1, 1975, p. 91.
176 Co-ordinating study group on the physical development of children and adolescents and Institute of Paediatrics of the Chinese Academy of Medical Science, Peking, Studies on physical development of children and adolescents in New China, 'CMJ', 26, November 1977, pp. 364-72.
177 J.D. Wray, Child care in the People's Republic of China: 1973, 'Pediatrics', 55, 1975, pp. 724-34.
178 Tao Jen and Shen Uo, Twenty-two years investigation of infant deaths in textile workers' families, 'CMJ', 92, 2, February 1979, pp. 107-17.
179 Dazhai Production Brigade, Upholding the dictatorship of the proletariat and deepening the revolution in health work 'CMJ', 2, 2, March 1976, p. 80.
180 Lim Khati, Obstetrics and gynaecology in the past 10 years 'CMJ', 79, 3, November 1959, pp. 375-83.
181 Fu Shigui and Shen Quinge, Operative treatment of female urinary fistulas, 'CMJ', 92, 4, April 1979, pp. 263-8.
182 H.S. Kaplan and P. Tsuchitani (eds), 'Cancer in China', Report of the American Cancer Delegation, New York, Adan Liss, 1978, p. 222.
183 First, second and third Hospitals of the Shanghai Textile Bureau, Mass survey and treatment of carcinoma of the cervix - a retrospective report, 'CMJ', 1, 6, November 1975 pp. 413-18.
184 Ibid.
185 Robert W. Miller, Cancer of the uterine cervix, in Kaplan and Tsuchitani, op. cit., p. 141.
186 G.W. Pinker and D.W.T. Roberts, 'A Short Textbook of Gynaecology and Obstetrics', London, English Universities Press, 1975, p. 27.
187 Robert W. Miller, Epidemiology, in Kaplan and Tsuchitani, op. cit., p. 51.
188 Shanghai Co-ordinating group for research on Liver Cancer Diagnosis and Treatment of primary hepatocellular carcinoma in early stage, 'CMJ', 91, 11, 1979, pp. 801-6.
189 News, Cancer Research, 'CMJ', 3, 6, November 1977, p. 42
190 L. Ackerman et al., Cancer of the oesophagus, in Kaplan and Tsuchitani, op. cit., p. 125.
191 S.M. Hillier, travel notes, 1978. Visit to Linhsien county.
192 L. Ackerman, op. cit., p. 115.
193 S.M. Hillier, interview files 10 and 11.
194 C.K. Chu and T.S. Sze, The Patriotic Health Campaign,

'CMJ', 4, 4, July 1978, p. 254.
195 News and notes, China holds first meeting of revised
sanitation movement committee, 'CMJ', 4, 4, July 1978,
p. 328.
196 Chu and Sze, op. cit., p. 254.
197 Tachai (Dazhai) Production Brigade Party Branch of
Hsiyang County, Shansi, Upholding the dictatorship of
the proletariat, op. cit., p. 78.
198 Chu and Sze, op. cit., p. 256.
199 Ibid.
200 Ibid.
201 News and notes, Spring health movement in full swing in
China, 'CMJ', 4, 4, July 1978, p. 328.
202 'NCNA', 7 August 1977, 'SWB'/FE/W943/A1.
203 'NCNA', 16 April 1978, 'SWB'/FE/W979/A1.
204 'NCNA', 'SWB'/FE/W1097/A/1, 27 August 1980.
205 'Beijing Home Service', 'SWB'/FE/W979/A1, 10 May 1978.
206 'SWB'/FE/6534/C/4, 29 September 1980.
207 Chengdu 'Sichuan Provincial Service', 18 March 1980,
'SWB'/FE/6415/B, 9 May 1980.
208 'SWB'/FE/6478/B/7, 23 July 1980.
209 'SWB'/FE/6322/B/1, 18 January 1980.
210 'SWB'/FE/W1078/A1, 16 April 1981.
211 'People's Daily', 1 May 1980, 'SWB'/FE/6415/B11/3, 9 May
1980.
212 'Peking Home Service', 29 April 1980, 'SWB'/FE/6415/B11/1,
9 May 1980.
213 'People's Daily', 19 January 1980, 'SWB'/FE/6531/B11/7.
214 'Shandong Provincial Service', 12 September 1980.
215 S.M. Hillier, travel notes, March 1979.
216 'SWB'/FE/W1079/A/2, 23 April 1980.
217 'SWB'/FE/W1102/A/1, 1 October 1980.
218 'People's Daily', 9 November 1979.
219 P. Lindop, travel notes, 1980.
220 I. Weinstein, Etiology of lung cancer, in Kaplan and
Tsuchitani, op. cit., p. 72.
221 'Atlas of Cancer Mortality in the People's Republic of China',
Beijing, China Map Press, 1979, p. 53.
222 'SWB'/FE/ 7 March 1979.
223 'SWB'/FE/W977/A/1, 26 April 1978.
224 S.M. Hillier, travel notes, 1978.
225 'NCNA', 2 April 1980, 'SWB'/FE/W1092/A/3, 23 July 1980.
226 'NCNA', 19 July 1980, 'SWB'/FE/6478/B11/7, 23 July 1980.
227 'SWB'/FE/6478/B11/8, 23 July 1980.
228 'Hunan Provincial Service', 'SWB'/FE/6415/B11/13, 9 May
1980.
229 Environmentalists call for an end to work on Peking Cotton
Mill, 'NCNA', 4 August 1980, 'SWB'/FE/6494/B11/1, 11
August 1980.
230 Urban planning and sanitation deficiencies, 'SWB'/FE/
6534/C/4, 29 September 1980.

231 News and notes, 'CMJ', 93, 7, July 1980, p. 450.
232 Tao Jen and Shen Yu, Twenty-two years' investigation of infant deaths, op. cit.
233 News and notes, China to intensify environmental protection, 'CMJ', 93, 5, May 1980, p. 357.
234 'Guangxi Regional Service', 6 June 1980, 'SWB'/FE/6442/B11/6.
235 'NCNA', 6 April 1977, 'SWB'/FE/W925/A/1.
236 'NCNA', 23 January 1978, 'SWB'/FE/W971/A/1.
237 'Hsinhua News Agency', 5 September 1978.
238 'People's Daily', 21 October 1978.
239 'Kwangsi Regional Service', 3 October 1978, 'SWB'/FE/W1003/A/1, 25 October 1978.
240 'People's Daily', Firmly carry out schistosomiasis control to the end, 26 December 1979, 'SWB'/FE/6317/B11/5, 12 January 1980.
241 Ibid.
242 H.K. Hsu *et al.*, Schistosomiasis vaccination. Historical development, present status and future prospects, 'CMJ', 93, 5, May 1980, pp. 297-312.
243 Ma Jinxin and He Yixun, Scanning electron microscopy of Chinese (mainland) strain schistoma japonicum, 'CMJ', 94, 1, January 1981, pp. 63-70.
244 'SWB'/FE/W982/A/1, 31 May 1978.
245 Anti-epidemic station of Chishan County, Shansi, communicable disease control in Chishan County, 'CMJ', 3, 6, November 1977, pp. 358-60.
246 Ibid., p. 360.
247 Municipal sanitary and anti-epidemic station, Shanghai, An epidemiologic observation post for early detection of influenza epidemics, 'CMJ', 92, 1, January 1959, pp. 51-6.
248 S.M. Hillier, visit to Luwan Anti Tuberculosis Hospital, March 1981.
249 Ibid.
250 Peking Tuberculosis Research Institute, Tuberculosis control in New China, 'CMJ', 3, 4, July 1977, pp. 218-23.
251 News and notes, Malaria control, 'CMJ', 94, 3, March 1981, p. 156.
252 S.M. Hillier, travel notes, March 1981.
253 Chen Yaozhen, Ramble in Chinese Ophthalmology, 'CMJ', 94, 1, January 1981.
254 News and notes, Prevention and treatment of endemic diseases renewed, 'CMJ', 92, 8, August 1979, p. 588.
255 News and notes, China makes progress in treating goitre, 'CMJ', 94, 1, January 1981, p. 70.
256 News and notes, Prevention and treatment of endemic diseases, op. cit.
257 Keshan disease research group of the Chinese Academy of Medical Sciences, Observations on effect of sodium selenite in prevention of Keshan disease, 'CMJ', 92, 7, July 1979, pp. 471-6.

258 He Guanquing, On the etiology of Keshan disease, 'CMJ', 92, 6, June 1979, pp. 416-22.

259 Chen Xuean *et al.*, Pellegra prevention, 'CMJ', 93, 11, November 1980, pp. 785-8.

260 Shanghai diabetes Research Co-operative Group, Diabetes mellitus survey in Shanghai, 'CMJ', 93, 10, October 1980, pp. 663-72.

261 Some examples are: Anti-epidemic stations of Zhuang Autonomous Region, Qingzhou Prefecture, Be hai Municipality and Weizhou Peoples Commune Hospital Guangxi and National Vaccine and Serum Institute, Clinical reactogenicity and immunogenicity of 5 live measles vaccine strains, 'CMJ', 94, 4, April 1981, pp. 201-6. Wang Fu *et al.*, The laboratory and clinical studies of sulphonamides, 'CMJ', 93, 4, April 1980, pp. 207-16. Human Institute of Pharmaceutical Industries and Institute of Epidemiology of Chinese Academy of Medical Sciences, Ethyl 4, (5) Imidazole carboxylate as an orally effective chemotherapeutic agent against lepto- spirosis, 'CMJ', 93, 4, April 1980, pp. 217-20. Polio Type III Vaccine Co-operative Research Group, Institute of Medical Biology Chinese Academy of Medical Sciences, Kunming, Studies on new attenuated strains of Tyle III live poliomyelitis vaccine, 'CMJ', 93, 9, September 1980, pp. 583-91. Yun Guilang *et al.*, Alum solution for prevention of dermal maceration and erosion among rice farmers in Shanghai districts, 'CMJ', 92, 7, July 1979, pp. 509-11. Li Chi, Toxicity and side effects of bepnerium, 'Clin. Pharm. Bull', 15, 3, 1980, p. 27.

262 'People's Daily', 11 February 1980. It is imperative to control population growth in a planned way, 'NCNA', 'SWB'/FE/6347/B17, 16 February 1980.

263 'NCNA', 'SWB'/FE/6313/B1/5, 8 January 1980.

264 Importance of quality of childbearing, 'SWB'/FE/6511/BII/1, 1 September 1980.

265 Ge Quinsheng *et al.*, Sex chromosome and chromatin examination in gynaecology, 'CMJ', 92, 5, May 1979, pp. 310-20.

266 'NCNA', 'SWB'/FE/W1103/A/1, 8 October 1980.

267 I. Chalmers, Better perinatal health - Shanghai, 'Lancet', 19.1.1980, pp. 137-9.

268 S.M. Hillier, travel notes, March 1978.

269 'Shenyang Liaoning Provincial Service', 2 April 1980, 'SWB'/FE/6415/A/4, 9 May 1980.

270 S.M. Hillier, travel notes, March 1981/March 1978.

271 S.M. Hillier, data from Shanghai First Maternity and Children's Hospital, March 1981.

272 S.M. Hillier, travel notes, March 1981.

273 Chang Juinru *et al.*, A study of the etiology of winter infantile acute gastro enteritis in Chengdu-rotavirus, 'Acta Academic Medicinae Sichuan', 12, p. 56.

274 Co-ordinating study group on the physical development of children and adolescents and Institute of Paediatrics of

the Chinese Academy of Medical Science, Peking, Physical
development of children and adolescents in New China,
'CMJ', 3, 6, November 1977, pp. 364-72.
275 'Shanghai City Service', 25 May 1979, 'SWB'/FE/6129/B11/1.
276 Child care in Shanghai, 'Xinhua News Agency', 10 April
1979.
277 S.M. Hillier, travel notes, March 1981.
278 'NCNA', 11 October 1980, 'SWB'/FE/6552/B11/8, 19 October
1980.
279 Chinese minister on better student health work, 'Xinhua
News Agency', 16 March 1979.
280 Number of cases and deaths due to infectious disease. All
China 1978, 'WHO Division of Health Statistics', Geneva,
1980.
281 'National Atlas of Cancer Mortality', op. cit., p. 52.
282 Tang Zhaoyou *et al.*, Evaluation of population screening
for hepatocellular carcinoma, 'CMJ', 93, 11, November
1980, pp. 795-9.
283 I. Weinstein, in Kaplan and Tsuchitani, op. cit., p. 68.
284 Su Delong, Drinking water and liver cell cancer. An
epidemiologic approach to the etiology of this disease, 'CMJ'
92, 1979, pp. 748-56.
285 B. Armstrong, The epidemiology of cancer in the People's
Republic of China, 'Int. J. of Epidemiology', 1980, 9,
pp. 305-15.
286 News and notes, Nationwide cancer mortality survey, 'CMJ',
93, 7, July 1980, p. 450.
287 Wu Yingkai *et al.*, A five-year report on community control
of hypertension, stroke and coronary heart disease in
Shijingshan People's Commune, Beijing, 'CMJ', 94, 4,
April 1981, pp. 233-6.
288 Campaign against smoking, 'NCNA', 29 July 1979,
'SWB'/FE/6184/B11/10, 3 August 1979.
289 Ibid.
290 Peking meeting warns against smoking, 'Peking Home
Service', 'SWB'/FE/6236/B11/9, 4 October 1979.
291 Antismoking campaign in Shanghai, 'NCNA', 16 April 1980,
'SWB'/FE/6406/B11/4.
292 Co-operatives in cigarette production, 'NCNA', 9 July
1980, 'SWB'/FE/W1090/A/15, 23 July 1980.
293 'SWB'/FE/6534/C/4, 27 September 1980.
294 'NCNA', 17 April 1980, 'SWB'/FE/6406/B11/4, 28 April 1980.
295 'NCNA', 27 September 1980, 'SWB'/FE/W1103/A/11, 8
October 1980.
296 Wu Yingkai, Epidemiology and control of hypertension,
stroke and coronary artery disease in China, 'CMJ', 92,
19, October 1979, pp. 665-70.
297 Ibid., p. 666.
298 Ibid.
299 Ibid.
300 Ibid.

301 Wu Yingkai *et al.*, A five-year report on community control of hypertension, stroke and coronary heart disease in the Shihjingshan People's Commune, Beijing, 'CMJ', 94, 4, April 1981, pp. 233-6.

# Part Three

# TRADITIONAL MEDICINE

# 7 THEORETICAL BASIS OF CHINESE TRADITIONAL MEDICINE

J.A. Jewell

Chinese medicine is not the world's earliest recorded medical system: Egyptian and Babylonian medicine outdate it by perhaps a millennium! It is, however, the oldest continuous surviving tradition, rivalled only by Ayurvedic medicine in India.(1)

## ANCESTRAL HEALING AND DEMONIC MEDICINE

Since the earliest days human societies have developed concepts about the causes and treatment of disease. In China these can be traced back at least 3,500 years to the Shang dynasty (-1520 to -1066). Tortoise shells, ox and sheep scapulae with inscriptions dating back to -1300 have been found. These appear to have been used for divination in the practice of ancestral healing which seeks for harmony between the living and the dead. Ancestral wrath could lead to crop failure or personal illness but the inscriptions on the bone and shells also contain references to natural causes of disease such as wind, snow and phases of the moon.(2)

The notion developed of 'demonic spirits' who were constantly on the move seeking to attack humans. There were also postulated to be spirits within human beings who could protect against these marauders, but who often had to make alliances with others in the spiritual hierarchy. The cure of illness by the use of spiritual defences was aided by talismans, amulets, exorcistic spells and some drugs.

Wang Ji Min (Chimin Wong) tells of one naive concept of disease: 'the demons of malaria, three in number, one with a bucket of cold water to give the chills, another with a stove to set up the fever, and a third with a hammer with which to knock the head producing headaches'.(3)

Examples of superstitious practices have been present up to the twentieth century and Edward Hume, who was in China in the 1930s, records:

Calling for the return of the soul is something that may be witnessed everywhere in China. Of one who is in a fainting fit it is often said: 'His soul is not united with his body.' When for example a baby is seized with convulsions the frightened mother hastens up to the roof of the house, waves a bamboo pole to which is fastened a garment of the sick child and calls aloud. . . . Meanwhile another member of the family beats a gong loudly to get the attention of the missing soul.

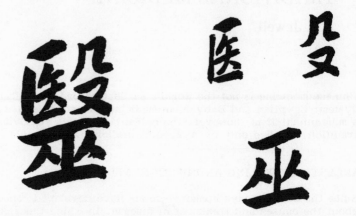

(a)   This is an early and rare form that appeared on oracle
      bones and the bottom radical means a shaman or sorcerer.
      (Calligrapher, Mr S.K. Ho)

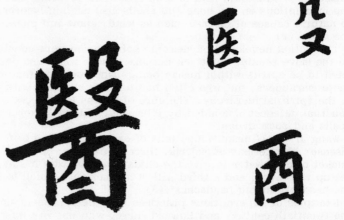

(b)   This is the common form and was the one listed in the Han
      dynasty Shuo wen dictionary (+100). The bottom radical
      here means wine. (Research, Frances Wood and calligraphy,
      Mr S.K. Ho)

Figure 6   Chinese character meaning medicine/doctor divided
into its component parts

Hume notes that 'many believe that convulsions are due to the mischievous prank of some ghost who is fond of coaxing vital spirits away from children'. These unseen beings are described as 'celestial agents astride galloping horses'.(4)

The ancient character 'Yi' for doctor is made up of three component parts. At the top of the left corner is the radical for a quiver of arrows or chest of arms; at the right-hand corner a hand grasping a weapon and below the symbol for sorcerer or priest. The complete character may denote that the priest or shaman employs strong weapons to kill or drive away the demons of sickness. Later however the third part of the symbol was changed to wine, signifying that the practice of medicine was no longer confined to the priests but had been taken up by doctors who administered elixirs or wines to their patients.(5) Needham suggests that these arrows may indeed represent acupuncture needles and notes that arrows or needles appear also in the bone or bronze forms of the characters denoting illness. He feels however that rather too much has been read into the early ideogram.(6)

The Zhou dynasty (-1066 to -221) was the transition period during which the functions of priest and physician began to be separated, and by the late Zhou a class of secular physicians emerged clearly distinct from priests and sorcerers.(7) It was during the Spring and Autumn period (-770-476) that a secular medical tradition and profession emerged. The Zuo Zhuan, collection of myths, records for instance that two famous physicians treated Prince Jin in the -sixth century. One of them, Yi He, spoke of six atmospheric influences (Yin/Yang; wind, rain, gloom and brightness) that can produce six types of illness if found in excess.(8)

Folk medicine can be found in every traditional society and can be defined as 'popular ideas about the causes and treatment of disease usually with relatively simple remedies applied on a generally empirical basis often by non-professional practitioners'. A distinct medical system on the other hand means 'a theoretically articulated body of ideas about disease causation and treatment contained in a written tradition and practiced by men whose knowledge of that tradition causes their society to recognise them as medical specialists'.(9) Chinese traditional medicine qualifies by this definition from the time of the Spring and Autumn period in having a predominantly rational theoretical basis, a large corpus of medical classics and a secular class of physicians. An important development was its early separation from the magico-religious tradition, although these influences remained important and for practitioners at one end of the spectrum superstitious practices were still the major therapeutic effort. It is interesting to note that these practices still survive in China today. Recent reports describe cases of exorcism and witchcraft.(10)

## DAO-YIN AND YANG

There were however some philosophical precepts that developed
during the earlier period. During the Shang dynasty there
evolved one of the most influential of all concepts - that of the
oneness of all life (the Dao). Later in the Zhou these ideas
were developed.(11) One of the basic concepts of the Dao lies
in the word itself which means 'the way'. The Way is the method
of maintaining harmony between this world and beyond. These
conceptions are based on the original theory of creation, which
for one early source, Lieh-tze;

> starts from chaos, in which the three primary elements of the
> universe - force, form and substance - were still undivided.
> The first stage is followed by a second, the great inception
> when force becomes separated, then by a third, the great
> beginning, when form appears and a fourth, the great
> homogeneity, when substance becomes visible. Then the
> light and pure substances rise above and form heaven, the
> heavier and coarser sink down and produce the earth.(12)

This description was an early example of the division of substance
into lighter and heavier parts which is basic to the Chinese belief
in duality. The Yin and Yang are the elementary terms used to
express this fundamental polarity in life, while the Dao is the harmony. The Yi Jing (Book of Changes) notes that: 'yi yin, yi yang
zhi wei dao' (one yin and one yang being called the tao).(13)
    Importantly, the concepts of Dao and Yin and Yang predate
the Daoist philosophies, and Hackman points out that

> The word Tao, which later became the shibboleth of a separate
> creed Taoism, is basically a concept common to all Chinese and
> therefore retains its validity also in Confucianism and even
> Buddhism. Tao is the key to the mysterious intermingling of
> 'heaven and earth'. Tao means the way and the method of
> maintaining the harmony between this world and the beyond,
> that is by shaping earthly conduct to correspond completely
> with the demands of the other world.(14)

The Dao and the Yin and Yang play an important part in early
Chinese medical thought. The Dao as the supreme regulator of
the universe represents a code of conduct in which health and
longevity depend on the individual's behaviour. Thus the earliest
extant and complete book on Chinese Medicine, the Huangdi
Neijing, notes: 'Those who follow Tao achieve the formula of
perpetual youth and maintain a youthful body.'(15)
    Yin and Yang are the primogenial elements from which the
universe was evolved. Originally these ancient terms referred
to the sunny and shady side of the hill(16) although other early
analogies may have been between sun and moon, fire and water,
male and female.

Yang stands for sun, heaven, day, fire, heat, dryness, light and tends to expand and flow upwards and outwards. Yin stands for moon, earth, night, water, cold, dampness and darkness and tends to contract and flow downward. As Heaven Yang sends fertility in the form of sun upon the earth; hence heaven's relation to earth is like that of man to woman – the man being Yang and the woman being Yin. All events in life were thought to be conditioned by the dynamic relationship between these two cosmic forces. Perfect harmony between the two meant health; disharmony or undue predominance of one brought disease and death. From about the -fourth century onwards the Chinese theory of nature was dominated by the Yang-Yin dualism.(17) The diagram of the 'Supreme Pole'(18) represents the division of the cosmos into these forces. Note that the smaller codes represent 'yin within yang' and 'yang within yin', reminding us that it is a relative concept and one cannot exist without the other.

*Diagrammatically:*

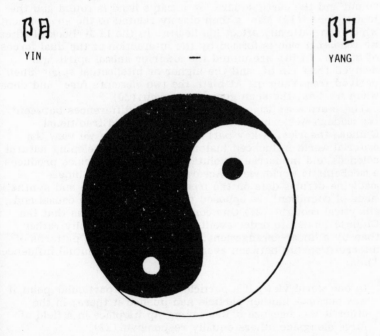

YIN  —  YANG

Figure 7  The supreme pole representing yin and yang

It is difficult to give accurate analogies to explain Yin/Yang. One useful one is the example of a lighted candle. The candle-stick represents the Yin, being solid, cool and tends to flow

downward. The flame is the Yang, being insubstantial, hot and
has an upward direction. Their interdependence is self-evident
The more difficult 'Yin within Yang' concept is analogised to
the day/night cycle. Midday represents Yang and midnight Yin.
The transition to both through sunrise and sunset is a process
of expanding of 'Yang within Yin' and 'Yin within Yang' respectively.

Similarly the four seasons represent the polarity of midsumme
heat and midwinter cold with spring and autumn phases of
change. The water cycle from solid ice to the liquid state,
evaporation and condensation is another example of natural
polarity separated by different phases in the aggregation of
matter-energy. Modern concepts that reflect the universal
polarities are that of positive/negative, hyperactivity/hypo-
activity, sympathetic/parasympathetic, excitation/inhibition,
centrifugal/centripetal and even the concept of cyclic AMP/ATP
(adenosine monophosphate/adenosine triphosphate).

A further idea was that man is a 'miniature heaven and earth'
and is therefore a microcosm. 'Thus we read that as heaven is
round and the earth square, so a man's head is round and the
foot square.'(19) Man is then closely related to the environment
which can naturally affect his health. In the Li Ji 'Book of Rites
we read that man is formed by the interaction of the dual forces
of nature. In him are united the lower or animal spirit 'gui'
derived from Yin qi, and the higher or intellectual spirit 'Shen'
derived from Yang qi. At birth the two elements fuse, and depa
when he dies, the shen going to heaven.(20)

There are some important philosophical differences between
the modern Western scientific perspective and traditional
Chinese theories. A key part of this is the way we view the
material world influenced historically by the developing natural
sciences and industrial revolution. Newtonian physics produces
a mechanistic world view. According to Porkert 'Chinese
medicine defines data on the basis of the inductive and syntheti
mode of cognition', as opposed to modern scientific causal and
analytical thought.(21) One consequence of this was that the
Chinese tended to order events and objects cyclically rather
than by a linear arrangement, and they perceived patterns of
interrelationship between events in a sphere of mutual influence
Thus:

> In one world view, if a particle occupied a particular point it
> was because another particle had pushed it there; in the
> other it was because it was taking up its place in a field of
> force alongside others equally responsive.(22)

The measurement of time is another example. Eastern Mediter-
ranean countries acquired a system of chronology with fixed
starting-points allowing the calculation of years backwards and
forwards. China however used a chronology of compartments,
a series of temporal cycles shut off from each other, the longest

of which were the dynastic periods, but extending to seasons, days and smaller units of time.(23) 'To the Chinese numbers are cyclic signs, concerned to indicate position rather than order and able to lead to combinations rather than totals.'(24)

As a result of this perspective Chinese medicine tends to stress the qualitative rather than the quantitative, and the functional as opposed to the structural. When we consider for instance the 'anatomical' descriptions used by traditional physicians in the light of modern scientific descriptive anatomy it is clear that the latter has a more functional application, the former starts from an accurate structural description. Indeed descriptive anatomy based on dissection and applied in surgery was poorly developed in China. One reason for this may have been the reluctance, in a Confucian society oriented toward filial piety and ancestor worship, to dissect bodies. Similarly the scientific subjects of physiology and pathology that developed rapidly in the industrial-ising West were more speculative in China. Nevertheless Chinese medicine is a rich source of clinical experience and therapeutic achievement.

## WU XING

The Wu Xing or 'law of the five elements' was a later development, probably of Eastern influence from the school of Cu Yan in the -4 century.(25) They are the basic materials of life which were meant to have been generated by the two cosmic forces and were regarded as affecting one another according to two main cyclical successions:

1   Mutual production - each element was regarded as generat-ing the next one in a series.
2   Mutual conquest order - each element was believed to conquer or destroy the other in sequence.

The rather complex relationship can be shown diagrammatically (Figure 8).

In pathological states there is a relative excess or deficiency of one element and the normal balance is upset. For instance if wood is in excess it overacts on earth and counteracts on metal. If deficient the reverse relationships follow. Each main internal organ is correlated with an element and thus basic physiological and pathological relationship can be surmised.

The use of the word element has been criticised as being a rather static concept. The translation of Xing is literally 'passage'(26) and it is thought that the Wu Xing are best con-ceived of as 'five phases of change' in order to develop the idea of interdependence, mutual interaction and systematic corres-pondence.(27) In modern traditional Chinese medicine the law of the five elements still holds its place but is not as central a concept as for instance that of the Yin/Yang and Qi.

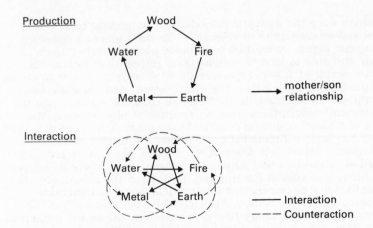

Figure 8   The five elements
Example:  Wood promotes fire
Wood acts on earth
Wood is acted on by metal
Wood is counteracted by earth
Wood can counteract metal

## QI

A fundamental concept of Traditional Chinese Medicine (TCM)
is the qi which is all-pervading. It has been interpreted as
representing 'life energy' or 'vital breath' and is analogous to
the Greek concept of 'pneuma', the Indian 'prana' and the Latin
'spiritus vitalis'.(28) The Chinese character for qi has the
radical for 'grain' or 'rice' under the one for 'vapour' or 'gas'
incorporating both the concept of substance and function. (29)
    Modern traditional Chinese medicine has differentiated
different aspects of the qi. The first is 'congenital qi' which is
inherited from the parents and is related to the reproductive
function. Acquired qi comes from food and the so-called 'clean
qi' is that derived from the air. These two meet in the chest region
to form the essential qi which nourishes the heart and lung and
promotes their function of dominating blood, vessels and
respiration. The nutrient qi circulates in the vessels and supplies
the viscera while the defensive qi circulates outside the vessels
in the skin and muscles nourishing the subcutaneous tissues and
defends the body from exogenous pathogens. Both in the lungs
and kidneys there is the notion of excretion of waste qi.(30)
    This conception allows both a substantive mode for qi as well
as its functional role. Thus blood (Xue) is part of the nutritive
qi and helps to nourish the body and promotes the functional
metabolic activities of the organs and tissues. The concept of
metabolism is perhaps a close modern equivalent. The free

circulation of the qi and blood involves the Zang Fu organs, channels and collaterals. Stagnation or deficiency can lead to pathological states. For health the qi must be able to flow freely around the body and this notion is central to both TCM and the related areas of massage, gymnastics (such as Taijiquan) and breathing techniques. These are techniques for maintaining and promoting the free flow of qi around the body.

## NEIJING

'Huangdi Neijing' ('Yellow Emperor's Manual of Internal Medicine') is the earliest complete book on traditional Chinese medicine, although earlier literary references to medical techniques and experiences exist. The important texts on silk and bamboo slips unearthed from the Han dynasty tomb of Mawangdui are said to be earlier than the Neijing but are not complete.(31) The Neijing is divided into two sections – the Su Wen (Questions and Answers about Living Matter) and the Ling Shu (vital axis). Needham dates them as -2 and -1 centuries respectively and considers the work to be a compilation.(32)

The Su Wen is the main theoretical text and the Ling Shu is concerned with practical medicine, acupuncture and moxibustion in particular. What follows is largely drawn from this work and the modern interpretations of traditional Chinese medicine. Inevitably this ignores all the historical adaptations to the basic theory that have taken place since the classical period.

## ANATOMICAL AND PHYSIOLOGICAL CONCEPTS

The heart, liver, spleen, lung and kidney are the five main Zang organs and their physiological functions are to manufacture and store essential substances. (The pericardium was a later addition to make six Zang organs but is of less importance.) The six Fu organs include the stomach, small intestine, large intestine, gall bladder, urinary bladder and the 'san jiao' or 'triple burner'. Their function is to receive and digest food, absorb nutrients, transmit and excrete waste material. The Zang-fu have a close interaction and functional connection, e.g. liver and gall bladder; kidney and urinary bladder. They also are linked to the system of channels and collaterals which helps to integrate the bodily functions and provides a connection between the external and internal. Each Zang organ relates also to a sense organ and particular tissue group, e.g. liver connected to the eye and ligaments (see Table 7.1).

Each Zang organ has its particular physiological function that is described in traditional terms. For instance the liver stores blood, maintains the free flow of qi and controls the tendons.

Table 7.1 The correspondence between the five elements and the human body

| Five elements | Zang | Fu | Sense Organ | Tissues | Emotions | Tast |
|---|---|---|---|---|---|---|
| Wood | Liver | Gall-Bladder | Eye | Tendon | Anger | Sour |
| Fire | Heart | Small intestine | Tongue | Vessels | Joy | Bitter |
| Earth | Spleen | Stomach | Mouth | Muscle | Meditation* | Sweet |
| Metal | Lung | Large intestine | Nose | Skin and hair | Grief and melancholy | Punge |
| Water | Kidney | Urinary bladder | Ear | Bone | Fear and fright | Salty |

(From 'Essentials of Chinese Acupuncture', op. cit.)
*Meditation in this context means 'overthinking'.

Emotional factors can influence its function and a fit of anger can damage the liver and conversely dysfunction of the organ leads to irascibility. The zang organs also relate to each other and the liver helps to harmonise the function of the spleen and stomach system responsible for digestion and absorption. If the qi stagnates in the liver, this will affect the stomach causing symptoms of distention and belching. The liver by way of the gall-bladder has a role in the excretion of bile. These physiological interactions can become quite complex but the main physiological functions of the zang organs can be summarised:

Heart:  1 Houses the mind
        2 Controls blood and vessels
        3 Opens to the tongue
Liver:  1 Stores blood
        2 Maintains patency for the flow of qi
        3 Controls the tendons
        4 Opens to the eye
Spleen: 1 Governs transformation (digestion and absorption) and transportation
        2 Controls the blood in the vessels
        3 Dominates the muscles
        4 Opens to the mouth
Lung:   1 Dominates qi (air) and respiration
        2 Regulates water passages
        3 Dominates skin and hair
        4 Opens into the nose
Kidney: 1 Stores essence and dominates reproduction, growth and development

    2  Produces marrow, forming the brain, and
       dominates the bones and manufacturing of blood
    3  Dominates water metabolism (clear and turbid
       water)
    4  Receives the qi (air)
    5  Opens to the ear

(From Academy of Traditional Chinese Medicine, 'Essentials of
Chinese Acupuncture', Beijing, Foreign Languages Press, 1980).
No doubt these physiological relationships sound strange to
the Westerner and space does not permit a more detailed explanation. The relationships are extremely complex and demonstrate
the very functional nature of traditional medical explanations.
A typical question from a sceptic is what happens after the
spleen, for instance, is surgically removed? This question, while
betraying the assumptions of Western medicine, is nevertheless
valid. The response is that the 'spleen' in TCM is not only
located in the organ of the spleen itself. It is a functional concept that is closely related to the 'stomach' and 'pancreas' and is
involved with digestion and absorption of nutrients and their
transportation in the blood-vessels to the body. Thus a splenec-
tomy will have some adverse effects on the system but the
function of the spleen is not located purely in the structure that
we call the spleen.
The 'San jiao' or 'triple burner' is another aspect of the
Zang-fu that is difficult for Western trained doctors to grasp.
It is suggested that there are three main areas of the body -
above the diaphragm, between diaphragm and umbilicus, and
below the umbilicus. Each zone has distinct metabolic activities
that involve absorption and elimination. For instance, in the
chest clear air qi is absorbed and waste eliminated. In the
third Jiao the kidney receives the qi and filters waste qi separ-
ating clean and turbid water. There are disputes about the
exact meaning of the 'San jiao' but the above is one reasonable
suggestion of metabolic functions at different levels of the
body.
The Zang-fu are connected through the channels and
collaterals to each other and the rest of the body to provide an
integrated whole. There are twelve paired regular channels
representing each Zang and Fu system with eight extra channels.
The collaterals link each channel and provide a branch network
to cover the body. The function of the channels and collaterals
includes the circulation of qi and blood, warming and nourishing
the tissues and linking up the whole body to keep the Zang-fu,
four limbs, skin, muscles, tendons and bone intact. It is
interesting to note that the brain was thought to be a reservoir
of bone marrow and knowledge of a distinct nervous system was
absent although the channels and collaterals provide an integrative network. The Neijing however did postulate the circulation of blood centuries before it was discovered by Harvey.
The Neijing notes that: 'All the blood is under the control of

the heart' and 'the blood current flows continuously in a circle and never stops'.(33) Another example of traditional physiology that has been demonstrated by modern science is the far from obvious association between the kidney and the control of marrow and bone. We now know of the involvement of the kidney in stimulating blood formation in the marrow through erythro-poietin and of affecting bone and calcium metabolism through Vitamin D metabolism.

The Neijing also relates the function of the Zang-fu to the feudal-bureaucratic state structure:

> The heart is the Prince of the body, the seat of the vital spirit. The lungs are the ministers who regulate one's actions The liver is the general, the abode of stratagem. The gall bladder is the central office, courage dwells in it. The pericardium is the ambassador who brings joy and happiness. The spleen and stomach are the granaries, the five tastes emanate from them. The large intestine is the organ of communication where matters are undergoing changes. The small intestine is the receiving organ, the place of digestion. Skill proceeds from the kidney, the seat of vigour and strength. The san chiao [jiao] constitutes the sewerage system which drains off fluids. The bladder is a reservoir storing up the secretions which pass out having been interacted upon by vapour.(34)

## PATHOLOGICAL CONCEPTS

Traditional Chinese medicine teaches that the phenomena that contribute to health or disease are related to the universe as a whole. Balance or imbalance of the living forces which make up the world lead to health or disease respectively. The implication here is that prevention is all-important and illness is often the result of lack of moderation. In the Yi Jing (Book of Changes), the basic text of which dates from -seventh -eighth century there is a fundamental statement: 'The great souled man always meditates on trouble in advance and takes steps to prevent it.'(35)

Confucius' analects state: 'If a man is irregular in his sleep, intemperate in his eating and immoderate in his work, sickness will kill him.'(36)

It was no accident that the Zhou Li (Record of Institutions of the Zhou dynasty), dated from about -2, records an Imperial Dietician (Shi Yi) as a senior and important minister of the Imperial Medical staff.(37) His job was to provide a balanced diet for the Imperial household properly adapted to the seasons. Later the Taoists who believed in the possibility of attaining a material immortality took preventive medicine particularly seriously and used all kinds of techniques in addition to the development of alchemy.(38) At the beginning of the Neijing it is stated: 'Regimen being adopted and the mind and emotions being guarded, how could diseases arise at all?'(39)

The following quote from the Neijing has a definite contemporary significance and summarises the basic orientation:

> *Yellow Emperor:* 'I have heard that in ancient times the people lived (through the years) to be over a hundred years, and yet they remained active and did not become decrepit in their activities. But nowadays people reach only half of that age and yet become decrepit and failing.'
> *Ch'i Po answered:* 'In ancient times those people who understood Tao (the way of self cultivation) patterned themselves upon the Yin and Yang (the two principles in nature) and they lived in harmony with the arts of divination. There was temperance in eating and drinking. Their hours of rising and retiring were regular and not disorderly and wild. By these means the ancients kept their bodies united with their souls, so as to fulfil their allotted span completely, measuring unto a hundred years before they passed away.
>
> 'Nowadays people are not like this; they use wine as beverage and they adopt recklessness as usual behaviour. They enter the chamber (of love) in an intoxicated condition; their passions exhaust their vital forces; their cravings dissipate their true (essence); they do not know how to find contentment within themselves; they are not skilled in the control of their spirits. They devote all their attention to the amusement of their minds, thus cutting themselves off from the joys of long (life). Their rising and retiring is without regularity. For these reasons they reach only one half of the hundred years and then they degenerate.'(40)

Pathological theory also proposes a division between internal and external causes of disease. A modern interpretation lists the following:

| External factors | Internal factors |
| --- | --- |
| Cold | Joy |
| Heat | Anger |
| Summer Heat | Meditation |
| Excessive dryness | Grief |
| Damp | Melancholy |
| Wind | Fear |
| | Fright |

(From 'Essentials of Chinese Acupuncture', op. cit.)

These factors provide the means with which to interpret disease states. There is also a category of miscellaneous factors such as irregular food intake, excess sexual activity, overwork, lack of physical exercise and trauma.(41) Understanding is based on the relationship between the resistance of the human body and external adversaries or internal psychic disorders. These are then interpreted in terms of Yin and Yang and qi. The Neijing states:

> Nature has four seasons and five elements. In order to grant a long life the four seasons and the five elements store up the power of creation within cold, heat, excessive dryness, moisture and wind.
> Man has five viscera in which these five climates are transformed to create joy, anger, sympathy, grief and fear.
> The emotions of joy and anger are injurious to the spirit. Cold and heat are injurious to the body. Violent anger is hurtful to Yin, violent joy is hurtful to Yang. When rebellious emotions rise to heaven, the pulse expires and leaves the body
> When joy and anger are without moderation, then cold and heat exceed all measure and life is no longer secure. Yin and Yang should be respected to an equal extent.(42)

The pathogenic factors relate to external influences which can be both physical (e.g. damp and cold) as well as internal psychosocial factors. These factors can influence the internal functioning of the body and this depends on the state of health and thus the body's defences. It is interesting to note that the perspective of strengthening resistance rather than attacking a pathogenic invader is more in tune with our traditional perspective of vis medicatrix naturae which has been overwhelmed by the antiseptic method derived from modern bacteriology.(43) Modern immunology is correcting the bias by emphasising the importance of the body's defences both for infectious diseases as well as other categories such as cancer.

## TRADITIONAL DIAGNOSIS

The classical consultation would involve four main steps toward a diagnosis:

1  Inspection.
2  Listen and smell.
3  Question.
4  Palpate – particularly the pulses.

The traditional physician would take note of the patient's facial expression and general appearance and would then make a specifi visual inspection. This would include the colour and lustre of the skin and particularly the state of the tongue.

Tongue diagnosis has been elevated to an important place in TCM and it is interesting to compare this to the interest shown by nineteenth century Western physicians in the tongue compared to their twentieth century successors. Chinese medicine recognises a close connection between the tongue and the internal functioning of the Zang-fu organs. An indication of the disease can be learned by observing the colour, form, mobility, moistness and tongue coating. The two main categories are tongue 'proper' and 'coating' and some examples are summarised below:

Table 7.2 Connection between tongue and internal functioning of Zang-fu organs

| Tongue proper | Significance |
| --- | --- |
| Pale | Deficiency state or cold type; insufficient qi or blood; invasion by pathogenic cold |
| Red | Excess syndrome, e.g. invasion by pathogenic heat |
| Purple | Stagnation of qi and blood |
| Flabby | Internal phlegm-damp |

| Tongue coating | | |
| --- | --- | --- |
| White | Thin | - Normal or wind-cold |
| | Thick | - Retention of food |
| | Sticky | - Exogenous cold-damp Internal phlegm-damp |
| | Dry | - Pestilential factor |
| Yellow | Thin | - Wind-heat |
| | Thick | - Accumulation of food |
| | Sticky | - Damp heat |
| | Dry | - Accumulation of heat |
| Greyish black | Moist | - Cold-damp |
| | Dry | - Consumption of body fluid by excess heat |

(From 'Essentials of Chinese Acupuncture', op. cit.)
The tongue relates to the Zang-fu organs through the channels and collaterals and the heart, spleen and kidney channels all connect to it. The root of the tongue is said to relate to the kidney; the centre to the spleen/stomach; the tip to the heart/lung; and sides to the gall-bladder/liver.

These few examples demonstrate some aspects of tongue diagnosis which itself can be extremely complex. Generally observation of tongue proper helps to differentiate between whether the internal organs and body fluids are in a state of excess or deficiency while the coating indicates the state of the pathogenic factors. The findings must be related to the clinical picture generally and not taken in isolation.

The traditional physician would then listen to the sound of the patient's voice or the quality of the respiration, groans, sighs, coughs and hiccoughing. For instance, a feeble voice or weak breathing indicates a deficiency type of illness. The smell of the breath, body and excretions would be noted. Thus thick sputum with a foul smell indicates phlegm-heat, while if it is dilute, clear and odourless, this would be cold-phlegm. Specific questioning would then be made with special attention being paid to the time of onset of symptoms, events leading up to this, sexual, sleep and dietary habits, and many other variables Direct questioning would ask about chills and fever which may indicate wind-cold or wind-heat respectively. Similarly perspiration, defecation and urination are important. Constipation due to dryness of stool for instance would point to an excess type illness and internal heat. Pain that responds to pressure suggest a chronic deficiency state while if heat helps then a cold factor is involved. Fixed pain is associated with destruction by cold-damp while migrating pains are due to pathogenic wind. In this way the clinical picture is formed. Palpation would follow which often was limited to pulse-taking but did sometimes include examination of wounds, swellings and occasionally abdominal palpation. Pulse-taking is a central feature of Chinese medicine, and is developed to a very high level of skill.

*Pulse diagnosis*
Bian Que, who lived c. -255 was the first exponent of pulse diagnosis.(44) In +280 Wang Shu-he during the Jin dynasty wrote the 'Mai Jing' or 'Pulse Classic'.(45) A twentieth-century author Wang Ji Min, describes the method:

> Chinese pulse lore is extremely complicated and in practice constitutes a most detailed procedure amounting almost to a solemn rite. The examination is made upon both the right and left wrists, the physician using his right hand for the left pulse and his left hand for the right. The middle finger is first laid on the head of the radius, then adding the index and ring fingers whilst the thumb rests upon the dorsum of the carpus. The physician should keep cool, first noting if his own breathing is in order. One inspiration and one expiration constitutes one cycle of respiration. The normal ratio is four beats to one respiration.(46)

The pulse is divided into three parts called Cun or inch, Guan or bar and Chi or cubit. Each of these divisions has two different and distinct pulses, one internal and one external, making altogether twelve pulses.

A normal pulse is of medium frequency (four to five beats per breath), of regular rhythm and is even and forceful. Abnormal pulses can be summarised as follows:

| Pulse | Description | Syndrome |
|-------|-------------|----------|
| Superficial | Easily palpable but weak with heavy finger pressure | Early stage of exogenous disease |
| Deep | Felt only on heavy pressure | Internal syndromes |
| Slow | Less than four beats/breath | Cold syndromes |
| Rapid | More than five beats/breath | Heat syndromes |
| Xu type | Weak and forceless and disappears on heavy pressure | Deficient syndromes |
| Shi type | Forceful and felt even on deep pressure | Excess syndromes |
| String taut (or wiry) | Taut and forceful | Hyperactivity of Yang of liver, and insufficient Yin |
| Rolling or slippery | Smooth, flowing and forceful | Excessive phlegm or retention of food. Pregnancy |
| Thready | Rather 'fine' pulse | Deficient of qi and blood |
| Short | Uneven and of short duration. Irregular missed beats | If 'shi type' indicates hyperactivity of heat, excessive phlegm, stagnation of qi and blood and retention of food. If 'Xu type' is a sign of collapse. |
| Knotted | Slow and gradual with irregular missed beats | Endogenous cold or retention of cold-phlegm and stagnant blood |
| Intermittent | Slow and gradual with missed beats at regular intervals | Impairment of qi and blood and declining Yang qi |

(From: 'Essentials of Chinese Acupuncture', op. cit.)

This list is not complete and is an example of 'pulse generalisation' which modern Chinese doctors of TCM have rationalised. Clearly the old traditional doctors used to have many different ideas and subtle variants based on the teaching they had as apprentices and on their own experience. There has also been some dispute about the pulse location and the relationship with the internal organs. A modern authoritative Chinese source describes them as:

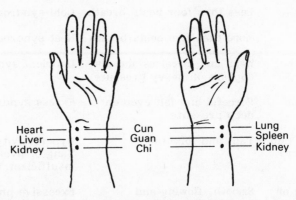

Figure 9   Location of pulses on the radial artery

> Point guan is on the radial artery opposite the styloid process of the radius. The middle finger locates this and the index and ring fingers palpate the cun and chi respectively. The kidney pulse on the right is the kidney yang or vital gate.

Source:   'Essentials of Chinese Acupuncture', op. cit.

Other sites can be used to palpate the pulse, e.g. on the head, neck and legs. Classically at least twenty-eight qualities of the pulse are distinguished. Pulse-taking could be complicated

> In order to find an auspicious moment for his undertaking he had to decide which of the two celestial stems had started the first month of the year because their constellation determined the day on which the examination was to take place. The best time of the day for taking the pulse was considered to be early in the morning, when the physician himself was still cool and collected and 'when the breath of Yin has not yet begun to stir and when the breath of Yang has not yet begun to diffuse, when food and drink have not yet been taken, when the twelve main vessels are not yet abundant . . . when vigor and energy are not yet exerted'.(47)

The seasons influenced the pulse as did age, sex and 'constitution'.

Although modern physicians may find some of this rather fanciful it must be noted that the real pulse masters can obtain an enormous amount of clinical information from the pulse. They view invasive modern investigations with some dismay.

*Diagnosis: differentiation of syndromes*
Having taken the history and examined the patient the doctor
would summarise the finding and make a diagnosis. This process
is referred to as the 'differentiation of syndromes' and takes
three main forms. The first is according to the eight principles:

|                   |              |
|-------------------|--------------|
| Internal          | / External   |
| Cold              | / Heat       |
| Xu (deficient)    | / Shi (excess) |
| Yin               | / Yang       |

The first category refers to the depth of the disease and thus
the common cold would be external while if it developed into
bronchitis this would mean it had become internal. The second
subdivision refers to the nature of the disease and thus acute
fevers will be under 'heat', while cold illnesses lead to cold,
numb and painful limbs, chill shivering, diarrhoea and a large
urine output. Xu and Shi are an indication of the state of
struggle between the pathogenic factors and the bodily resistance. Thus 'excess' states mean the resistance is still strong
whereas 'deficiency' states imply a chronic condition with
lowered resistance. The Yin/Yang category is the principal
generalisation and external, heat and excess types will be
defined as Yang while interior, cold and deficient will be Yin.
Clinically of course there are intermediate, e.g. half internal/
external, states that can be recognised and match the progress
and natural history of the disease.
The second means of differentiation is according to the Zang-
fu, for instance syndromes of the Zang organ 'lung':

| Invasion of lung by pathogenic wind | Itching throat and cough with possible fever and chills |
|---|---|
| Retention of damp-phlegm in lung | Cough, shortness of breath and expectoration of dilute white frothy sputum |
| Retention of phlegm – heat in lung | Cough, shortness of breath, wheezing. Thick purulent yellow-green sputum. Haemoptysis. |
| Insufficiency of Yin of lung | Dry unproductive cough, scanty sticky sputum, blood-streaked |

This method takes account of the effect the pathogenic factor
has on the physiological functions of the Zang-fu organs.
The final method is to assess the effect the disease is having

on the channels and collaterals. Each channel has a specific course through the body for the circulation of qi and blood and links to the Zang-fu organs. The symptoms and signs of the disease may indicate that a particular channel is being affected, e.g. lateral aspect of the lower legs may indicate problems in the gall-bladder channel, or the sciatic radiation down the posterior aspect of the leg a problem in the urinary bladder channel. Some diseases that are not yet internal may only be a disease of the channel which is of course the pathway connecting external with internal.

Having defined the symptom-complex and located its site in the body the physician can plan a course of treatment which would aim both to eliminate pathogenic factors and tonify the bodily resistance.

NOTES

1 R. Croizier, 'Traditional Medicine in Modern China', Cambridge Mass. Harvard University Press, 1968, p. 13.
2 P. Unschuld, 'The Cambridge Encyclopedia of China', Cambridge University Press, 1982, p. 139.
3 Chimin Wong and Wu Lien-teh, 'History of Chinese Medicine', Tientsin Press, 1932, p. 4.
4 E., Hume, 'The Chinese Way in Medicine', Baltimore, Johns Hopkins Press, 1940, p. 21.
5 Wong and Wu, op. cit., p. 7.
6 Joseph Needham and Lu Gwei-djen, 'Celestial Lancets. A History and Rationale of Acupuncture and Moxa', Cambridge University Press, 1980, p. 78.
7 Croizier, op. cit., p. 15.
8 'Common Terms of Traditional Chinese Medicine in English', Peking Medical College, 1980, p. 423.
9 Croizier, op. cit., p. 5.
10 'Guardian', 28 February 1980. Report of a case in Hainan Island when an attempt to exorcise a monkey spirit crippled a patient.
11 Hume, op. cit., p. 15.
12 I. Veith, 'The Yellow Emperor's Classic of Internal Medicine' Los Angeles, University of California Press, 1966, p. 13.
13 M. Porkert, 'The Theoretical Foundations of Chinese Medicine' Cambridge, Mass. MIT Press, 1974, p. 9.
14 Veith, op. cit., p. 11.
15 Ibid., p. 12.
16 Ibid., p. 14.
17 Joseph Needham, 'Clerks and Craftsmen in China and the West', Cambridge University Press, 1970, p. 340.
18 Porkert, op. cit., p. 34.
19 Wong and Wu, op. cit., p. 12.
20 Hume, op. cit., p. 20.
21 Porkert, op. cit., p. 13.

22 Joseph Needham, 'Science and Civilisation in China', vol. 2, Cambridge University Press, 1956, p. 285.
23 P. Huard, and Ming Wong, 'Chinese Medicine', London World University Library, Weidenfeld & Nicolson, 1968, p. 9.
24 Ibid., p. 64.
25 Needham, 'Clerks and Craftsmen', op. cit., p. 341.
26 Porkert, op. cit., p. 45.
27 Ibid., p. 43.
28 See J. Needham and Lu Gwei-djen, Problems of translation and modernisation of Ancient Chinese technical terms, 'Annals of Science', vol. 32, no. 5, September 1975, p.495-6.
29 Kao and Kao, 'Recent Advances in Acupuncture Research', Institute for Advanced Research in Asian Science and Medicine, New York, 1979, p. 14.
30 Academy of Traditional Chinese Medicine, 'Essentials of Chinese Acupuncture', Beijing, Foreign Languages Press, 1980, p. 36.
31 Study group for Han silk manuscripts from Mawangdui, 'Transcriptions of the silk manuscripts of medical treatises from the Tomb No. 3 at Mawangdui, Changsha, Wen Wu', 6, 1-6, 1975.
32 Needham, 'Clerks and Craftsmen', op. cit., p. 296.
33 Wong and Wu. op. cit., p. 20.
34 Ibid., p. 19.
35 Needham, 'Clerks and Craftsmen', op. cit., p. 343.
36 Wong and Wu, op. cit., p. 27.
37 Needham, 'Clerks and Craftsmen', op. cit., p. 346.
38 Ibid., pp. 316-339.
39 Ibid., p. 353.
40 Veith, op. cit., pp. 97-8.
41 Academy of Traditional Chinese Medicine, op. cit., pp. 45-6.
42 Veith, op. cit., p. 117.
43 Needham, 'Celestial Lancets', op. cit., p. 7.
44 Wong and Wu, op. cit., p. 39.
45 Ibid., pp. 39-40.
46 Ibid., p. 40.
47 Veith, op. cit., p. 43.

# 8 TRADITIONAL THERAPIES I: ACUPUNCTURE AND MOXIBUSTION

## J.A. Jewell

ACUPUNCTURE AND MOXIBUSTION (Zhen Jiu)

Acupuncture and moxibustion are two of the most ancient
therapeutic techniques of Chinese traditional medicine with a
recorded history of over 2,000 years and a legendary one of
3,500 years.(1) They have the same theoretical basis and are
considered to be two different methods of effecting the same
cure. The Chinese word for acupuncture is Zhen Jiu. Zhen
literally means to 'prick with the needle' and Jiu to 'sear with a
burning object'.(2) In the early period (up to the Spring and
Autumn period, -770-476) needles were made of stone, bone and
bamboo. These were subsequently replaced by metal needles.(3
Many kinds of combustible materials were used in ancient times
for Jiu but moxa (Artemisia vulgaris or mugwort) has remained th
most generally used cauteriser. Acupuncture techniques have
been thought to be most valuable in the treatment of acute illnesses, those of moxa in chronic cases.(4)

*Acupuncture*
Needham defines acupuncture as 'the implantation of needles to
different depths at a great variety of points on the surface of
the human body, points gathered in connected arrays according
to a highly systematised pattern with a complex and sophisticate
if still essentially medieval physiological theory behind it'.(5)
In keeping with traditional Chinese theory there is the concepti
of a continuous circulation of qi and blood (xue) around the
body. The channels (Jing) and their collaterals (Luo) are
passages distributed in the body in which the qi and xue circu-
late. They form a network connecting the superficial and interi
parts of the body, regulating its function.(6)

*The regular channels* (Jing) There are twelve main channels
running through the body (see Figure 10). They are symmetri-
cally distributed, one side being the mirror image of the other,
and connect the internal viscera with the four extremities, the
skin and the sense organs. This creates the organic whole
between the internal zang-fu organs, the skin and sensory syst
and environment. The channels are named in accordance with:

1  Hand or foot (extremities)
2  Yin or Yang (qualities)
3  Zang or Fu (organs)

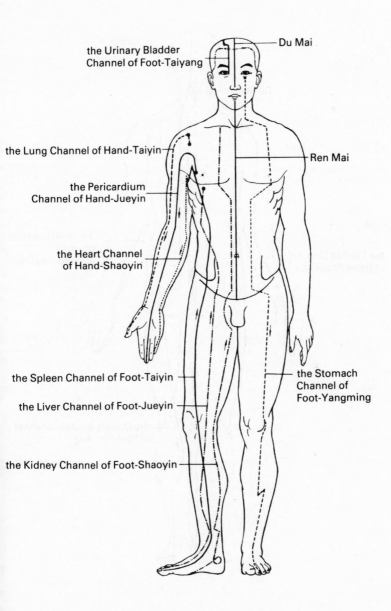

Figure 10(a) Distribution of the fourteen channels (anterior view)

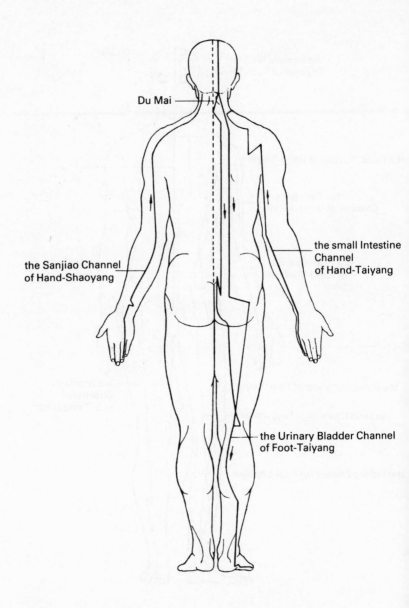

Figure 10(b) Distribution of the fourteen channels (posterior view)

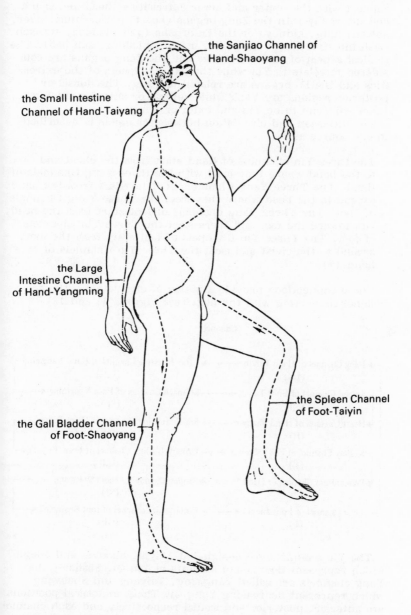

Figure 10(c) Distribution of the fourteen channels (side view)

The twelve channels in their course of circulation superficially connect with the upper and lower extremities, head and trunk and internally with the Zang organs (heart, pericardium, liver, spleen, lung, kidney) or the Fu organs (gall-bladder, stomach, small intestine, large intestine, urinary bladder, san jiao). The medical aspect of the extremities and the Zang organs are considered to relate to Yin while the lateral aspects of the extremities and the Fu organs are related to Yang. The dorsal or posterior regions are Yang while ventral or anterior are Yin. Inner will tend to be Yin and exterior Yang.

The direction and circulation between channels is described in one source as:

> The three Yin channels of Hand start from the chest and flow to the hand where they meet with the three Yang Channels of Hand. The Three Yang Channels of Hand start from the hand, ascend to the head where they meet the Three Yang Channels of Foot. The Three Yang channels of foot start from the head, run toward the foot and there meet the Three Yin Channels of foot. The Three Yin Channels of foot start from the foot, ascend to the chest and meet the Three Yin Channels of hand.(7)

These connections provide a notion of circulation with each channel connecting with the next (see Figures 11 and 12).

Channels

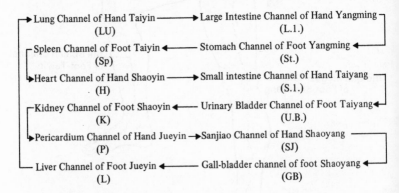

The Yin channels are designated Taiyin, Shaoyin and Jueyin which represent decreasing amounts of Yin Qi. Similarly the Yang channels are called Yangming, Taiyang and Shaoyang which represent decreasing Yang Qi. Their anatomical positions are anterior, posterior and medial respectively and each channel is paired externally/internally as shown, e.g. lung channel and large intestine channel.

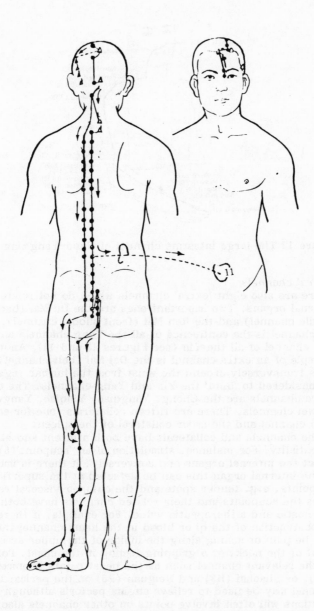

Figure 11 The urinary bladder channel of Foot-Taiyang showing connections with kidney and bladder

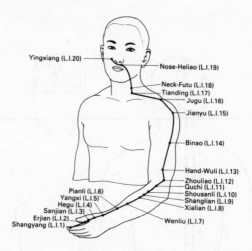

Figure 12 The large intestine channel of Hand-Yangming

*'Extra' channels*
There are also eight 'extra' channels which do not relate to the internal organs. Two important ones are the Du Mai (back middle channel) and the Ren Mai (front middle channel). The Du channel is the confluence of all the Yang channels and the Ren channel of all the Yin (see Figures 13 and 14). Another example of an extra channel is the Dai Mai (belt channel). It runs transversely around the waist from the lumbar region and is considered to 'bind' the Yin and Yang channels. The other extra channels are the Chong, Yangqiao, Yinqiao, Yangwei and Yinwei channels. There are fifteen collaterals; one for each main channel and the major collateral of the spleen.

The channels and collaterals have both afferent and efferent potentiality. For instance, stimulation of an 'acupoint'(8) can affect the internal organs and conversely, if there is imbalance in the internal organ this can be detected at the superficial acupoints, e.g. tender spots and the cutaneo-visceral reflex. Thus the acupoints and their related channels have both a diagnostic and a therapeutic value. For example, if there is an obstruction of the qi or blood in the heart channel there may be pain or aching along the inside of the upper arms, front of the neck, or a gripping feeling in the chest. Points on the relevant channel such as the heart points Shenmen (H7), or Shaohai (H3) and Neiguan (P6) on the pericardium channel may be used to relieve angina pectoris although prescriptions will often involve points on other channels also. (9) An example in Western medicine that has some similarity with these concepts is 'carotid sinus massage which stimulates the sinus reflex to slow the heart and decrease blood pressure. An acupuncture point, Renying (St. 9) is located at this spot and one of its indications for use is in the control of blood pressure. Eyeball pressure is a less commonly used method to stimulate vagal nerve slowing of the heart through the autonomic nervous system. This manoeuvre to slow the heart in cases of simple tachycardia is used quite frequently by modern scientific physicians. Similarly surgeons are familiar with shoulder-tip pain and tender spots on

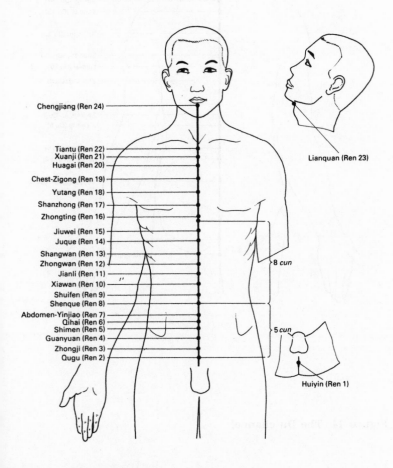

Figure 13  The Ren channel

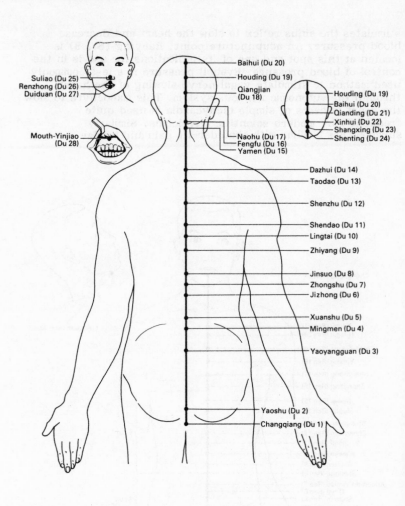

Suliao (Du 25)
Renzhong (Du 26)
Duiduan (Du 27)

Mouth-Yinjiao
(Du 28)

Baihui (Du 20)
Houding (Du 19)
Qiangjian
(Du 18)

Houding (Du 19)
Baihui (Du 20)
Qianding (Du 21)
Xinhui (Du 22)
Shangxing (Du 23)
Shenting (Du 24)

Naohu (Du 17)
Fengfu (Du 16)
Yamen (Du 15)

Dazhui (Du 14)
Taodao (Du 13)

Shenzhu (Du 12)

Shendao (Du 11)
Lingtai (Du 10)
Zhiyang (Du 9)

Jinsuo (Du 8)
Zhongshu (Du 7)
Jizhong (Du 6)

Xuanshu (Du 5)
Mingmen (Du 4)

Yaoyangguan (Du 3)

Yaoshu (Du 2)
Changqiang (Du 1)

Figure 14  The Du channel

the back with gall-bladder disease. The therapeutic basis in traditional terms of acupuncture stimulation is that by restoring the flow of qi and xue within the channels, the 'vital energy' of the viscera is regulated (reinforced or reduced) and thus restores balance, improves body resistance, and helps to eliminate pathogenic factors.

The selection of points and the formulation of a prescription is the key to acupuncture therapy. 'Essentials of Chinese Acupuncture' lists 361 regular points and 20 extraordinary points. There are five main groups of points used by modern Chinese acupuncturists:

1 Distal points: After determining which channel or organ is involved, points on the extremities below the elbow or knee of the involved channel are selected, e.g. Zusanli (St 36) on the leg for diseases of the upper abdomen; Hegu (L.I.4) on the hand for diseases of the face and mouth.
2 Local points: These are points in the local area, on the affected channel, related ones or sensitive spots, e.g. Zhongwan (Ren 12) and Tianshu (St 25) in abdominal pain which are located near the umbilicus.
3 Symptom points: Special points used for particular symptoms such as fever, shock or insomnia, e.g. Renzhong (Du 26) on the philtrum in shock. Dazhui (Du 12) between C7-T1 spinous processes for fever.
4 Specific points: Each of the Zang and Fu organs' corresponding points on the front and back channels. e.g. Weishu (UB 21) for stomach Feishu (UB 13) for lung which are located parallel to the spine in the appropriate dermatome lateral to T12 and T3 respectively (Wei means stomach, Fei-lung and 'shu' point).
5 Nerve points: These are points relating to local spinal nerve roots and are used for the corresponding dermatome,(10) e.g. Huatuo jiaji points along the lateral borders of spinous processes T1-L5 (extra points) and the organ-specific points on the urinary bladder channel running parallel to the spine.

Having selected the points to be used their exact location is aided by 'rule of thumb' techniques which incidentally are early examples of the 'modular system'. An example of such a technique is the method of proportional measurement (cun). On the forearm the distance from the crease of the wrist to the cubital crease is equivalent to twelve cun. Point Neiguan (P.6) is therefore located on 'the medial aspect of the forearm 2 cun above the midpoint of the wrist crease'(11) (see Figures 15 and 16). Thus the distance is always proportional to the patient and explains how points in babies and adults can be located.

The acupuncture needles are of many different types and sizes. The Neijing records nine different ones which have been described as 'arrow-headed, blunt, puncturing, spear-pointed, fusiform, round, capillary, long and great',(12) and are of

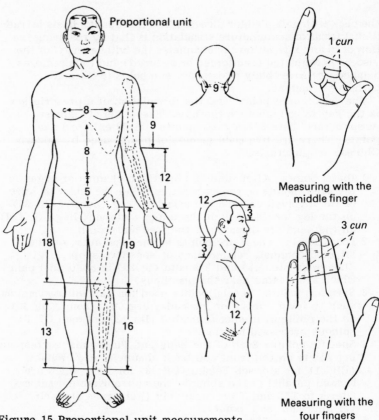

Figure 15 Proportional unit measurements

varying length. They are divided into three main categories for (1) scratching the skin; (2) piercing and bleeding; (3) piercing hypodermic and deep-lying tissues. The third category is most commonly used and is typically a steel filiform needle which is inserted to a given depth under the skin.

When the needle is manipulated the patient may experience the 'de qi' which means 'obtaining the qi' (responding to the needle). Typical responses are warmth, soreness, numbness or distension around the needle.(13) These sensations travel up and down the body and may have been the means by which the channels were traced(14) (known as propagating sensation of channel - PSC). The 'de qi' is an important indication as to therapeutic effect and the depth will vary from point to point and according to patient response. Special types of needle are the 'three edge needles' for drawing small drops of capillary blood, and the 'plum blossom' seven-star needles which have five to seven needles and are used to tap the skin, either on the local area or along the course of the channel.

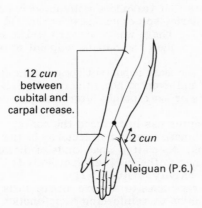

12 *cun*
between
cubital and
carpal crease.

*2 cun*

Neiguan (P.6.)

Figure 16  Location of point Neiguan

Point Neiguan is on the pericardium channel of Hand-Jueyin. It is located two cun above the transverse crease of the wrist between the tendons of M. Palmaris Longus and M. Flexor Carpi Radialis.

More recently long-term point stimulation has been achieved by implanting foreign bodies such as catgut sutures or injecting substances such as vitamin B12. Electro-acupuncture has been used since the 1930s in China(15) and a source of DC current is used. This delivers biphasic pulses with a variable frequency from one to several hundred cycles per second. This technique has been particularly useful in acupuncture analgesia when a number of points are used for long periods of time.

*Therapeutic application*  For many people in the West acupuncture means the use of needling to relieve pain in conditions such as migraine or 'lumbago' and the extraordinary use of acupuncture analgesia for surgery in China. However, acupuncture and moxibustion have been used for centuries prophylactically, symptomatically and therapeutically for almost all known diseases. Recent studies within China have shown its efficacy for instance in the treatment of bacillary dysentery, acute appendicitis, gallstones, coronary heart disease, deafness and some forms of paralysis.(16) Felix Mann, a Western acupuncturist, notes that: 'Theoretically it is possible to help or cure by acupuncture any disease that can be affected by a physiological process.'(17)

Before giving a specific example of acupuncture treatment it is important to stress the preventive aspect again. Modern practitioners urge regular 'check-ups' in order to detect early changes that will lead to specific disease states.(18) Early acupuncture to restore balance or general advice about diet and life style will be prophylactic. Needham records the use of unhealed moxa spots that travellers maintained in order to protect against 'malaria, epidemics, pestilences and infectious ulcerating sores'.(19) There was a proverb which said: 'If you wish to be safe never allow the San-Li acupoint to become dry.'(20)

Moxa was one of the most important components of first aid kits for travellers and even at home the careful scholar would apply moxa at three or more points after each ten-day period of good health.

The previous chapter has introduced the concepts of disease process used by Chinese traditional doctors: in the Su Wen of the Neijing it states: 'No matter what kinds of diseases they are bound to relate either to the xu [deficient activity] nature or the shi [excessive activity] nature.'(21)

Acupuncture therapy aims to restore 'homeostasis' by either reducing hyperfunction or reinforcing hypofunction, and it is interesting that both high and low blood pressure can be treated by the same points. The Neijing Ling Shu points out: 'In the case of xu apply the reinforcing method and in the case of shi apply the reducing method.'(22)

An example of acupuncture therapy is the treatment of 'Bronchial Asthma' as given in the Academy of Traditional Chinese Medicine's textbook 'Essentials of Chinese Acupuncture'.

*Asthma*  There are two main types of asthma: the xu type and the shi type. Shi type is due to invasion of exogenous wind-cold or disturbance of phlegm-heat. Xu type is due to deficiency of the lung or kidney. (The differentiation of the syndromes has been outlined in the next chapter 'Traditional therapies II: Chinese Materia Medica', pp. 284-8.)

  *Treatment*
  1 Shi type: wind-cold
    Points on the lung channel are taken to eliminate wind and
      cold. Reducing method is used and moxa may be added:
    Local points: e.g. Feishu (UB13) - located on upper back
    Distal points: e.g. Lieque (Lu7), Hegu (L.1.4) - on wrist
      and hand
  2 Shi type: phlegm-heat
    Points on the stomach channel are taken as the main points
      to resolve phlegm, using reducing method.
    Local points: e.g. Dingchuan (Extra 17) - back of neck
      Tiantu (Ren22) - front of chest
    Distal points: e.g. Fenglong (St.40) - lower leg Chize
      (Lu5) - front of elbow
  The specific properties of these points are:
    Feishu: reinforces the Qi of the lung
    Lieque and Hegu: eliminate wind and cold
    Fenglong and Tiantu: pacify breathing and resolves phlegm
    Chize: reduces heat in the lung

treatment description continues p. 257

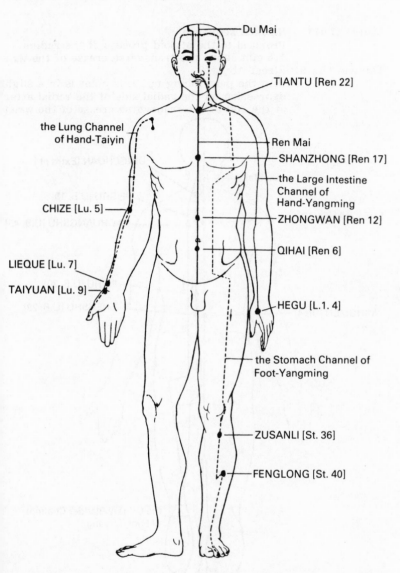

Figure 17(a)  Some acupuncture points commonly used for asthma (anterior view)

*Examples of point location:*
Hegu (L.I.4)      'Adjoining valleys'
                  Located on the index side of the prominence of
                  the dorsal aspect of the Ist interosseus muscle
                  at the midpoint of the second metacarpal bone.

Lieque (Lu7)   'Broken sequence'
               Proximal to the styloid process of the radius.
               1.5 cun above the transverse crease of the wrist

Taiyuan (Lu 9) 'Great Abyss'
               With the palm facing up, this point is in a slight
               depression on the radial side of the radial artery
               at the end of the transverse crease of the wrist.

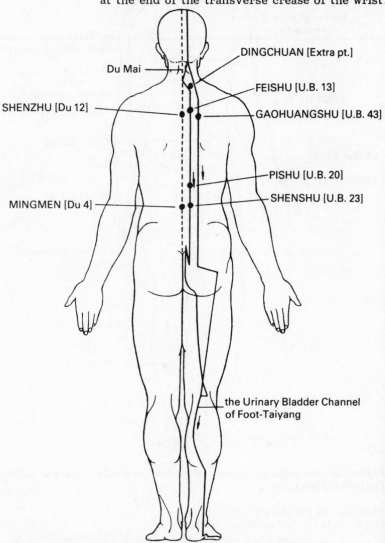

Figure 17(b)  Some acupuncture points commonly used for
asthma (posterior view)

Examples of point location:
Dingchuan (Extra pt.) 'Stop wheezing'
>> 0.5 cun lateral to the lower end of the spinous
>> process of the seventh cervical vertebra.
Feishu (U.B.13) 'Lungs hollow'
>> One and a half cun lateral to the lower end of the
>> spinous process of the third thoracic vertebra.
Shenzhu (Du 12) 'Body's pillar'
>> Between the spinous processes of the third and
>> fourth thoracic vertebrae.

Source: for point locations 'Essentials of Chinese Acupuncture',
FLP, 1980. Translation of point names from 'Acupuncture - A
Comprehensive Text' Shanghai College of Traditional Medicine,
translated and edited by John O'Connor and Dan Bensky,
Eastland Press Chicago, 1981.

Asthma treatment contd

3 Xu type: deficiency of lung
>  Local: Feishu (UB13) - upper back
>  Distal: Taiyuan (Lu9) - wrist; Zusanli (St36) - lower leg
4 Xu type: deficiency of kidney
>  Local: Shenshu (UB23) - lumbar region; Mingmen (Du4)
>  - lumbar region; Qihai (Ren6) - abdomen;
>  Shanzhong (Ren17) - anterior chest.
Specific properties of points:
>  Feishu: reinforces the qi of the lung
>  Shenshu and Mingmen: reinforce the qi of kidney
>  Taiyuan and Zusanli: strengthens the lung (metal) by
>  invigorating the spleen (earth) and stomach
>  Qihai: strengthens qi.
>  Shanzhong: an influential point dominating qi (respiration)
Other points that can be used for specific purposes include
>  Shenzhu (Du12) - on back; Gaohuangshu (UB43) - on back
>  for chronic asthma; Zhongwan (Ren12) -abdomen;
>  Pishu (UB20) - on back for spleen deficiency.
>  Also ear acupuncture points on lung, kidney, adrenal,
>  sympathetic nerve or ear asthma (Dingchuan) points.
Source: Academy of Traditional Chinese Medicine, 'Essentials
of Chinese Acupuncture', Beijing, 1980, pp. 347-8.

This example illustrates how the acupuncturist needs first to
make a formal traditional diagnosis. Having done this his point
selection will be guided by general principles as above as well
as any specific symptoms given by the patient that may affect
his prescription.

*Ear Acupuncture* Auriculotherapy has developed rapidly since
1956 following the work of Nogier in France,(23) although the
relationship between the ear, internal organs and channels were
noted in the Neijing. For instance, the Ling Shu section notes

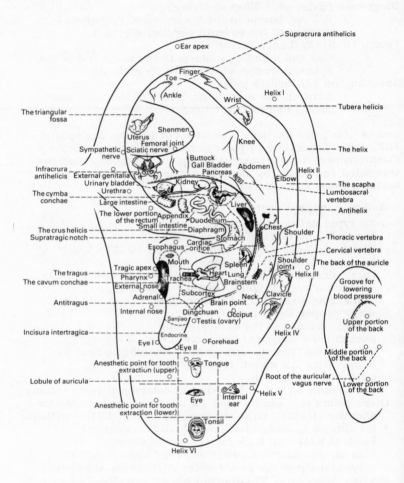

Figure 18  Distribution of auricular points

that: 'The ear is the place where all the channels meet.'(24)
In a similar way to other areas pathological changes in the
internal organs manifest themselves in various points on the
auricle and can themselves be influenced by stimulation of these
spots. Discolorations, tenderness or increased electrical con-
ductivity are signs of point activity. The acupoints are distributed on the ear in a representative way that stimulates zones
of an inverted foetus (see Figure 18).

Clearly accuracy of point selection is crucial as there are now
more than 200 acupoints on the ear: hence the use of special
electrical detectors and fine needles. One commonly used form of
needle is the thumbtack one, which can be left in place for
longer periods of time.

It is interesting to note that the innervation of the ear is
extremely complex. The main nerves are the great auricular and
lesser occipital nerve derived from the second and third cervical
spinal nerves, the auriculo-temporal branch of the trigeminal
nerve, the posterior auricular branch of the facial nerve, the
mixed branch of the vagus and the glossopharyngeal nerves.
There are also three arteries supplying the ear which may also
be an important factor. This anatomy is very unusual and would
explain how numerous pathways may be involved. The vagus has
the longest course of all cranial nerves passing down the
oesophagus, and chest, into the abdominal cavity. The ear is the
only place that it connects with the skin surface.(25) In traditional Chinese theory the 'kidney opens to the ear' and it is
interesting to relate this to the congenital abnormality of Potter's
syndrome. These babies have renal agenisis and have low-set
ears which are also abnormal anatomically.

*Surgical acupuncture analgesia* This is another modern development of acupuncture that was in a sense a logical progression
from the long-standing use of acupuncture analgesia. This new
application was first recorded in 1957 from different centres in
Shanghai and Xian(26) which having used acupuncture for the
treatment of post-operative pain, were bold enough to experiment its use during operations. The early work was done for
ear, nose and throat (ENT) surgery and tonsillectomies in
particular. After this initial success surgeons, anaesthetists and
acupuncturists experimented its use in many different operations
and perhaps the high point was reached in the late 1960s when
one report quoted its use in 60 per cent of all operations.(27)
In general acupuncture analgesia is the method of choice in 15
to 30 per cent of cases(28) and is used particularly with surgery
of the head, neck, chest and gynaecological operations. In some
procedures such as thyroidectomies the vast majority of patients
achieve satisfactory analgesia. The most astonishing application,
first used in 1972, must be the use of acupuncture analgesia for
cardiac operations using extracorporeal blood circulation.(29)

Acupuncture analgesic efficacy was shown to be approximately
70 per cent in a series of 80,000 operations carried out in Shanghai

hospitals(30) (see Table 8.1). They used a four-grade assessment:

I  Excellent analgesic effect. Patient calm and feels only slight pain. Blood pressure (BP), Pulse (P) and respiratory rate (RR) normal.

II  Good analgesia effect. The patient may groan occasionally as if with dull pain. Slight changes in BP, P and RR. Local analgesia may be used.

III  Fair analgesia, but patient feels some pain though not enough to interrupt surgery or require systemic analgesia. Local analgesia given.

IV  Poor analgesia with marked changes in physiological function requiring general anaesthesia.

Table 8.1 Effectiveness of acupuncture analgesia expressed as average percentages from series of 80,000 different operations

| % | I | II | I & II | III | IV | III & IV |
|---|---|----|--------|-----|----|----------|
|   | 37.3 | 38.25 | 75.45 | 17.0 | 7.8 | 24.8 |

Source: Needham and Lu Gwei-djen, 'Celestial Lancets', 1980, pp. 224-5.

Usually patients are given the choice of using acupuncture analgesia. If they want acupuncture, they are admitted to hospital a little earlier to meet the acupuncturist and are shown the operating theatre. Pre-operative injection of small amounts of sedatives (e.g. phenobarbitone) and analgesics (e.g. pethidine) are commonly given. The patient is then mildly sedated but fully conscious and co-operative. The acupuncturist inserts the needles and usually links them to an electrostimulator approximately fifteen to twenty minutes before incision. Routine vital signs such as blood pressure, pulse and respiration are recorded throughout the operation. Increasingly local acupuncture points that relate to the relevant spinal roots and subcutaneous needles along the incision are being used and there has been a tendency to decrease the number of points used even to the extent that some thoracotomies have been done with the one acupuncture insertion.(31) Below are listed some of the advantages and disadvantages of the method:

*Advantages:*
Patient conscious and can co-operate (e.g. squint and some neurosurgical operations).
Safe - no deaths or serious complications have been recorded with its anaesthetic use.
Fewer drugs with less side effects (e.g. Caesarian section).
Prolonged post-operative analgesia noted (up to 24 hours).
Few post-operative side effects commonly seen with general anaesthetics such as nausea and vomiting, respiratory

problems, retention of urine and ileus.
Early mobilisation and feeding.
Suitable for poor anaesthetic risks such as the elderly or
debilitated.
Little interference with physiological function such as cardio-
pulmonary, digestive or fluid and electrolyte balance (the
physiological effects are regulatory and positive such as
blood pressure regulation and immunological stimulation
effects).
Simple technique with little equipment.
Cheaper than conventional general anaesthesia.
Readily adaptable technique suitable for use in remote areas
and in time of war.

*Disadvantages:*
Incomplete analgesia, a degree of visceral pain experienced.
Incomplete control of visceral reaction.
Unsatisfactory muscle relaxation (e.g. for abdominal surgery).
Less useful for operations necessitating more than three hours.

It is recognised that for acupuncture to be used successfully
the patient's orientation and relationship with the acupuncturists
and surgical team is important. However, suggestions that
analgesia is purely a psychological effect, do not explain why
the technique is successful in a high percentage of cases on
babies, young children and animals.(32) Hypnosis and mesmerism
are other postulated explanations, but Needham points out:

What is certain is that under acupuncture analgesia a patient
shows none of the trance-like or somnambulistic states
characteristic of hypnosis; he is alert to a normal or almost
normal degree, he can co-operate actively with the surgeons
and converse with the anaesthetist, he can ingest liquids for
refreshment or medication and can tell those around him
exactly what he is feeling and finally at the conclusion of the
operation he can in many cases get off the table unaided and
walk back to his bed.(33)

*Mechanism*
Research into the mechanisms of acupuncture analgesia has
expanded rapidly both within China and in the West. The neurophysiological theories and evidence are extremely complicated
but in general there appear to be afferent and efferent
mechanisms involved. The afferent messages are transmitted
from the needle point up the peripheral, sensory nervous system
to the spinal cord and higher centres. At the spinal cord level
a mechanism like the 'gate theory' of Melzach and Wall (Melzach,
R. and Wall, P., Pain mechanisms, a new theory, 'Science',
150, 3699, 1965, p. 971) is probably applicable with the
suggestion that the acupuncture sensory stimulation probably
from deep receptors blocks the pain input. At the higher levels

and in particular with the thalamic/hypothalamic axis neuro-
humoral mechanisms are probably at work. The recent work on
the 'endorphins' which are endogenously produced morphine-
like substances found in the cerebro-spinal fluid would suggest
their involvement in the acupuncture effect. The specific opiate
antagonist Naloxone has been shown to reverse analgesia in
some cases.(34) They may have an 'efferent' action on lower
brain levels or even on the spinal cord. Other neurotrans-
mitters have also been shown to be involved and these neuro-
humoral effects may explain the fifteen to twenty minutes'
delay before acupuncture analgesia takes effect. There may also
be substances carried in the bloodstream as animal cross-
circulation experiments demonstrate that the acupuncture effect
can be transferred. Other general metabolic effects of acupuncture have been an increase in circulating steroids, increased
antibody formation and regulation of blood pressure. There is
then an enormous amount of research that is beginning to
explain in modern scientific terms the evident efficacy of this
ancient therapy.(35) One important area is its effect on the
autonomic nervous system.

*Moxibustion*
'Moxibustion therapy means treating diseases with ignited
"moxa wool" to produce heat on the points or certain locations
of the human body.'(36)
   The moxa 'wool' is made of dry moxa leaves (Artemisia vulgaris)
ground into a fine powder. It can be used in the shape of a
cone, the size varying from that of a grain of wheat to 1 cm in
height by 0.8 cm in diameter, or more commonly in the shape of
a cigar (20 cm long by 1.5 cm wide). The burning moxa produces an even and dry heat and the smoke is thought to have
therapeutic affects.

*Techniques of moxibustion* There are three methods; with
moxa cones, moxa sticks and with 'warming needle'.
   'Direct moxibustion' is when the cone is placed onto the skin
and ignited. In non-scarring moxibustion the cone is removed
when the heat becomes uncomfortable. The scarring method
allows the cone to be completely burnt and between three to
seven cones are used. The resultant blister develops into a
scar. This method is rarely used now because of the pain and
the fact that the acupoint cannot be used again.
   'Indirect methods' use slices of ginger, garlic or salt over the
point with the cone lying on them. These materials provide a
physical barrier but also have their own properties, e.g. hot
and Yang qualities of ginger.
   The moxa sticks are ignited and held just above the skin to
produce a local inflammatory response. Moxa boxes are sometimes used and can cover a wider area, e.g. over the lumbar
region or abdomen.
   The warming needle is quite commonly used and is another

method of needle stimulation. The moxa is put on the handle of
the needle and ignited. This is typically used for painful joints
due to cold and damp.(37)

   Moxibustion has, in addition to stimulating acupoints, obvious
counter-irritant effects useful for analgesia. The heat itself
probably has antibacterial effects and must have been useful in
the past for the treatment of skin ulcers. It has Yang and heat
qualities and is typically used for chronic diseases related to
the cold and 'Xu' types of disease, e.g. asthma, chronic
diarrhoea and indigestion.

*Cupping*   Cupping was called the 'horn method' in ancient times
and is a method of counter-irritation and acupoint stimulation.
The effect is achieved by using a small jar, in which a partial
vacuum is created by flaming, which is then attached to a
selected area of the skin. This produces a local inflammatory
response. The position may be chosen over specific acupoints
or along channels. Glass, ceramic or bamboo jars or cups are
used. Commonly alcohol is used to flame the jar and produce the
relative vacuum. This treatment is used especially for musculo-
skeletal disorders such as sprains, and arthritic joint pain, but
also commonly for bronchitis and asthma. The practitioner needs
to be careful not to burn the skin or use the cup on ulcerated
skin.(38)

*Massage*   This is another ancient technique intrinsic to traditional
medicine and features in the Neijing. Unguents are used and in
some cases a small wooden mallet replaces the hand. Its application is based on the 'Jing Luo' system and the massage actions
can be either finger pressure on acupoints, or broader movements along the channels. Stimulation or dispersal effects can
be achieved by different actions such as rolling, rubbing or
kneading. Massage and manipulation techniques are commonly
used in orthopaedic clinics.

*Breathing exercises and gymnastics*   These widely practised
techniques are an integral part of Chinese theory and culture.
Hua Tuo (+136-208) was the father of physical culture with his
'five animal' method (bear, tiger, stag, monkey and crane), the
detailed record of which has been lost.(39) Important findings
from the Han tombs at Mawangdui (c. -168) show illustrations
of an ancient form of physical exercise called Daoyin which
probably dates to the period before the Neijing.(40)

   There are two complementary aspects to breathing exercises
and gymnastics - one prescribes immobility with the emphasis
on breathing, and the other uses movement. The Buddhist
influence must have been important in contributing to the
breathing techniques, although before this the Neijing described
the potential of respiratory exercises. Gymnastics took its name
from the 'Tai Qi' (Supreme Pole) symbol and means to maintain
life by keeping up a healthy movement of the breath and blood

within the body. The idea is to facilitate the smooth circulation
of qi around the body relieving any 'obstructions' or 'stasis'
there might be. Regular exercising maintains the harmony and
is prophylactic in keeping the body healthy and encourages
'healthy respect'. The popularity of physical exercises and
Taijiquan in particular in China is obvious to the visitor and is
practised by all age-groups. Taijiquan itself is a relatively
recent form probably dating from some 300 years ago(41) and
a simplified form has been adopted for mass appeal. Other
martial arts are also practised and relate to traditional concepts
in for instance their identification of danger or vital spots on
the body.

NOTES

1 The earliest extant work, the 'Huangdi Neijing', is dated
   from the second century BC and contains in the Ling Shu
   part treatises on acupuncture and moxibustion. Huangdi or
   the Yellow Emperor was supposed to have reigned between
   2696 and 2598 BC (see Ilza Veith, 'The Yellow Emperor's
   Classic of Internal Medicine', Los Angeles, University of
   California Press, 1966, p. 5).
2 Chu Lien, 'Chinese Chen Chiu Therapy', People's China,
   no. 23, 1954, p. 12. The word acupuncture is Latinised from
   acus (needle); punctura (puncture). Moxibustion is thought
   to have been derived from Kaempfer (1712) of the Dutch
   East India Company from its Japanese term for 'burning
   herb' - mokusa.
3 Academy of Traditional Chinese Medicine, 'An Outline of
   Chinese Acupuncture', Peking, Foreign Languages Press,
   1975, p. 3.
4 Needham and Lu Gwei-djen, 'Celestial Lancets, A History
   and Rationale of Acupuncture and Moxa', Cambridge
   University Press, 1980, p. 3.
5 Ibid., p. 1.
6 Needham uses the analogy of modern urban underground
   railway systems.
7 'An Outline of Chinese Acupuncture', p. 55.
8 As used by Needham in 'Celestial Lancets', op cit., p. 23.
9 'An Outline of Chinese Acupuncture', pp. 127-30 and 232-3.
10 Ibid., p. 218.
11 Ibid., p. 91
12 Chimin Wong and Wu Lien-teh, 'History of Chinese Medicine',
   Tientsin Press, 1932, p. 29.
13 Academy of Traditional Chinese Medicine, 'Essentials of
   Chinese Acupuncture', Beijing, Foreign Languages Press,
   1980, p. 307.
14 Suggestion by Needham in 'Celestial Lancets', p. 192 -
   'acutracts' derived from sensation secondary to acupuncture.
   A great deal of research on the 'propagating sensation of

channels' is being undertaken in China.

15 1934 is the date given in 'An Outline of Chinese Acupuncture',
   but Needham notes that the Frenchman Chevalier Sarlandière
   used an electrical stimulation in 1825 ('Celestial Lancets',
   p. 188).
16 Advances in acupuncture and acupuncture anaesthesia,
   'Abstracts of papers presented at the National Symposium of
   acupuncture, moxibustion and acupuncture anaesthesia',
   Beijing, 1-5 June, 1979, Beijing, People's Medical Publishing
   House, 1980.
17 Felix Mann, 'Acupuncture, Cure of Many Diseases', London,
   Heinemann Medical, 1971, p. 87.
18 Ibid., pp. 100-4.
19 Needham and Lu Gwei-djen, op. cit., p. 181.
20 Ibid.
21 'An Outline of Chinese Acupuncture', p. 13.
22 Quoted from Neijing (Ling Shu) in 'An Outline of Chinese
   Acupuncture', p. 14.
23 Nogier in France (1956) introduced some 48 ear points and
   described the relationship between the ear and the body.
   This influenced the Chinese who introduced it by 1958 and
   developed its use.
24 'An Outline of Chinese Acupuncture', p. 269, from Ling Shu.
25 'Essentials of Chinese acupuncture', p. 400, and 'Textbook
   of Human Anatomy', Hamilton (ed.) London, Macmillan, 1966,
   p. 853.
26 'Acupuncture Anaesthesia', Peking Foreign Languages Press,
   1972, p. 4. H. Agren notes reports of this in 1957 in
   Patterns of Tradition and Modernisation in Contemporary
   Chinese Medicine, in Kleinman (ed.) 'Medicine in Chinese
   Cultures', Fogarty International Centre, DHEW PHS, ed.
   Kleinman 1975, p. 43.
27 Work of Tobimatsu et al. quoted in 'Celestial Lancets', p. 221
28 Needham and Lu Gwei Djen, op. cit., p. 221.
29 Acupuncture anaesthesia in open heart surgery with heart
   lung machine on the home front, 'Peking Review', no. 20,
   1973. Also see series reported in 'Advances in acupuncture',
   op. cit., pp. 17-20.
30 Needham and Lu Gwei-djen, op. cit., p. 225.
31 'Advances in acupuncture', p. 10.
32 Needham and Lu Gwei-djen note in 'Celestial Lancets', p. 6,
   that veterinary medicine has used acupuncture since the
   Yuan Dynasty (AD 1260-1368).
33 Ibid., p. 226.
34 'Advances in acupuncture', pp. 479-86.
35 See 'Celestial Lancets' pp. 184-262, for a very comprehensive
   review of the physiological mechanisms involved.
36 'An Outline of Chinese Acupuncture', p. 28.
37 'Essentials of Chinese Acupuncture', pp. 314-17.
38 Ibid., p. 317.
39 Pierre Huard and Ming Wong, 'Chinese Medicine', World

University Library, London, Weidenfeld & Nicolson, 1968, p. 223.

40 Personal communication, Dr Ma Kan Wen, Academy of Traditional Chinese Medicine. Other details of the tomb from 'Out of China's Earth – Archaeological discoveries in the People's Republic of China', London, Frederick Muller, 1981.

41 'Simplified Taijiquan', Beijing, China Sports Editorial Board, 1980, p. 1.

# 9 TRADITIONAL THERAPIES II: CHINESE MATERIA MEDICA

J.A. Jewell

The Chinese Materia Medica is a vast subject with a long and complicated history. I will attempt to highlight some important historical details, describe the elementary principles of treatment and give some examples of remedies and their modern application.

Tortoiseshell inscriptions some 3,000 years old suggest that the ancients used to brew medicinal liquor with tulips and other herbs to cure disease.(1) The Herbal (Ben Cao Jing) attributed to the legendary Shen Nong symbolically lists 365 drugs, divided into superior, common and inferior. The superior or high-grade drugs are meant to be non-toxic and have rejuvenating properties; the medium or common drugs are said to be tonics and used for deficiency states while the inferior or low-grade ones are used for curing disease, being toxic, and are not to be given for a prolonged period of time.(2) Shen Nong's Herbal is dated to the -1 century.(3) He was traditionally worshipped by the drug guilds as their patron god and each month offerings and incense were laid by his shrine.(4)

In AD659 the Tang dynasty court promulgated the First Pharmacopoeia called the 'Revised Compendium of Materia Medica'. This listed 844 medicinal substances and is probably the earliest State Pharmacopoeia in the world.(5) Later during the Song dynasty (+10-13th century) there are records of some fifty-eight kinds of traditional herbs being exported abroad,(6) an indication of China's medical ascendancy.

In the early period the use of drugs was pragmatic, based on empirical experience, with an important 'magico-religious' input. It was not until the Jin-Yuan period (+1175-1368) that the classic 'system of correspondences' was incorporated. This means that the medicines were differentiated into their qualities, i.e. taste and energy, and applied rationally to diseases analysed in the traditional syndromes, e.g. hot or cold, excess or deficiency, Yin or Yang. It was during the Ming dynasty (+1368-1644) that the pharmacopoeia developed in this way. Li Shi-Zhen's 'The Compendium of Materia Medica' (Ben Kao Gang Mu) was the most outstanding and comprehensive work. It was published in AD1590 in fifty-two volumes and listed 1,892 medicinal substances.(7) There were more than one thousand illustrations and over ten thousand prescriptions with detailed descriptions of the appearance, properties, method of collection, preparation and use of each substance. It is arranged into sixteen classes; water, fire, earth, metals, minerals, herbs,

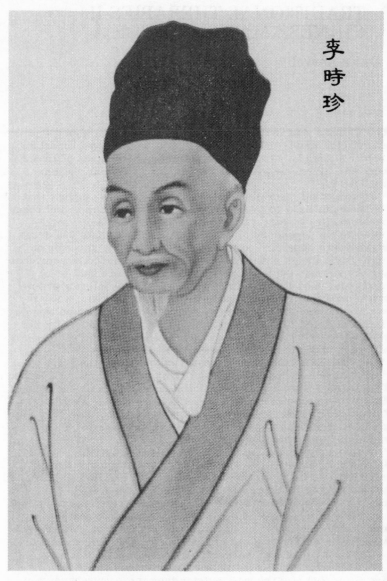

李時珍

Figure 19  Li Shi-zhen (+1518-93)

grains, vegetables, fruits, trees, garments and utensils, insects, fishes, molluscs, birds, beasts and man. His work is a classic and is still studied today by traditional practitioners:

Li Shi Zhen (+1518-93) was the son of an accomplished physician who failed three times to gain the higher civil service exam. He then decided to concentrate on medical studies and in addition to the 'Compendium' wrote the 'Pulse studies of Bin-hu' and 'A study on the eight extra channels'.(8)

It is interesting to note that although a Chinese Pharmacopoeia was issued in 1930 which included some traditional drugs, it was not until the late 1970s that a new Pharmacopoeia of traditional Chinese medicine was produced. This book lists 5,767 traditional medicinal drugs.(9)


DRUG PROPERTIES

Broadly speaking traditional drugs are categorised into four 'energies' and five tastes. The four energies are: cold (Han); hot (Jeh), warm (Wen); cool (Liang).

There are also a group of balanced or neutral drugs (B'ing). The energies are judged by the body's reaction to and the therapeutic effect of the drug. In general terms drugs used to treat fevers fall into the 'cold' or 'coolness' category, e.g. the cooling nature of dandelion tea for inflammed throats associated with thirst and fever. Conversely if the patient is suffering from a cold, chills and headache the warming quality of fresh ginger brew is used symptomatically.

The five tastes can be summarised as follows:

| Taste | Correspond-ance | | Action | | e.g. |
|-------|-----|--------|--------|------|------|
| Sour | Yin | Liver | Astringent | e.g. | Magnoliavine (Schizandra Chinensis Baill) |
| Bitter | Yin | Heart | Antipyretic and moisture drying | e.g. | Rhubarb (Radix Rhei) |
| Sweet | Yang | Spleen | Soothing and tonic | e.g. | Licorice (Glycyrrhiza uralensis) |
| Pungent | Yang | Lung | Dispersing and stimulating (carminative) | e.g. | Perilla leaf (Perilla Frutescens) |
| Salty | Yin | Kidney | Purgative | e.g. | Sodium sulphate (Sodii sulfas) |

There is also a group of bland and tasteless drugs which include talcum and pearl barley. These are supposed to have diuretic effects which in traditional terms means 'cleaning internal damp' and they have Yang qualities.

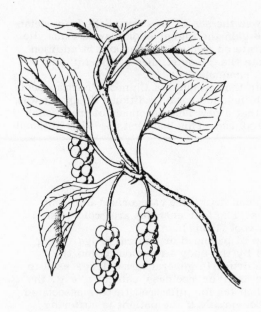

Schizandra
Chinensis. Baill.
(Magnoliaceae)
Chinese magnolia vi
an aromatic woody
vine. The dried
berries are used.

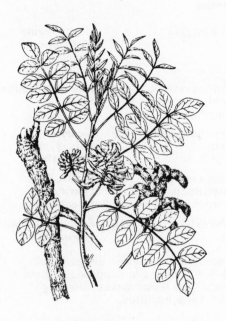

Glycyrrhiza
Uralensis. Fisch.
(Leguminosae)
Chinese licorice.
The root is used.

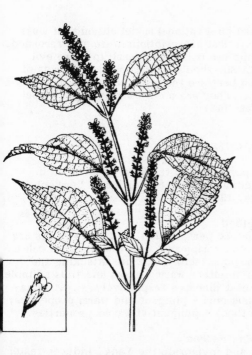

Perilla Frutescens.
Britt. (Labiatae)
An annual herb. The
leaves and seeds are
used.

Energy and taste are interrelated. Different drugs may fall
into the same energy category but taste differently or vice
versa. Guidelines for their use warn that excessive use of
bitter and cooling drugs are harmful to the stomach and spleen;
pungent and hot drugs should be given with care to patients
with deficient and heat-dominating constitutions; purgatives
that disrupt energy and blood should be avoided by pregant
women and used with care.(10)

Drugs can also be classified according to the channel on which
their therapeutic action is manifest, e.g. Balloon-flower root
(Radix Platycodi) under the lung channel because of its
antitussive effect.(11) There is also a notion of direction of
action. The so-called 'ascending and floating' drugs have an
upward and outward effect and are used for activating vitality,
inducing sweat and dispelling cold. Descending and sinking
drugs have a downward and inward effect and are used for
tranquillising, causing contraction, relieving cough and vomiting while promoting diuresis and purgation.(12) In addition to
this there is of course the basic principle of circulation of blood
and qi and the need to overcome stasis or obstruction if this
exists.

It is by this method of describing the different qualities of
drugs, i.e. taste, energy, related organ, direction of action
and therapeutic effect that the Materia Medica could be systematised in the terms of traditional Chinese medical theory. Thus

treatment could be based on a rational model although it must
be noted that certain mystical prescriptions were still recorded.
For instance the symbolic use of a cock's comb to scare evil
spirits is recorded in Li Shi-zhen's Materia Medica: 'Heads of
cocks kill spectres. The best are those of cocks that have stood
above doors on the east. They are a cure for sorcery, dispel
evil and overt pestilence.'(13)


## THERAPEUTIC APPROACHES

There are eight main approaches to therapy; as detailed in
'Common Terms of Traditional Chinese Medicine in English',
(Peking Medical College, 1980)

### 1 *The perspiration method*
Diaphoresis means to induce perspiration, and these drugs are
used for 'exterior-symptom complexes' with the object of releas-
ing externally the pathogenic factors that are attacking the
body. Diaphoretics can be either warm or cool and thus suitable
for wind-cold or wind-heat illnesses respectively, e.g. Cinnamon twig (Ramulus Cinnamoni) - pungent and warm properties;
Peppermint (Herba Menthae) - pungent and cold properties.

### 2 *Stimulation or warming method*
To dispel internal cold and invigorate the Yang. Induces restoration of vital function from collapse, warming the spleen and
stomach and the channels. Use warm or hot drugs e.g. Aconite
root (Radix Aconiti Praeparata). Note that the root is specially
processed as the fresh form is extremely toxic.

### 3 *Heat reduction method*
This is a febrifugal method of administering medicines of cold
property to treat acute febrile diseases and other conditions
with internal heat. There is a sub-classification:

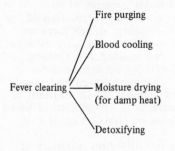

| Fever clearing | | |
|---|---|---|
| Fire purging | — | for solid heat fever with thirst, stupor, delirium, dry throat, etc. e.g. Gypsum. |
| Blood cooling | — | for febrile diseases with petechial eruptions, such as measles, e.g. Horn of Asiatic Rhino (Cornu Rhinoceri). |
| Moisture drying (for damp heat) | — | for moist fevers of internal organs, such as dysentery and jaundice, e.g. Coptis root (Rhizoma Coptidis). |
| Detoxifying | — | for febrile diseases with pyogenic inflammation such as abscesses, e.g. Weeping Forsythia (Fructus Forsythiae) and Honeysuckle flower (Flos Lonicerae). |

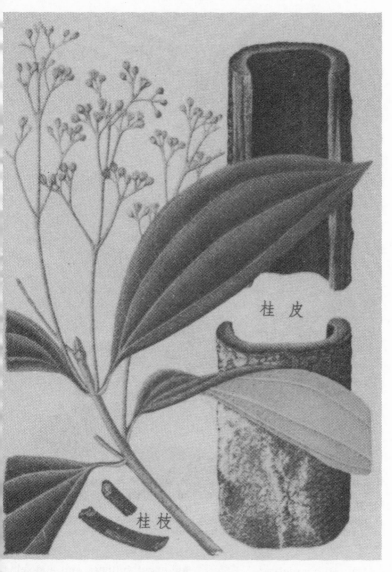

桂皮

桂枝

Cinnamomum Cassia. Blume, (Lauraceae)
Chinese cinnamon tree. The dried bark and twigs are used.

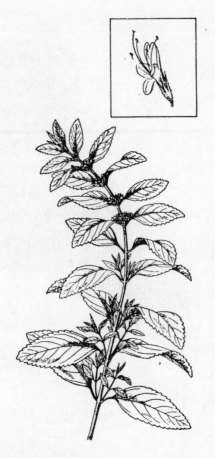

Mentha Arvensis. L. (Labiatae)
Peppermint a perennial herb. The leaves are used.

## 4  *Dispersing method*
This method is used to correct energy/blood circulation by overcoming channel stagnation and loosening sputum. There is a sub-classification:

(i)   Qi correcting
- for chest fullness and abdominal distension, hiccoughs, nausea, regurgitation, irregular menstruation.
- aim to get a smooth normal circulation of qi, e.g. liver qi stagnation, Thorowax root (Radix Bupleuri).

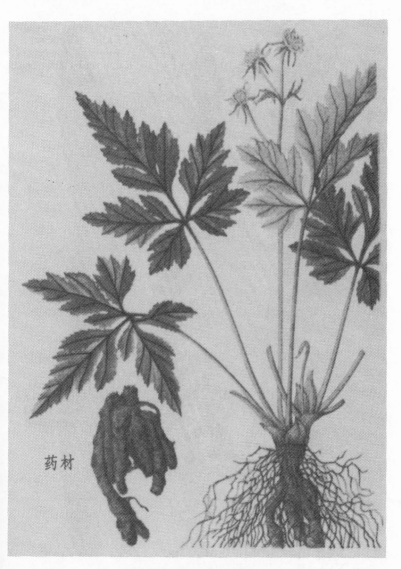

药材

Coptis Chinensis. Franch. (Ranunculaceae)
Chinese goldthread, a perennial herb. The root is used.

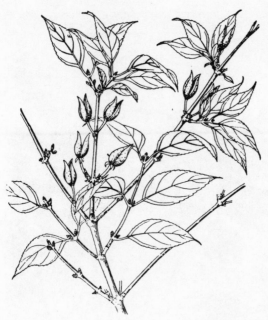

Forsythia Suspensa,
Vahl. (Oleaceae)
Weeping forsythia,
a shrub. The fruit
is used

Lonicera Japonica.
Thunb.
(Caprifoliaceae)
Honeysuckle. The
stem, leaves and
flowers are used.

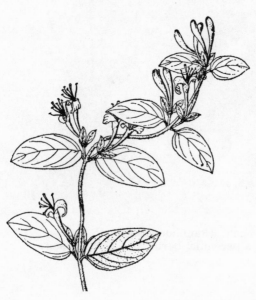

(ii)  Blood correcting        –   for irregular menstruation, tumours, bruises, abscesses and rheumatoid arthritis.
                              –   aim to eliminate blood stasis, e.g. Safflower (Flos Carthami).

(iii) Digestion promoting     –   for abdominal pain, acid regurgitation, indigestion, nausea and vomiting, diarrhoea.
                              –   aim to restore proper functioning of liver and spleen/stomach with stomachics, e.g. Tangerine peel (Pericarpium Citri Reticulatae).

(iv)  Sputum liquifying       –   for productive coughs, asthma, epilepsy, convulsions, scrofula, e.g. Jack-in-the-Pulpit Tuber (Arisaema Tuber).

(v)   Moisture converting     –   for oedema, urinary problems such as polyuria, e.g. Water Plantain (Rhizoma Alismatis).
                              –   aim to dispel dampness, e.g. Eupatorium (Herba Eupatorii)

## 5 *Tonic method*
Drugs that can supplement the Yin/Yang, imbalance of qi and blood and treat deficiency diseases. There are four main types of tonic:

(i)   Yang supplementing      –   especially in cold deficient illness, e.g. Radix Ginseng.

(ii)  Yin supplementing       –   in fever caused by Yin deficiency, e.g. White Peony root (Radix Paeoniae Alba).

(iii) Qi supplementing        –   used for convalescent weakness and fatigue exhausting the spleen, e.g. Astragalus root (Radix Astragali) or Ginseng.

(iv)  Blood supplementing     –   used for blood deficiency, e.g. human placenta (dried).

## 6 *Emetic method*
To expel noxious substances with emetics or mechanical stimulation to induce vomiting.

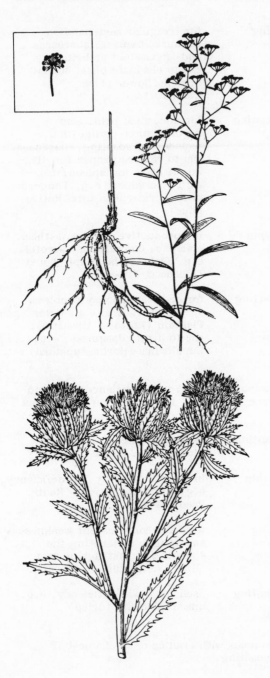

Bupleurum Falcatum
L. (Umbelliferae)
Thorowax root,
a perennial herb.
The root is used.

Carthamus
Tinctorius. L.
(Compositae)
Safflower, an annual
herb. The flowers
are used.

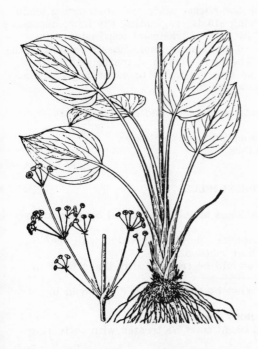

Alisma Plantago-
aquatica. L.
(Alismaceae) Water
plantain, a perennial
herb. The tuber
is used.

## 7 *Purgative method*

To relieve constipation, clear stagnation of food or blood and expel internal heat and excessive fluid. Mild laxatives are used for the older, weaker and chronically ill, e.g. Hemp seeds (Fructus Cannabis), Bush cherry seed (Semen Pruni). Stronger purgatives include Rhubarb (Radix et Rhizoma Rhei), Croton bean (Fructus Crotonis) or Senna (Folium sennae).

## 8 *Mediation method*

To use drugs of regulating or intermediate action to restore normal balance between the internal organs or to eliminate pathogenic factors from the part exterior/interior of the body. For example, co-ordinating the liver/spleen when the stomach/ spleen are being affected by the disordered liver energies. Also the example of febrile illnesses when the pathogenic threaten to invade the interior of the body.

These therapeutic approaches reflect the basic orientation of traditional Chinese medicine. One cause of disease are the pathogenic factors such as 'wind-cold' and words such as expel and eliminate refer to dealing with these. The other main factor is the body's resistance to disease and an important aspect is concerned with nourishing, tonifying, warming-up, invigorating the organ system and the qi (vital energy). The qi and blood are circulating freely in the normal state and obstruction leads to disease and so removing stasis, regulating the flow, become important objectives. The plan of treatment emphasises the conception of the body as an organic whole closely related to the external environment. Therapy is aimed at treating the root cause, which could be an internal factor or external pathogen. Thus the therapeutic aims are to:

strengthen the patient's resistance and consolidate his constitution;
restore the normal functioning of the body;
dispel pathogenic factors.

## TWELVE TREATMENT PRINCIPLES

Excessive symptom-complexes should be treated by purgation and reduction.
Deficiency symptom-complexes should be treated with re-inforcing or replenishing methods.
Cold symptom-complex should be treated with drugs warm or hot in property.
Heat symptom-complex must be treated with drugs cold in property.
External pathogenic factors must be removed.
Sluggish flow of qi and blood must be treated with activating method.
Dryness must be cured by moistening method.
Dampness must be removed.
Prolapse and ptosis must be treated with the lifting method.
Upward reversed action, e.g. cough, hiccough, must be suppressed.
What has become loose must be consolidated (e.g. nocturnal emission).
Debilitated and exhausted must be nourished (e.g. with warm-natured tonics).

Using these criteria traditional prescriptions can become extremely complicated especially as they take into consideration the state of the patient, the drug interactions and subsequently the observed response. Zhang Zhong Jing (+150-219), the author of 'Treatise on Febrile and Miscellanous Diseases' and 'Synopsis of Prescriptions of the Golden Chamber', stated:

Individual therapeutics imply not only a special consultation for each patient carried out according to one's own opinion; the treatment and prescriptions will be constantly modified in accordance with the pathological change if necessary several times in the course of a day. (14)

Such prescriptions are still commonly used today in a decoction.

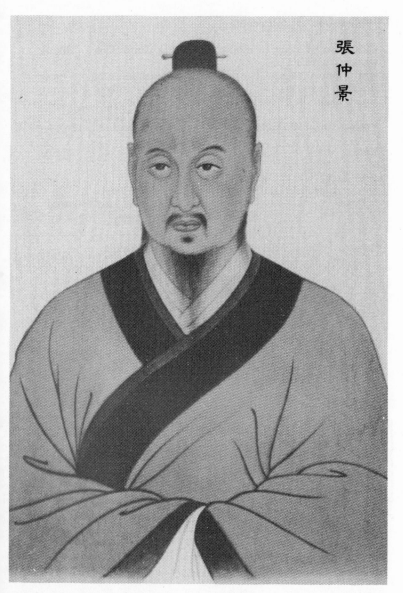

張
仲
景

Figure 20  Zhang Zhong Jing (+150-219)

The ingredients are weighed as per prescription, boiled together and the residue discarded. An example of a classic Zhang Zhong Jing prescription is:

'Cinnamon Cassia decoction'

| Cinnamon (Cassia branch without bark) | Ramulus Cinnamoni | 3 liang |
| White peony (wash in wine) | Radix paeoniae alba | 3 liang |
| Roasted licorice | Radix Glycyrrhizae | 2 liang |
| Raw ginger in slices | Rhizoma Zingiberis recens | 3 liang |
| Peeled Chinese dates | Fructus Ziziphi jujubae | 12 pieces |
| Water | | 7 pints |

(1 liang = 31.25 grams)

Instructions:  Boil mixture over a slow fire.

Dose        :  One pint to be taken warm and followed by a pint of hot thin congee (rice soup). If necessary repeat.

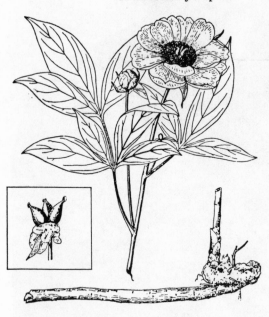

Paeonia Albiflora. Pall. (Ranunculaceae). Chinese peony, a perennial herb. The root is used.

This prescription is used as a 'diaphoretic' for dispelling external pathogenic factors such as feverish illness caused by the invasion of wind-cold. It also helps to restore the body's defences and is typically used for 'exterior-symptom complexes' including headache, fever, sweating and 'intolerance of wind'. It is well balanced and tasty, utilising the warming and pungent properties of the cinnamon and ginger which stimulate and cause perspiration. The white peony is both an analgesic and a 'heat clearing', cool drug. Licorice is a neutral drug which is pleasant to taste and has some supplementary properties such as invigorating the heart and spleen; spasmolytic and antitussive; anti-inflammatory and antitoxicant. The Chinese dates are also neutral and pleasant to taste. They help to strengthen the spleen-stomach and low-energy states. Some of these descriptions of the drug actions such as 'anti-inflammatory' reflect the 'integration' of concepts of Western and traditional medicine. 'Inflammation' in modern scientific medicine has a specific meaning but its origin in traditional European medicine refers to the red heat of the flames of fire.

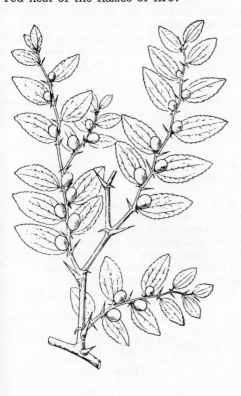

Zizyphus Jujuba. Mill. (Rhamnaceae) Chinese dates, a deciduous shrub. The date fruit is used.

Probably decocting, which is still widely used, is not a very efficient way to extract the active principles and it necessitates the consumption of very large volumes of fluid. Infusing or decocting have the disadvantage of losing volatile oils that will tend to evaporate. Methods such as macerating or making tinctures using alcohol overcome this problem and also prevent ingredients being damaged by heat. Both methods are known to traditional practitioners.

The decoction method is laborious and a recent report describes the benefits of the more modern drug formulations:

> To deal with my chronic diarrhoea and neurasthenia I used to go to the medicine shop once a week and bring home several packets of dry herbs, each packet was as big as a medium sized loaf of bread, having several or over a dozen ingredients I boiled a whole package of them in the evening, first over a high fire, then a low fire, for about an hour. Then I gulped down a bowl of this bitter decoction while it was still warm. The whole lot had to be boiled again and strained through a cheese-cloth sieve. The liquor was left for the next morning, when it had to be warmed again before I took it. I was quite fed up with the whole business. Now I am gratified to see on the market many herbal medicines in pill form which can be taken right away after mixing with some wine or boiled water.(15)

There have been traditionally many forms of drug prescriptions - as pills pasted with water, honey and flour, coated sometimes with wax, powder, plaster, ointments, medicinal wines, teas, eyedrops, enemas as well as the more usual decoctions.

## TREATMENT OF DISEASE: THE EXAMPLE OF ASTHMA

'Asthma' is not a term used in traditional Chinese medicine but a clinical state of difficulty in breathing with cough sputum and noisy breath sounds would be recognised. In Western medicine different causes of asthma are accepted such as emotion, exertion, cold air, allergies, infection and genetic predisposition. There is also the notion that asthma is a syndrome and not a specific disease and that there are extrinsic and intrinsic factors. Similarly in TCM it is differentiated into external and internal causes:

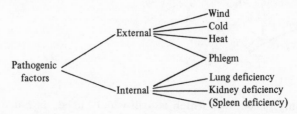

The pathogenesis in TCM is commonly the invasion of the lungs by wind-cold which leads to the lungs becoming obstructed by phlegm. This prevents the lungs from taking in the 'air qi' and passing it downwards for the kidneys to receive. Phlegm is a sign of dysfunction of water metabolism which is controlled by the lungs, kidneys and spleen. Phlegm-damp causes excessive sputum which in combination with pathogenic heat is characteristically thick and yellow. Both wind-cold and phlegm-heat cause excess (Shi) syndromes. Deficient (Xu) syndromes develop when the problem becomes chronic and organs dysfunctional.

The symptoms will vary for each category and can be summarised:

| | | |
|---|---|---|
| 1 | Wind-cold | Cough with thin sputum, shortness of breath. Fever and chills, white coating on tongue, superficial pulse with no sweating. Fear of cold, headache and pain in body. |
| 2 | Phlegm-heat | Rapid and coarse breathing, stifling sensation in chest, thick purulent and sticky sputum, thick yellowish coating on red tongue, rapid rolling and forceful pulse. Fever, fear of wind, sore throat, headache and thirst. |
| 3 | Xu lung | Short and rapid breathing. Weak and low voice, sweating with weak pulse. Prolonged cough with feeble sound. Tongue pink and not coated. |
| 4 | Xu kidney | Shortness of breath worse on moving, chilliness with cold extremities, deep, thready and feeble pulse. Pain in loins and prolonged expiration. No coating on tongue. |

There can be combinations of the above, e.g. lung and kidney deficiency or the addition of spleen deficiency which is associated with the control of phlegm. Phlegm refers to body fluid formed when normal water metabolism is disrupted. The spleen is the source of phlegm which in the lung presents as sputum. Western medicine used to refer to cardiac and renal asthma when difficulty in breathing was related to dysfunction of these organs. Even now the shortness of breath of heart failure is treated with diuretics acting on the kidney to increase the output of the body fluid. The treatment principles adopted can be broadly summarised:

Wind-cold ⟨ — Eliminate wind and cold
⟨ — Promote function of lung

Phlegm-heat ⟨ — Eliminate heat
⟨ — Reduce phlegm
⟨ — Make lung qi go downwards

Deficiencies ⟨ — Nourish organs and reduce shortness of breath
⟨ — Nourish spleen and reduce phlegm
⟨ — Nourish kidney and help it receive the qi

Examples of herbal medicines given for the four major categories are as follows:(16)

1   Wind-cold

| | |
|---|---|
| Eliminate external cold wind and disperse qi of lung | – Ephedra (Herba Ephedrae) (warm-pungent) |
| | Perilla seed (Fructus Perillae) (warm-pungent) |
| Eliminate phlegm stop shortness of breath and assist the downward direction of qi | – Platycodon root (Radix Platycodi) |
| | – (Neutral-sweet) |
| | – Licorice root (Radix Glycyrrhiza) (Neutral-sweet) |
| | – Bitter apricot kernel or seed (Semen Armeniacae amarum) (Neutral-sour) |

2   Phlegm-heat

| | |
|---|---|
| Eliminate heat of lung | – Mulberry bark (Cortex Mori Radicis) (cold-pungent) |
| | Wolfberry bark (Cortex Lycii Radicis) (cold-bitter) |
| | Stemona root (Radix stemonae) (slightly warm-bitter) |
| | Scutellaria root (Radix Scutellariae) (cold-bitter) |
| Reduces phlegm and assists qi to go down | – Loquat leaf (Folium Eriobotryae) |
| | – (neutral-bitter) |
| | Hogfennel root (Radix Peucedari) (cold-bitter) |
| | Platycodon root (Radix Platycodi) (warm-pungent) |

3   Xu lung

| | |
|---|---|
| Reinforce qi of lung | – Ginseng (Radix Ginseng) (neutral-sweet) |
| | Gecko (dried lizard) |
| Nourish spleen and lung | – White Atractylodes (Rhizoma Atractylodes macrocephalae) |

(warm-bitter sweet)
Poria (Poria cocos) (neutral-
    sweet)
Licorice root (Radix Glycyrrhiza)
    (neutral-sweet)

4  Xu kidney
   Reinforce qi         -  Ginseng (Radix ginseng) (neutral-
   of lung                 sweet)
                       -  Gecko (dried lizard)
   Nourish kidney      -  Human placenta (Placenta hominis)
                         Psoralea fruit (Fructus Psoraleae)
                             (warm-pungent)
                         Rehmannia root (Radix Rehmanniae
                             praeparata) (cool-sweet)
   Help kidney to      -  Magnoliavine fruit (Fructus
   receive qi             Schizandrae) (warming-sour)

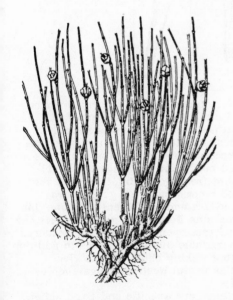

Ephedra Sinica,
Stapf. (Gnetaceae)
An undershrub. The
roots and stem are
used.

The traditional physician would diagnose the principal condition causing the asthma and prescribe the drug with the
appropriate action as the 'master' drug. Depending both on the
other clinical aspects of the case and the anticipated side effects
of the main drug other 'adjuvants' would be added. The Shen
Nong Herbal actually arranged the drugs in a hierarchy of Ruler,
Minister, Assistant and servant.
Although this may seem extremely complicated there is a basic
pattern. The principles of treatment are the elimination of

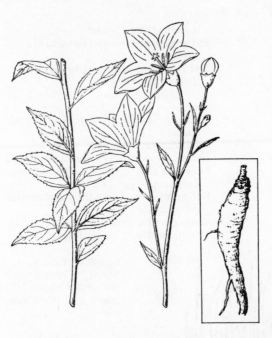

Platycodon Grandi-
florum, D.C.
(Campanulaceae)
Balloonflower,
a perennial herb.
The root is used.

external pathogens and the reinforcement of internal organs
related to the respiratory function. The Hunan 'Barefoot
Doctors' Manual' divides asthma into broadly similar cold,
feverish, mucus and deficiency states. Some of the more fascinating ingredients they recommend include; toasted grass-
hoppers (those with pointed heads and long legs the best),
white-necked earthworms and fresh goat's bile! Many of the
above prescriptions are also recommended, e.g. Ephedra,
powdered placenta, loquat leaves and the patent medicine 'Liu
wei ti huang tang' which contains Rehmannia glutinosa. Rather
characteristically the manual recommends preventive measures
such as avoiding smoking, irritable dusts and gases in addition
to keeping warm and avoiding 'taking chill'. It also gives
acupuncture points as well as useful Western drugs such as
ephedrine and caffeine.(17)
   Traditional herbs do not have one specific and fixed action.
For instance one report notes that rhubarb if steamed with wine
can alleviate its purgative function, easing fever and inflammation, promoting blood circulation and 'relieving stasis'. Char-
coalised rhubarb can be used in cases of internal bleeding.
Lime-soaked rhubarb helps to stop external traumatic bleeding.
Prepared with vinegar it is more efficient at promoting blood
circulation and relieving stasis. It should be noted that rhubarb
in this context is not the common garden rhubarb but the root
of the Chinese and Tibetan plant. Also Ephedra can be used
in treating common colds but if mixed with cinnamon stem acts as

a diaphoretic. It can be used in asthma if prepared with bitter almond and gypsum. With ginger and atractylodes root it makes a prescription for detumescence.(18)

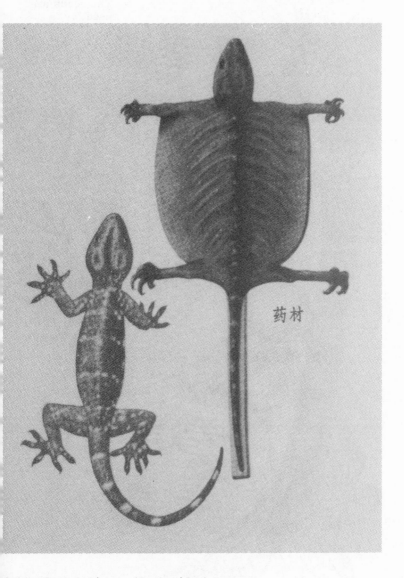

药材

Gekko Gecko. Linne. (Geckonidae)
The dried lizard is used.

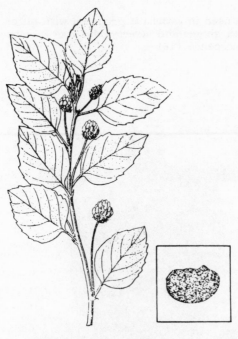

Psoralea Coryli-
folia. L.
(Leguminosae)
An annual plant.
The seeds are
used.

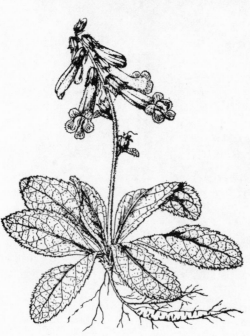

Rehmannia
Glutinosa. Libosch
(Scrophulariaceae)
A perennial herb.
The root is used.

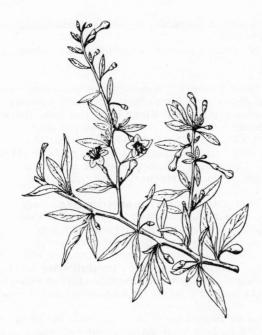

Lycium Chinese.
Mill. (Solanaceae)
Chinese Wolfberry,
a shrub. The fruit
and root are used.

## PATENT MEDICINES

It has been reported that the varieties of traditional medicines
in clinical practice has reached over 5,000, of which more than 90
per cent are plant drugs. The use of pharmacies as a source of
primary medical care is widespread in China and their contribution should not be underestimated. Many of the drugs bought
in these shops will be patent medicines – for colds, constipation,
diarrhoea, headache, and fever. In China, unlike in the West
today, the majority of the medicines purchased will be herbal
although both have in common their wide application and
promised efficacy.

However, there is something special about the Chinese
patents. For instance, the advertisement for Royal Jelly reads:

> Royal Jelly is a precious substance produced by the worker
> bees from their salivary glands exclusively for the nutrition
> of the Queen Bee. This nutritious food enables the Queen Bee
> to lay at the height of the laying season 2,000 to 3,000 eggs
> in twenty-four hours. It also gives her the vitality to live for
> more than five years while the worker bees could only live for
> two to four months.(19)

Royal Jelly is recommended for a wide range of conditions
including: conditions of underdevelopment, senility, general

weakness, convalescence, depression, hepatitis, rheumatoid
arthritis, and gastric ulcer.

In the promotion of another famous compound, Tiger Bone
pills, we are told:

> The use of Tiger bone for curing diseases has been recorded
> in Chinese medical classics as far back as the Tang dynasty
> (+618-907) which also certify that Tiger bone has good thera-
> peutic effect in treating muscular, osseous and flatulent
> pains and relevant ailments. The Pen Tsao Kang Mu, the
> master work of Li Shih Chen of the Ming dynasty (1368-1644)
> again asserts that Tiger bone is efficaceous for expelling
> flatulence, relieving pains and strengthening bones.(20)

Anxieties over sexual potency provide another large market
for patent medicine. Ginseng is marketed for 'lack of sexual
power and weakness' while Red Antler Horn capsules are
'widely acknowledged as a very good drug for increasing
vitality and virility'. It is recommended for: 'impotence and
premature ejaculation, nocturnal pollution, involutionary issue,
as well as loss of memory'. Other tonics include chicken essence,
'sugar coated placenta tablets', 'cerebral tonic pills' and 'birds'
nest pear syrup'.

In addition to these medicines there is also a wide range of
medicinal plasters such as Dog Skin plaster, many of which are
counter-irritants much as the Western embrocations. You can
of course also buy 'stomachache pills' and 'toothache lotion'.
The bewildering number of natural products that are used in
traditional Chinese medicine is demonstrated by the following
list of some 'exotic' substances in use:

| | | |
|---|---|---|
| Cockroach | Donkey-hide gelatin | Black nightshade |
| Scorpion | Mother of pearl | Haematite |
| Centipede | Oyster shell | Musk |
| Gadfly | Dragon bones | Cinnabar |
| Silkworm excreta | Anteater scales | Amber |
| Egg case of pray-<br>ing mantis | Aloes | Frankincense |
| Wasps' nest | Betel nut | Myrrh |
| Bears' gall-bladder | Pumpkin seed | Calomel |

This selection confirms that the traditional Materia Medica makes
use of minerals and animals in addition to the more commonly
referred to herbs or plant drugs.

*Scientific evaluation*
One popular patent medicine and regularly prescribed treatment
is 'Liu wei ti huang tang' (Pills of Six Drugs with Rehmannia)
whose formula is:

| | |
|---|---|
| Radix Rehmannia praeparata | 25.0g |
| (Rehmannia glutinosa root) | |
| Dogwood fruit - Fructus Corni | 12.5g |
| (Cornus officinalis fruit) | |
| Chinese yam - (Rhizoma Dioscoreae) | 12.5g |
| (Dioscorea batatas root) | |
| Water plantain - (Rhizoma Alismatis) | 9.4g |
| (Alisma plantago aquatica var. orientale tuber) | |
| Tuckahoe - (Poria) | 9.4g |
| (Pachyma cocos tuber) | |
| Tree peony bark - (Cortex Moutan Radicis) | 9.4g |
| (Paeonia suffructicosa root) | |

These tablets are supposed to 'replenish vital essence of both
the liver and kidney for the treatment of its deficiency in
chronic diseases with symptoms of asthenic fire such as dizziness, tinnitus, sore throat, tidal fever, nocturnal emission'.(21)
The principal ingredient is Rehmannia glutinosa and a generalisation of the principal actions of the six drugs is:

| | |
|---|---|
| Rehmannia glutinosa - kidneys | Alisma pl. - disperse fire on kidney |
| Cornus officinalis - liver | Paeonia suff. - disperse fire on liver |
| Dioscorea batatas - spleen | Pachyma coc. - absorbs spleen humidity |

Theoretically by dispersing the fire from the kidneys the plantain gives the kidneys the full advantage of the Rehmannia's
action. The cornel has a tonic effect on the liver while the peony
disperses the liver fire and the same complementation applies
for the spleen. The prescription then is balanced in such a way
as to maximise the therapeutic properties of the drugs used by
combining a tonic with a dispersive. This prescription has
traditionally been used for treating kidney problems and
recently was subjected to a controlled experiment.(22) Renal
hypertension was induced in rats and a control group was
untreated while the experimental group was given the decoction.
This was shown to improve the renal function, lower the elevated
blood pressure and decrease the mortality rate. These effects
were probably related to improvement of the renal blood circulation. This is one of many examples of traditional prescriptions
'proving' their efficacy on the basis of modern scientific methods.
It is interesting to note that the *Rehmannia glutinosa* tuber root
contains mannitol, glucose and cardiac active glycosides.(23)
Mannitol is a recognised Western medicine treatment for acute
renal failure, helping renal circulation.

Traditionalists, however, feel that the search for the 'active
agent' reflects the causal and analytical methodology of modern
science and that Chinese medicine needs to be evaluated 'on its

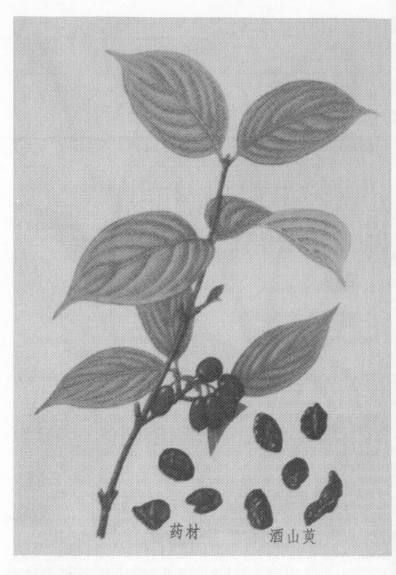

药材            酒山萸

Cornus Officinalis. Sieb et Zucc. (Cornaceae) Dogwood fruit,
a deciduous shrub. The fruit is used.

own terms'.(24) In analysing traditional remedies it is necessary
to test their biological activity, prepare them as prescribed and
recognise that they may only be effective in combination. Despite these strictures most research in China is aimed at evaluating

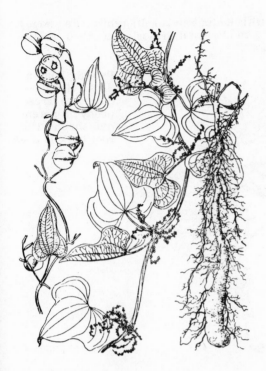

Dioscorea Batatas.
Decne. (Dio-
scoreaceae) Chinese
yam. The tubers
are used.

in a modern scientific way traditional prescriptions that appear
to be effective. A recent example is the isolation of an effective
antimalarial 'Qinghao'. A report in the 'Chinese Medical Journal'
noted that chloroquinine-resistant parasites made the discovery
of a new antimalarial drug important. Research work started in
1967 and investigated Quinghao (Sweet wormwood, Artemisia
annua) which had been used in China for some two thousand
years. Records of its use have been found in the 'Fifty-two
prescriptions' unearthed at the Han tomb at Mawangdui (c. -
168). It was also noted in the Shen Nong Herbal (-1 to -2
century) as well as the 'Handbook of Prescription for Emergencies' written in +341. Li Shi-Zhen also said that chills and fever
could be treated with it in his 'Compendium of Materia Medica'
of 1596. Its antimalarial activity was rediscovered in 1971 and
the crystal was isolated in 1972 and named Qinghaosu. It has a
direct parasiticidal action on plasmodium in the erythrocyte
stage and promises to be a useful addition to antimalarial
work.(25)

Another example of traditional therapies that have been shown
to be clinically effective and have been studied both in traditional categories and by modern scientific techniques is in the

treatment of angina with Radix Salvia miltiorrhiza (Red Sage).
Earlier studies used a fundamental prescription called 'Ershen
tungmai tang decoction'.

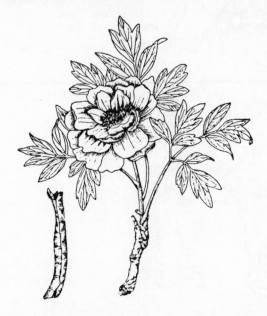

Paeonia Moutan.
Sims. (Ranun-
culaceae) Tree
peony, a peren-
nial shrub. The
root bark is used.

The prescription is decocted and administered orally once
a day. The syndrome of 'angina pectoris' was differentiated by
this group into the following main categories:

1  Lowered chest function;
2  Stagnation of vital function and blood;
3  Sputum obstruction;
4  Debility of Yin 'body fluids and blood' and liver hyperactivity;
5  Insufficiency of cardiac vital function.

The fundamental prescription was modified in each case. For
instance in the case of 'stagnation of vital function and blood'
which is recognised by symptoms such as: chest pain, pale and
dark lips and tongue, petechiae on both sides of the tongue and
a sluggish or taut pulse, other herbs, e.g. Rhizoma ligustici
wallichii (ligusticum) were added:
The initial experience with 112 cases showed that 34.8 per
cent markedly improved, 56.2 per cent improved and 9 per cent
remained unchanged. Investigation of these patients demonstrated some lowering of blood fats, improvement of micro-
circulation and improvement in their electro-cardiograms.(26)

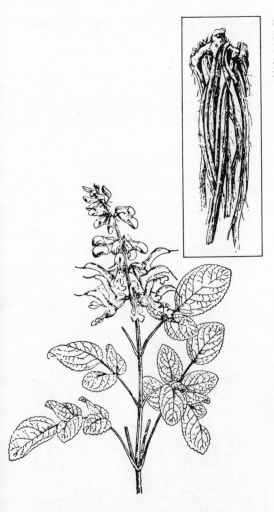

Salvia Miltiorrhiza, Bunge. (Labiatae) Red sage, an annual herb. The root is used.

Another study used only two of these drugs: Radix Salvia miltiorrhiza and Rhizoma Ligustici wallichii and administered them as an intramuscular injection of the raw extract. Animal experiments showed that the injection increased coronary blood flow and also showed 'anti-thrombotic' activity. A clinical trial on 150 cases demonstrated that 37.1 per cent of the cases had a good therapeutic response and another 58.1 per cent obtained some relief. In this experiment the blood fats remained unchanged as did the blood pressure and heart rate.(27) Further studies identified the contents of Radix Salvia miltiorrhiza (various Tanshinones ($C_{18}H_{12}O_3$)) and tested its anti-coagulant properties finding that it had a strong fibrinolytic action.(28) This would go some way to explaining its activity against the formation of 'thrombus', an important cause of angina and heart attacks because it obstructs the arteries.

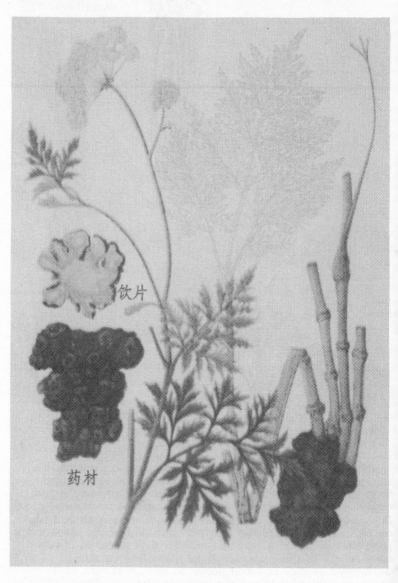

Linusticum Wallichii, Franch. (Umbelliferae)
The dried rhizome and root are used.

This example shows how investigations of traditional therapies
an be conducted. The original experiments used the formal-
raditional differentation of syndromes and the full traditional
rescription. One particular aspect was identified - the dis-
ersion of blood stasis - and two herbs in the prescription
nalysed on their own. One was finally tested as an active
rinciple and its efficacy was confirmed in a way that is com-
rehensible in modern scientific and traditional terms. This
solation of the active principle however does not explain the
hole effect of the prescription nor begin to analyse possible
esults of the combination together. The difficulties in
esearching such prescriptions should not be underestimated.

Other drugs that have been studied include the demonstration
hat Fructus Schizandrae lowers the raised liver enzyme (SGPT)
1 patients with hepatitis and in experimental animal models.(29)
ngelica sinensis has a good effect on stroke patients and has
een shown to have anti-coagulative activity particularly on
lood platelets.(30) Scopolia tangutica contains Anisodamine
hich is an atropine-like drug and Anisodine which is like
copolamine.(31) Both these can be used as intravenous
naesthetics and are similar to the legendary Hua Tuo anaesthetic
rescriptions used some one thousand years ago as Flos
aturae has been found to contain scopolamine.(32) Farrerol,
n extract from 'Rhododendron dauricum', has been shown to be
n effective expectorant(33) in animal experiments.

Other lines of research are not based on folk or traditional
rescriptions but investigate natural products for uses.
ossypol, which is still being investigated as a male contra-
eptive, was derived from cotton-seed oil.(34) The cotton-seed
il was used by peasants as cooking oil in some parts of China
nd their diet was being investigated in order to explain an
utbreak of an unrelated disease. The incidental finding of
elative infertility of the male population led to the isolation
f gossypol. Similarly screening natural products for antibiotic
nd anticancer properties continues as in the West, e.g. the
solation of the anti-cancer drugs vincristine and vinblastine
rom the Madagascan periwinkle developed by Western pharma-
eutical companies was an unexpected discovery while research-
ng its supposed anti-diabetic properties surmised from
olk-tradition. In China researches on alkaloids from a plant
pecies Cephalotaxus have identified Harringtonine as one
onstituent effective against some leukaemia and lymphoma
ells.(35)

## OMBINED TREATMENTS

n important use of traditional medicines in China is in combin-
tion with Western medical treatment. Such integration has
eveloped rapidly since 1958.(36) Attempts at combined treat-
ent have been applied in a wide variety of cases from acupunc-

ture 'analgesia' to the use of herbal decoction in acute myocardi
infarction,(37) crush syndrome,(38) and burns.(39) There has
been enormous progress in the treatment of acute abdominal
diseases by combined methods.

Conditions that have been managed in this way include acute
appendicitis, perforation of peptic ulcers, intestinal obstruction
pancreatitis, biliary tract infection, gallstones and ectopic preg
nancies. Large series of cases have shown that between 70 to 8(
per cent of cases were managed successfully without operation.(
Research is aimed at improving the diagnostic criteria that will
indicate accurately those cases that require surgery as well as
improving the treatment given. An example of integrated manag
ment is that of 'acute perforation of peptic ulcers'. There are
three stages of treatment following diagnosis:(41)

1  a.  Acupuncture - for pain relief and other therapeutic
       effects.
   b.  Gastric suction and intravenous infusion for twenty-
       four to forty-eight hours.

2  Traditional herbal medicines (e.g. tachai-hu-tang) after
   spontaneous closure of perforation. Liquid diet.

3  After peritoneal exudates were resolved, the ulcer was
   managed in out-patients' department by combined treatments (e.g. Kuiyang wan ulcer pills).

The Nan Kai Hospital in Tianjin has been a 'pace-setter'. The
abstract of one of their series published in the 'Chinese Medical
Journal' notes:

> 170 cases of acute perforation of peptic ulcer were treated
> with combined traditional Chinese and Western medicine. Of
> these, 137 (80.6 per cent) underwent non-operative treatment
> and 33 (19.4 per cent) immediate surgery. The treatment of
> patients in the non-operative group was successful, a success
> rate of 87.6 per cent. The remaining 17 cases failed to respon
> and were transferred for operation, a transfer rate of 12.4
> per cent. The overall mortality was 2.9 per cent and morbidit
> 1.8 per cent. . . . Oral administration and local application of
> traditional herbal medicine were considered essential in the
> prevention of complications.(42)

In the West, contemporary treatment consists of immediate
surgical intervention unless the patient is a poor anaesthetic
risk, when conservative management is used. In the past before
anaesthesia improved conservative treatment was recommended.

In the management of these acute abdominal conditions traditional diagnoses are also made and the 'medicinal herbs' used
are categorised into four main groups.(43) Their functions are:

1 Promotion of intestinal peristalsis and enhancement of bowel movement;
2 Activation of blood circulation to end stasis;
3 Regulation of vitality to end stagnation;
4 Detoxification and inhibition of the growth of bacteria.

Examples of drugs that increase peristalsis are Rhubarb (Rhizoma Rhei) and Kansui Root (Radix Euphorbiae kansui). They are the main ingredients of the frequently used 'ta chengchi tang' and 'kansui tung chieh tang' decoctions. They have been shown to increase intestinal peristalsis in experimental dogs.(44) Drugs that improve the circulation, reduce capillary permeability of the small intestine and mesentery and promote absorption of peritoneal exudate include peony root (Radix Paeoniae) and tree peony bark (Cortex Moutan radicis). Drugs that have a regulatory effect include white peony (Radix Paeoniae alba) which has been shown to have an antispasmodic action, and Thorowax root (Radix Bupleuri) decreases gastric acid secretion.(45) The detoxificants and bacteriostatic agents include honeysuckle (Flos Lonicerae) and weeping forsythia (Fructus Forsythiae) which have been shown to inhibit growth of intestinal bacterial flora (E. coli) and detoxify endotoxins (from B typhosus in rabbits.(46)

In another study, of 500 cases of acute appendicitis, 425 cases were managed non-operatively. Of these patients 93.4 per cent were cured with traditional medicine; 3.8 per cent with a combination of traditional drugs and antibiotics and 2.8 per cent required surgery. About thirty cases (7 per cent) had a relapse shortly after recovery. The 'anti-appendicitis' mixture contained Flos Lonicerae, Herba Taraxaci, Herba Patriniae, Fructus Forsythiae, Herba Hedyotidis diffusa, Semen Benincasae, Semen Persicae, Radix Saussureae, Fructus Meliae toosendan, Radix Paeoniae rubra and Rhizoma Rhei.(47) In another series of 1,200 patients with acute appendicitis 94.2 per cent were managed non-operatively and there were only two deaths in the series giving a mortality rate of 0.17 per cent. In 400 cases followed up after this 14.5 per cent had a recurrence which led to operation.(48)

This type of research is aimed at testing the efficacy of combined treatments - Western, traditional herbal and acupuncture. In addition some manipulative techniques are used such as the 'jolting method' which attempts at a manual non-operative reduction of volvulus (twisted intestines). This is ultimately the aim of the Chinese: to take the best from both systems and literally 'walk on two legs'. The importance of such research is the scientific evaluation of the combined therapies and it is hoped that more research will use control groups and do direct comparisons with standard Western treatments. It is quite likely that some combined treatments or predominantly traditional herbal therapy will prove more effective and for the Western doctor it is always surprising to read reports of the traditional

treatment of for instance childhood pneumonia without
antibiotics.(49)

There is a real difficulty in trying to relate the use of 'herbal
medicine' in China to the situation most of us experience in the
West. Our health care systems are dominated by mainstream
scientific and orthodox medicine, while herbalists for instance
are pushed into the 'fringe'. It is chastening for the practitioners of scientific medicine, however, to remember that it
was only about sixty years ago that 90 per cent of prescriptions
were of plant origin. It has only been over this half century
that the 'therapeutic revolution' has brought hundreds of
synthetic chemical drugs into the modern armamentarium. The
sulphonamides, originally, were linked to chemical dyes and are
the classical example of synthetic origin although as early antibiotics it is worth recalling the later and naturally derived
penicillins. The number of drugs which had plant origins still
in common use is quite impressive and the following list is not
exhaustive:

| | | | |
|---|---|---|---|
| Morphine | Scopolamine | Cocaine | Glycyrrhizin |
| Codeine | Pilocarpine | Vincristine | Salicylic acid |
| Hyoscine | Quinine | Vinblastine | Colchicine |
| Atropine | Quinidine | Curare | Ergotamine |
| Digoxin | Ephedrine | Caffeine | Ergometrine |
| Digitoxin | Pseudoephedrine | Podophyllum | Papaverine |
| Strophanthine | Reserpine | Croton oil | Bromocriptine |
| Theophylline | | | |
| Theobromine | | | |

*Crude plant extracts*
Belladonna (Atropa belladonna)
Opium (Papaver somniferum)
Rauwolfia (Rauwolfia serpentina)
Cascara (Rhamnus purshiana)
Digitalis (Digitalis purpurea)
Citrus bioflavinoids (Citrus sp.)
Veratrum (Veratrum viride)
Tincture of cannabis (Cannabis sativa)
Nux vomica (strychnos, nux-vomica)
Ipecacuanha (cephaelis ipecacuanha)

A national survey of prescriptions dispensed from American
community pharmacies during 1968 revealed that of 1.68 billion
prescriptions 25 per cent contained one or more active principals
from either a crude plant extract or purified principal from
plant material. (50)

This information gives an idea of the continuing contemporary
importance of 'plant drugs', but the potential is even more
impressive. At Harvard the botanic archives contain over two
and a half million specimen sheets. A team of researchers spent
four and a half years examining the records for plants recorded

s having some medicinal value. They have identified about
,000 of potential value. In Britain, at Kew and the British
Iuseum, there are about 8 million specimens, a legacy of our
nperial past.(51) This 'treasure-chest' has yet to be system-
tically researched for medicinal plants. One problem is the
ole of the pharmaceutical industry which on the one hand is
nterested in possible leads for new active principals but is
esitant about developing the natural product as plants cannot
e patented. A recent example of this type of consideration is
he development of a synthetic chemical with similar activity to
annabis. Because it is distinctive it can be patented by the
ompany and also presumably avoid the legal problems associated
'ith the use of cannabis. It is debatable, however, whether
he millions of dollars spent on developing Levonantradol can
e considered to be a socially useful expenditure given the long
xperience in the use of cannabis, its easy cultivation and
rocessing.(52) For Third World countries keen to cut down the
eavy expenditure on synthetic drugs, many but not all plant
rugs can be produced and processed far more cheaply that the
ost of importing expensive foreign drugs. This is why the
orld Health Organisation has been taking an interest in tra-
itional medical therapies in Third World countries and trying to
ncourage their study. In the West the potential application of
erbal medicines has reached a bizarre stage with official instruc-
ions as to their recognition and use in the event of nuclear
ar.(53) It is hoped that their value and potential can be recog-
ised early for the benefit of all peoples.

OTES

1   Traditional medicine in China, 'Beijing Review', 15.12.80.
2   'Common Terms of Traditional Chinese Medicine in English',
    Peking Medical College, 1980, p. 176.
3   Ibid., p. 467.
4   Chimin Wong and Wu Lien teh, 'History of Chinese Medicine',
    Tientsin Press, 1932, p. 5.
5   'Common Terms', op. cit., p. 468.
6   'Beijing Review', op. cit.
7   Wong and Wu, op. cit., p. 78.
8   'Common Terms', pp. 442-3.
9   News and Notes, 'CMJ', 4, 5, September 1978, p. 414.
10  'Barefoot Doctors' Manual', prepared by the Revolutionary
    Health Committee of Hunan Province, London, Routledge &
    Kegan Paul, 1978, p. 191.
11  'Common Terms', p. 175.
12  Ibid.
13  E.H. Hume, 'The Chinese Way in Medicine', Baltimore, Johns
    Hopkins University Press, 1940, p. 37.
14  P. Huard and Ming Wong, 'Chinese Medicine', World Univer-
    sity Library, London, Weidenfeld & Nicolson, 1968, p. 196.

15 'Beijing Review', op. cit.
16 Personal communication with Dr Gao Li-sheng and Dr Tian Conghuo at Guananmen Hospital, Beijing, 1981.
17 'Barefoot Doctors' Manual', pp. 122-3.
18 'Beijing Review', op. cit.
19 Product data from Peking Dietetic Preparation Manufactory.
20 From 'Fundamental knowledge of Chinese Herb Therapy', Lesson 6, Academy of Oriental Heritage Vancouver BC, North American College of Chinese Herbalism, 1977 Appendix
21 'Common Terms', p. 306.
22 Yi Ning-yu et al., Pharmacologic studies on Liu Wei Di Huangtang, 'CMJ', 84, July 1965, pp. 433-6.
23 'Barefoot Doctors' Manual', p. 343.
24 M. Porkert, The Quandary of Chinese Medicine, 'Eastern Horizon', December 1977, p. 19.
25 Qinghaosu Antimalaria Co-ordinating Research Group, Antimalaria Studies on Qinghaosu, 'CMJ', 92, no. 12, December 1979, pp. 811-16.
26 Coronary Heart Disease Group Traditional Chinese Medicine Hospital Peking, Traditional Chinese medicine treatment of angina pectoris, 'CMJ', 3, 3, May 1977, pp. 167-72.
27 Lu Chun-sheng et al., 'Radix Salviae Miltiorrhizae and Rhizoma Ligustici Wallichii in coronary heart disease', 'CMJ' 4, 1, January, 1978, pp. 43-6.
28 Wang Chen-sheng et al., In vitro Radix Salviae Miltiorrhizae action on blood anticoagulation and fibrinogenolysis, 'CMJ', 4, 2, March 1978, pp. 123-6.
29 Pao Tieng-tung et al., Protective action of Schizandrin B on hepatic injury in mice, 'CMJ', 3, 3, May 1977, pp. 173-8
30 Discussion with Dr Xu Li La, Institute of Materia Medica, Beijing, September 1981.
31 Ibid.
32 Dept. of Anaesthesiology, Fu Wai Hospital and Chinese Academy of Medical Sciences Beijing, Traditional Chinese Medicine balanced anaesthesia for open heart surgery, 'CMJ 2, 4, July 1976, pp. 273-8.
33 Chronic Bronchitis Research Group Dept. of Pharmacology, Institute of Materia Medica, Peking, Expectorant action of Farrerol, 'CMJ', 3, 4, July 1977, pp. 259-65.
34 National Co-ordinating Group on Male anti-fertility agents, Gossypol - a new anti fertility agent for males, 'CMJ', 4, 6, November 1978, pp. 417-28.
35 Dept. of Pharmacology, Institute of Materia Medica, Peking, The antitumour effects and pharamacologic actions of Harringtonine, 'CMJ', 3, 2, March 1977, pp. 131-6.
36 Editorial, Earnest implementation of the Party policy on Traditional Chinese Medicine, 'CMJ', 78, 1959, pp. 205-6.
37 Acute myocardial infarction treated with traditional and Western medicine, 'CMJ', 1, 1, 7 January, 1973, p. 7.
38 Crush syndrome team Liaoning College of Traditional Chinese Medicine, Shenyang, Treatment of crush syndrome by

traditional purging to end stasis, 'CMJ', 92, 9, September 1979, pp. 635-8.

9 Burn Department of Juchin Hospital and Burn Research Unit, Shanghai, 2nd Medical College, Studies on the toxic effects of certain burn escharotic herbs, 'CMJ', 4, 5, September 1978, pp. 388-93.

0 Institute of acute abdominal disease, Wankai Hospital Tientsin and Acute Abdominal Conditions Research Group, Tsunyi Medical College Kweichow, Treatment of acute abdominal diseases by combined traditional Chinese and Western medicine, 'CMJ', 4, 1, January 1978, pp. 11-16.

1 Nankai Hospital Tientsin, Further experience in treatment of acute perforation of peptic ulcer by combined traditional Chinese and Western medicine, 'CMJ', 4, 5, September 1978, pp. 379-82.

2 Ibid., p. 379.

3 Research Institute of acute abdominal disease Nankai Hospital, Tientsin, Treatment of acute intestinal obstruction by combined traditional Chinese and Western medicine. A report of 1006 cases, 'CMJ', 4, 6, November 1978, pp. 472-5.

4 Treatment of acute abdominal diseases, 'CMJ', op. cit.

5 Ibid., pp. 15-16.

6 Gossypol, 'CMJ', op. cit.

7 Pathologic Laboratory and Group for combined traditional Chinese and Western Medicine in acute abdominal diseases, Provincial Peoples Hospital Honan, Combined traditional Chinese and Western medicine in acute appendicitis, 'CMJ', 3, 4, July 1977, pp. 266-9.

8 Treatment of acute abdominal diseases, 'CMJ', op. cit.

9 Zhao Yuxian, Traditional Chinese in pneumonia of children, 'CMJ', 94, 9, September 1981, pp. 601-6.

0 'Herbal Pharmacology in the People's Republic of China', Washington, National Academy of Sciences, 1975, p. 7.

1 R. Eagle, 'Herbs, Useful Plants', London, BBC Publication, 1978, p. 21.

2 Ibid., p. 26.

3 East Anglia Regional Health Authority Circular, 'The Organisation of Health Services in a Time of War', quoted in A. Brown, 'War Games', 'Nursing Mirror', 19 March 1981, p. 8.

# 10 CHINESE TRADITIONAL MEDICINE AND MODERN WESTERN MEDICINE: INTEGRATION AND SEPARATION IN CHINA

S.M. Hillier and J.A. Jewell

> It has not been psychologically easy for any of the great high cultures of Asia to accept the necessity of borrowing so much of Western technology, institutions and values in order to survive in the modern world. This has been particularly true for those civilisations, like China, historically accustome more to the role of disseminators of culture than borrowers.(
>
> R.C. Croizie

Previous chapters have outlined the theoretical basis of the classical tradition of Chinese medicine and contain examples of traditional therapies. Clearly the integration of two such different systems of medicine as the traditional Chinese and modern Western is at best extremely difficult and perhaps even impossible. For Needham(2)

> What is at issue is the comprehension in modern terms of the quasi-empirical practices which grew up in China through the centuries. Since the theories of traditional Chinese medicine always remained relatively 'primitive' and 'pre-Renaissance' in type, there cannot be much future for them except in so far as they may be re-interpreted in modern terms.

## PRACTITIONERS IN ANCIENT TIMES

It was in the late Zhou dynasty (-722-221) that the process of differentiating a class of secular physicians distinct from pries and sorcerers began.(3) However, the 'practice of charms, incantations and invocatory prayers to deities persisted throug most of Chinese history, particularly among the poorer strata of society and in the exorcistic activities of Taoist adepts and Buddhist monks'.(4) Needham refers to these phenomena as the 'fringe activities' of Chinese traditional medicine.(5) The trans ition of the physicians from the status of Wu (sorcerers and magicians) to that of Shi which carried the dignity of a Confuc intellectual is crucial. This grouping places them in the tra- ditional division of Chinese society, which had four main ranks Shi (scholars); Nong (farmers); Kung (artisans); and Shang (merchants).(6) In the Qin (-221-206) there were court physicians and, following the Han (-206 + 220), there were offi medical posts attached to the court bureaucracy. Medical instruction was given at the Imperial Court during the Sui

Dynasty (+581-618) and, at least since the Tang (+618-907), at an Imperial College of Medicine in the capital. In +629 it was decreed that this be paralleled by medical colleges complete with certifying examinations in the provincial cities.(7) In the Tang dynasty medical students were beginning to be examined in general literature and the philosophical classics.(8) Gradually physicians were classified into three main groups: Ru-i ('Confucian physician'); Yong-i (common practitioner); Chuan-i or Ling-i (wandering medical pedlar).(9)

The highest prestige was given to those scholars who practised medicine from benevolent motives without pecuniary gain (Ju-i). Most of their knowledge was acquired from classical medical texts and the title was intended to distinguish them from those who practised without a literary background, or for money.(10) It appears that many scholars who failed their civil service examinations turned to medical practice.(11) One snag was that healing was considered 'artisan' - hence the aversion to manual operations and surgical skills and the reverence paid to textual authority.(12) A different and important group of doctors were those who came from a medical family or at least had been apprenticed to a respected doctor. In the 'Book of Rites' of the Zhou it states: 'The physic of a doctor in whose family medicine has not been practised for three generations at least should not be taken.(13)

Medical knowledge was 'private capital' and individual practitioners would keep their prescriptions secret from their professional rivals, perhaps only passing them on to a son or disciple. There were a large number of lower-grade doctors who had access to one of the medical classics and prescribed from that or used rather primitive acupuncture. Some of these would be the 'wandering medical pedlars'(14) who tinkled their bells on jingling staffs as they passed through the villages. At the lower level the range of 'healers' included 'herbalists, cuppers and barber masseurs as well as soothsayers, geomancers, fortune tellers, ocularists, aurists, dentists'.(15)

By the time of the Qing (+1644-1911) there were recognised to be three main categories of physician: (1) court physicians; (2) public physicians; (3) 'pavement' physicians.(16) Traditional medicine was in decline, having attained its maturity between the +7th and +14th centuries.(17) Spence notes that 'The Veritable Records of the Qing dynasty' (Da Qing Shi lu) of Emperor Kang Xi's reign (+1662-1722) present exorcism and black magic as factors in political life. At the same time the same Emperor's confidential edicts show him reading the Yellow Emperor's Classic of Internal Medicine, consulting Jesuits, and Taoist longevity adepts.(18) This was the medical culture that the surgeons of the East India Company who worked in Guangzhou (Canton) and Aomen (Macao) at the turn of the nineteenth century, and the ensuing medical missionaries, were to find. Western medicine of the same period had few effective therapies to offer apart from surgical skills and vaccination.(19) The use of ether and chloroform developed by 1840; Koch and Pasteur's work on 'germ' theory and Lister's use of antiseptics were beginning to be applied in the 1880s.(20) Thus even the surgical skills were pre-anaesthetic and pre-antiseptic. For Needham: 'If we judge strictly clinically the patient may not have been much better off in Europe than in China before the beginning of the twentieth century.'(21)

## EARLY WESTERN CONTACTS

The missionary Robert Morrison and John Livingstone, surgeon to the East India Company, set up a simple dispensary in Aomen in 1820.(22) In 1834 Peter Parker became the first full-time medical missionary in Guangzhou.(23) At first their activities were handicapped by limited money, manpower and Chinese suspicion and hostility. The restriction on foreign influence was smashed apart after the Opium Wars (1840-2) when four new treaty ports were opened. Under the terms of the Tianjin treaties (1858) the entire country was available for missionary work. Crozier says:

The medical missionary movement itself was of course closely tied to the exertion of Western military power which forced China to accept Western commerce, Western institutions and eventually Western culture. This association may have contributed to Chinese reluctance actively to accept a new medicine which came more or less in the same package with an unwelcome religion and an unwelcome culture.(24)

The expansion of Western imperialism was accompanied by growing medical missionary work. By 1889 the number of hospitals and clinics had risen to sixty-one and at the end of the century Western medicine had penetrated every province and major city in the Empire.(25) Growth reached a peak in the early 1920s when there were 326 hospitals and 244 out-patient clinics.(26)

The pneumonic plague epidemic of 1910-11, which left an estimated 600,000 dead, promoted an important shift in public consciousness, vis-à-vis Western medicine. Western medical principles such as isolation of cases, disinfection and quarantine were seen to be effective and prompted the viceroy of Manchuria to remark:

The lessons taught us by this epidemic have been great and have compelled several of us to revise our former ideas . . . if railways, telegraphs, electric lights and other modern inventions are indispensable to the material welfare of this country we should also make use of the wonderful resources of Western medicine for the benefit of our people.(27)

TRADITIONAL AND WESTERN MEDICINE IN THE
'NEW CHINA', 1911-19

The latter part of the nineteenth century and early part of the
twentieth saw the collapse of the Imperial order and the brief
inception of the Republic under Sun Yatsen in 1911. Despite
the degeneration of the Republic into warlordism, developments
culminated in China's first 'Cultural Revolution' of 4 May 1919.
By this time the Chinese intellectual world was dominated by a
new generation of intellectuals, who were prepared to denounce
every aspect of traditional culture, including Chinese traditional
medicine. One magazine article of the period stated:

> Our doctors don't know science. They don't understand human
> anatomy and what is more don't analyse the nature of medicine.
> As for bacteria and communicable diseases they haven't even
> heard of them. They only talk about the five elements, their
> production and elimination, heat and cold, yin and yang and
> prescribe medicine according to the old formulae. All these
> nonsensical ideas and reasonless beliefs must basically be
> cured by the support of science.(28)

When traditional doctors approached the Minister of Education
in 1914 seeking registration of their society the Minister is
reported as saying: 'I have decided to prohibit the native practice and do away with the crude herbs.'(29)
Later a Presidential Mandate of 30 September 1915 laid down
that candidates in medicine, pharmacy and veterinary science
should follow the same standards as in the other 'progressive
countries of the West'.(30)
Two interesting characters in this debate are Lu Xun, the
author and playwright much respected by the Chinese Communist
Party, and Guo Moro, the scientist and leading figure in the
post Liberation government. Both had gone to Japan to study
medicine but Lu Xun left before qualifying and Guo Moro never
practised.(31)
Lu Xun left his Japanese Medical College after deciding that it
was the Chinese national spirit rather than their physical health
that needed his revolutionary attention. One story, 'Medicine'
(1919), tells of a desperate parent paying an executioner to dip
steamed bread into the blood of an executed criminal. This was
to be a 'guaranteed cure' for his terminally sick child.(32)
The story was an attack more on general superstitious practices
than traditional medicine. However, the story 'Father's Illness'
(1926) is rather critical and he writes of the prescriptions he
had to collect:

> Most often it was 'a pair of crickets' with a note in small
> characters at the side: 'They must be an original pair, from
> the same burrow', so it seems that even insects must be
> chaste; if they marry again after losing their mates they for-

feit even the right to be used as medicine.(33)

He was antagonistic to traditional Chinese doctors who appeared to represent what was backward and unscientific in China. Mao was later to speak of Lu Xun's incorrect view on traditional medicine which he put down to the fact that the medicine failed to save his father.(34)

Guo Moro was to take a similar standpoint: 'The diseases Chinese medicine can cure anyway are diseases which can cure themselves.'(35) In the same article Guo criticised 'nonsensical theory' and said that 'old doctors' needed to be re-educated in modern medicine before being allowed to practise.

Despite the strictures of the modernists, there existed conservatives who were opposed to this pro-Western stance. Their view was that the Chinese 'essence' and national identity should be maintained. One proffered remedy to solve the conflict was to adopt the Western 'form' (Xing) while keeping the Chinese spirit (Shen).(36) In relation to medicine, a similar compromise held that Western medicine could be used for external diseases, and Chinese medicine retained to treat the more difficult internal problems. In fact this had been a long-standing practice and Chen records a newspaper editorial from 1881 which stated:

> Our view is that the Chinese and Western medical arts are different. Chinese physicians use plants and herbs whereas Western physicians use minerals and metals. The latter are strong drugs which the Westerners who eat strong meat like beef and mutton to strengthen their bodies can take without harmful effects. The Chinese however may not be able to withstand such potent substances because of their weak physique nourished on a daily diet of cereals which enfeeble their stomach and intestines . . . it might not be foolish for a Chinese to see a foreign doctor for skin, i.e. external disease; he would be stupid to do so for internal sickness.(37

## REPUBLICAN GOVERNMENT AND STATE REGULATION

After the modernising influences of the 4 May movement there was an increasing demand for regulations to govern and restrict traditional practice. In 1920 following a conference at the new Peking (Beijing) Union Medical College the Guomindang government was urged to 'regulate the practice of the doctors trained in the traditional way with a view to the unification of standards required of medical practitioners'.(38) In 1922 the Ministry of the Interior provided licences for the two types of practitioners with different standards of qualification. By 1929, however, when the Ministry of Health drew up 'provisional regulations for physicians' the dual status of 1922 was no longer recognised and the rules referred solely to Western-style doctors.(39) In the following month, to underline the point, the Ministry convened a public health conference, at which a resolution to 'Abolish traditional medicine' was proposed.(40) Such a resolution was too much for the traditionalists in the Guomindang, who strongly resisted abolition. The fight to retain traditional medicine continued successfully and at the Guomindang 5th Party Congress in 1935 a resolution backed by a petition from traditional medicine societies demanding equal status for Chinese and Western medicine, was passed.(41) The position of traditional medicine was further secured by the Nationalist Government in 1943, when the 'Physicians' Law' permitted traditional doctors to obtain a licence, equal in status to that of modern doctors, if they had received a diploma from a school of Chinese medicine; passed a government examination; had five years practice with a doctor of prominent reputation.(42)

Although the new law legalised the position of traditional doctors, the vast majority remained unregistered. There was a demand for their methods of treatment, so registration produced no particular advantages for them. In any case, the Nationalist government was ineffective in this as in other areas of its policy, and was not prepared to outlaw unregistered practitioners. There had been an attempt to modernise traditional medicine with the formation of an Institute for National Medicine, schools, hospitals and research centres, the publication of journals and formation of medical societies.(43) In 1930 Knud Faber, a League of Nations expert, noted fifteen schools of traditional medicine offering five-year courses which included modern physiology, anatomy and chemistry in their curriculum.(44) In general, however, the two systems remained divided with the Western-style doctors controlling the government health machinery and working in the large urban centres; and traditional doctors largely unchanged by modern science practising throughout the countryside.

## COMMUNISM AND TRADITIONAL MEDICINE

The increasingly influential Chinese Communist Party had been founded in 1921, and following the massacre of trade unionists and Communists in Shanghai and Canton in the 1926-7 period took to the countryside to form guerilla bases.(45) The CCP's attitude to traditional medicine is displayed in the little documentary evidence available. There are interesting parallels with the Guomindang disputes over legislation against traditional medicine. In 1929 at the First Central Hygiene Committee meeting of the Communist Party, Yu Yunxin and others proposed a 'plan to abolish old medicine and sweep aside the obstacles for a development of medicine and hygiene'.(46) This draft was opposed and never executed. The growing experience of the Communists in the type of medical care necessary under conditions of guerilla warfare crucially altered attitudes towards the utility of traditional medicine. Croizier quotes from some public health material from the Jiangxi Soviet which shows that 'while stress was put on modern medicine and basic public hygiene, the acute shortage of medical supplies forced some reliance on native herbals'.(47)

An article in the June 1933 issue of 'Red Hygiene' included the study and controlled use of traditional drugs as one of the suggested measures for coping with the nationalist blockade: 'Under enemy blockade in a situation of great difficulty regarding pharmaceuticals, we should all the more adopt Chinese drugs and process or screen them.'(48)

Both the Eighth Route Army and the Yanan Drug Co-operative maintained factories and manufactured 'native-style drugs'. Croizier quotes from Yang Shao in 1940 who proposed to 'scientificize, sinicize and popularize'(49) medicine in China:

> The old medicine confined within the scope of a feudal society, had been unable to avoid a 'mystical idealism' which vitiated any approach to science. But if the content of Chinese medicine was rejected as feudal and unscientific, the context of Western medicine was unacceptable as capitalist and imperialist. The present task was to build a 'new democratic medicine' in China by taking the latest scientific developments from abroad and assimilating them to Chinese conditions, while also using Western medicine's scientific basis to improve Chinese medicine and study Chinese drugs.(50)

Not all members of the Communist Party agreed with Yang Shao. Attitudes which had produced the 1929 resolution to abolish traditional medicine were still strongly held among those who opposed 'Confucian medicine'. 'The so-called rich national essence is just the collected garbage of several thousand years.'(51) Guo Moro, a leading party scientist, said: 'we have been slaves to the so-called national essence for several thousand years'.(52) Later as an official spokesman for the new Communist government he modified his views. At the National Health Conference of 1950 he stated: 'Chinese medicine must learn from the scientific knowledge of Western medicine; Western medicine must study the popular and widespread spirit of Chinese medicine.'(53)

Mao Zedong's influence in pressing for recognition of traditional medicine cannot be underestimated. As leader of the Communist Party both in the Yanan days, and after the Party's accession to power, his prestige and personal power were enormous. He threw all the authority of his position behind traditional medicine, and became one of its leading proponents. In an important speech in 1944, he said:

> Among the 1,500,000 people of the Shensi-Kansu-Ningsia border region, there were more than 1,000,000 illiterates, there are 2,000 practitioners of witchcraft and the broad masses are still under the influence of superstitions. . . .

The human and animal mortality rate are both very high. . . .
In such circumstances, to rely solely on modern doctors is no
solution. Of course modern doctors have advantages over
doctors of the old type; but if they do not concern themselves
with the sufferings of the people, do not train doctors for
the people, do not unite with the thousand and more doctors
and veterinarians of the old type . . . then they will actually
be helping the witch doctors and showing indifference to the
high human and animal mortality rates. . . . There are two
principles for the united front: the first is to unite and the
second is to criticise, educate and transform.(54)

*Chinese Traditional Medicine (TCM) in the early 1950s*
In 1949 when the Party assumed power unification had become
an even more urgent task and the call from the Party to a
conference on public health administration in October 1949 was
to unite the entire country's Chinese doctors and also help
Chinese doctors raise their level of techniques.

The Communist Party sought to achieve the objectives that
the Guomindang government had failed to reach in 1935; to
unify and regulate traditional practitioners and incorporate
them with doctors of Western medicine into a single federation
of medical workers under state control. Such unification was
necessary to utilise in the most efficient way every available
medical resource to combat the huge burden of infectious and
parasitic disease in China, to build up the ramshackle health
care system, and to exert ideological control over both the
'bourgeois' tendencies of modern doctors and the 'feudal superstitions' of the traditional ones.

*United clinics*
Under the banner of 'unite and reform' institutions such as the
Chinese Medicine Improvement Schools and the Chinese Medicine
Research Centres taught traditional doctors some basic tenets
of modern science and hygiene. Traditional doctors were urged
to work together in 'united clinics' and share their secrets. The
first clinic was started in Manchuria in 1949. In 1951 the
Ministry directed all local public health bureaux to set up united
clinics and by 1952 there were over 15,000.(55) These clinics
were group practices run on a co-operative basis with fees
pooled to meet expenses and pay salaries. They were government supervised but not funded and often consisted exclusively
of traditional doctors.

In the early 1950s power in the direction of health care lay
very much in the hands of the Western-style doctors who
dominated the Ministry of Health, the Academy of Medical
Science and Chinese Medical Association. The CMA had changed
very little after the liberation and in June 1949 had published
the 'outline of plans of future medical work in China' which
included the statement: 'The unscientific native medicine is to
be reoriented and duly abolished.'(56)

Traditional doctors did not belong to the CMA, had no government positions and were excluded from the large urban hospitals. Soviet medical professionals who were unsympathetic to traditional medicine held important positions in the Ministry of Health, in particular in the Medical Education Bureau.(57) A Ministry directive in May 1951 stated: 'Chung i (traditional medicine) must endeavour to incorporate the knowledge of scientific medicine and improve its methods of treatment.'(58)

The Ministry of Health's policy was basically at variance with the Communist Party's line and that of Mao Zedong. Although traditional doctors were working in the united clinics the integration was more organisational than professional. Their skills were to be brought up to an 'adequate level', and they were used as 'pairs of hands'. The CMA sought to introduce examinations and diplomas and set about the task of regulating traditional doctors. Regulation and exclusion rather than integration on an equal basis were the objectives which the Ministry followed. This was in direct opposition to Party policy. In July 1954, Mao complained: 'For a number of years there was no fastening of the medical heritage of the motherland. The directive of the Party Central Committee on integrating Chinese and Western medicine has not been carried out.'(59)

*A new direction for TCM*
Vice-Minister He Cheng, a Western-trained doctor, lost his position because of his opposition to Chinese medicine,(60) and new Party directives were issued to strengthen the position of Chinese traditional medicine. Most importantly, these directives stressed that Western doctors were required to study traditional Chinese medicine. By 1956, 5,000 Western doctors had enrolled in courses,(61) and 300 had a specialist course of two years. Traditional Chinese medicine occupied one month of the curriculum of third-year medical students.(62)

Traditional doctors, who had been looked down on in hospitals, were now to be regularly invited to give treatment. At Wuhan Medical College traditional doctors were given a twenty-two-bedded ward(63) and 'Full co-operation between the Chinese traditional doctor, and all Western trained doctors and nurses, is expected.' By 1956 government health departments had incorporated 30,000 traditional doctors.(64)

Chinese medicine was to be safeguarded and developed in three main ways: firstly by adequate training - there were 144 hospitals and four traditional medical colleges(65) running five-year courses at Chengdu, Beijing, Shanghai and Guangzhou and an Academy of Traditional Chinese Medicine was set up in Beijing. Apprenticeship training was tightened up. Secondly, pharmaceuticals and remedies were to be standardised and controlled. There was a crackdown on 'smuggling of fraudulent medicine, especially ginseng, cow bezoar and beeswax [which has] been rampant'.(66)

Thirdly, cases treated effectively by Chinese traditional

medicine were publicised, including 'hopeless' cases of B-encephalitis,(67) hypertension,(68) and, of course, schistoso-miasis.(69) The effectiveness of these actions by the Party was demonstrated by the growth of united clinics which incorporated the traditional doctors into government service and grew to 50,000 by 1957.(70) The number of publications on traditional medicine grew from 7 per cent of the total in 1953 to 27 per cent in 1955.(71) Most importantly, in 1957 the Bureau of Traditional Medicine was transferred from the Ministry of Commerce to the Ministry of Health,(72) thus giving traditional practitioners status in the health care system, and at the same time providing a means of controlling and integrating them. In 1955 the govern-ment reported the national total of traditional doctors as 486,700.(73) However, income disparities existed. The average income of a traditional doctor in 1956 according to one source was 30-40 yuan a month compared to 150-300Y for a veteran trained Western doctor.(74)

The attitudes of Western professionals could not readily be altered to accept traditional medicine. The instruction that Western doctors should study traditional medicine was thought to be particularly onerous. 'Busy medical personnel find it difficult to give four hours each week to study and practice traditional medicine and at the same time study textbooks and periodicals to keep up with Western medicine.'(75) Unqualified teachers 'do not know how to present their subjects system-atically in lectures. Frequent changing of teachers make the study of Chinese medicine chaotic'.(76) The inclusion of tra-ditional medicine into an already crowded undergraduate medical curriculum led to complaints: 'some feel that such an addition is unnecessary; others believe that only the most valuable data developed by Chinese traditional medicine should be taught to students'.(77)

During the 'Hundred Flowers' movement the encouragement of intellectuals to speak out led to outright criticism of tradi-tional medicine. The Dean of Pharmacy at Beijing Medical College claimed that: 'the Ministry of Health has dragged pharmaceuticals back into the eighteenth century'.(78)

The pressures for incorporation of traditional physicians into the health care system had led, it was felt, to the lowering of standards, which the opponents of traditional medicine were quick to seize upon:

> some Chinese traditional doctors have overreached themselves by taking on too many apprentices. Others have been totally unprepared to teach. . . . Prohibitively high fees are asked by some Chinese doctors for tuition . . . some doctors are only interested in making a quick profit by advertising 'short course training schools' for Chinese traditional doctors. The Peking Municipal Health Bureau is now cracking down on these 'fly by night' schools.(79)

Inexperienced poorly-trained novices were a danger,
especially in the use of acupuncture needles:

> For instance, one woman sought treatment to increase her flow
> of milk, and died after being treated with acupuncture by a
> trainee. She was punctured through the heart. Therefore it
> is dangerous for a novice to attempt acupuncture.(80)

Chinese traditional doctors also prescribed Western drugs
wrongly for the sake of profit:

> Many Chinese traditional doctors do not now prescribe
> traditional medicines because even the farmers believe in
> Western medicine, and there is more profit in Western
> medicine. . . . There was a case of a pregnant woman suffer-
> ing from a chronic disease whose death was caused by an
> overdose of antipyrin prescribed by a Chinese traditional
> doctor.(81)

The attempts of health officials to confine the practices of
Chinese traditional physicians in the united clinics to being
'epidemic prevention statistic clerks or educational propagandists
in health movements',(82) gave them no means of practising
their original craft, and affected their financial situation:

> Many Chinese traditional doctors who voluntarily joined train-
> ing classes for the prevention and treatment of epidemic
> disease have left because the cost of living allotments were
> unavailable for them or their families during the period of
> training.(83)

By the end of the 1950s attempts at integrating Western and
traditional practitioners were looking shaky. The inadequate
emoluments and low prestige offered to people who had previously practised privately led to lowering of standards, as
traditional practitioners sought to gain money in other ways -
by taking on too many apprentices, or wrongly prescribing
more expensive Western treatments. This gave already sceptical
Western physicians the opportunity to criticise them, and complain about the difficulties they themselves suffered from integration, while their real professional and intellectual interests
lay with better Western-style practice.

The traditional medicine establishment was not happy either.
The loss of independent status by integration had placed traditional doctors under the dominance of the Western trained
professionals of the Ministry of Health. Luan Zhiren, professor
at the Institute of Chinese Medicine, said:

> Work in traditional medicine in the last few years has actually
> shown no development. Traditional doctors have neither
> position nor power. The highest post held by a traditional

doctor in Peking is no more than deputy section chief. The society for Chinese medicine is only an empty vessel.(84)

Wang Leting of the Acupuncture Section of the Institute of Chinese Medicine complained: 'There is not one single principal of any college of traditional medicine who is himself a traditional doctor.'(85)

The fears of the traditional medical establishment about the attenuation of traditional knowledge due to excessive popular-isation and expansion were heightened during the Hundred Flowers Movement. Traditional medicine was not, after all, a systematic body of knowledge. 'There are many different branches of thought in traditional Chinese medicine due to the different interpretation of obscure terms in the medical classics',(86) and the Hundred Flowers debates emphasised the split within the rank of Chinese traditional doctors.

Under the direction of the Party, however, expansion in tra-ditional medicine continued. The expansion was twofold. On the one hand hospitals, clinics and colleges devoted entirely to Chinese medicine increased. By 1957 there were 144 traditional medicine hospitals (an increase of 77 from the previous year), 1,200 clinics and by 1958 13 traditional medical colleges (an increase of 9 from the previous year). There were 3,200 students of traditional Chinese medicine by 1958.(87) In this way the exclusive nature of Chinese traditional medicine was preserved. But in 1958, during the Great Leap Forward, rural people's communes, with their own health centres which replaced the united clinics, required staff. There were 24,000 such clinics, staffed by middle-level Western graduates, and by mid 1959 about half had functioning facilities.(88) In order to work, and reduce the burden on county hospitals, traditional medical doctors were brought in as manpower personnel, and the need for their services meant that the Ministry of Health now joined with the Party in backing their skills.

A Party directive therefore re-emphasised the need for Western doctors to study and respect traditional medicine, and perform joint hospital consultations. Examples of successful 'combined treatments' such as that for appendicitis were reported, and the prestigious China Union Medical College announced that cirrhosis of the liver and uterine prolapse had been successfully treated with traditional medicine.(89) As well as combination and integration 'separate development' also continued and at the end of 1959 students at traditional medical colleges amounted to some 5,000.(90) Politically, the popular and mass character of traditional medicine was emphasised; pro-fessionally, research into traditional pharmaceuticals and acupuncture analgesia increased.

The economic disasters following the Great Leap Forward, in particular the decline in grain output, greatly affected the progress of rural health care. Many commune clinics closed down, and traditional doctors returned to private practice. The prob-

lems of the Leap were partly due to the fact that Mao had
attempted, with some success, a rural transformation which was
not essentially supported by the urbanophile members of the
State bureaucracy. However, the overall temporary improvements in rural health wrought during the Leap when commune
clinics, doctors and medical graduates all increased in number,
were wiped out by the natural disasters of flood and famine in
China in 1960-2, as well as by the economic problems which had
hit the communes.

The early 1960s saw the organisation of health care move back
to the county hospitals, where the promotion of Western medicine
accompanied a national move in medical science towards world
levels of development. In Western medicine, higher standards
of training and medical school entry were enforced. The
numbers of Western trained doctors studying Chinese medicine
declined from 2,100 in 1959(91) to around 2,000 in 1961, but
by 1962 only reports of completed courses were given, with no
new signs of enrolment, the last intake having been in Shanghai
in 1960.(92) These Western doctors, 'Wen Hui Bao' remarked
lukewarmly, 'over the past three years have maintained a high
degree of enthusiasm for study. The greater part of the trainees
hear the lectures seriously, take notes carefully and persevere
in study; in general the results of study are good.'(93)

If the attempts to teach Western doctors traditional medicine
were meeting with little success, Party, and less enthusiastically,
Ministry, support for traditional medicine continued. However,
the tendency from the Ministry perspective was to stress traditional medicine's acceptability to the mass of the population,
and the cheapness of its remedies compared with Western
pharmaceuticals. At a time of financial shortage, the attempt to
maintain and improve health care in China required every existing resource both of money and manpower.

> Since, the 'folk methods' of treatment and 'folk medicine' are
> the treasures of effective values practised by the majority of
> the masses, they should be highly respected, generalised and
> earnestly increased and extended quickly and economically.(94)

The overall policy emphasis in the early 1960s on research
and development in all spheres produced a more tolerant attitude towards traditional medicine from professionals. Since
Western-style doctors were not under the patronage of the
Party, they no longer felt threatened by the image of Party
domination that traditional medicine had represented.

*Turnabout for TCM*
The traditional medicine establishment was eager to 'scientise'
traditional medical practices, although the equipment and
materials provided for research were inferior to those of
Western medicine research institutes.(95) This position was a
reversal: now traditional doctors would have to become more

expert in Western medicine, for in this lay their hopes of
acceptance and survival. One leading traditional doctor
remarked:

> Henceforth, the energetic development of Chinese traditional
> medicine skill depends upon overcoming the ideology of a
> section of the practitioners of Chinese medicine who consider
> that it is perfect – the conservative ideology and closed door
> mentality and of superstitious fidelity to antiquity. . . . To
> bring our medical science up to the level of modern science,
> it is imperative that it should be revised and supplemented
> with the methods of modern science.(96)

However, he implied that this should not involve a diminution
of Chinese medical theory:

> Some people have mistakenly viewed the diagnosis of diseases
> and discussion of treatment as the giving out of whatever
> prescription for whatever illness is in sight. This is a vulgar-
> isation of principle and a basic negation of the spirit of Chinese
> medical treatment.(97)

In keeping with the new emphasis on professionalising traditional medicine, by 1961 the number of Chinese Medical Colleges
increased to nineteen;(98) students were to study the rudiments
of Western medicine as well as TCM. Later during the Cultural
Revolution, Red Guards were to criticise the new elite and
scientific character of TCM.

> Ever since the counter revolutionary revisionist Kuo Tzu-hua
> took charge of the [traditional medicine] department he has
> placed the whole weight on nine research bases in this
> country. Famous old herbalists looked down on the herbalist
> teams dispatched to villages . . . and called them disrespect-
> ful names like 'charlatans' and dimwits.(99)

The 1963 international congress held in Beijing to acclaim the
world's first successful limb re-attachment by Chen Zhongwei
included a paper on the treatment of appendicitis with acupuncture.(100) The audience was informed that 'Many doctors of
traditional medicine avail themselves of scientific methods so
that their diagnosis can become more explicit.'(101) Other
traditional medicine treatments were also published – for fractures, brucellosis, goitre, spinal tuberculosis, tapeworms and
infantile paralysis.(102)
Graduates from the traditional medical colleges now began to
emerge. After their four or five-year periods of study the
majority were assigned to rural communes.(103) There was
consistent development, and by 1966 there were 10,000 students
and twenty-one colleges of traditional medicine.(104) Traditional
medical knowledge was becoming more standardised, as veteran

doctors with secure employment were able to write down and publish the 'secret remedies' of their families.(105) This expansion was not paralleled in other areas of medical education, which suffered some cuts. Traditional medicine had become respectable, institutionalised on a small enough scale to satisfy its own establishment and to prove unthreatening to Western trained professionals, and traditional doctors were a useful source of manpower. They were also acceptable practitioners in the xian hospitals and surviving commune clinics. Patients who might avoid Western doctors had the choice of traditional treatment and could be passed over for Western treatment if necessary.

As important as the traditional doctors themselves were the traditional pharmaceuticals which, if proved effective, could provide adequate substitutes for expensive Western drugs, as well as sources of revenue for communes.


## TRADITIONAL MEDICINE DURING
## THE CULTURAL REVOLUTION

The focus of the Cultural Revolution on rural health care was to have an effect on the future of traditional medicine. Although traditional medicine was not a focus of struggle in the way that Western style medicine was, it nevertheless enjoyed an ambiguous status at the outset of the Cultural Revolution. Having taken the same path as Western medicine during the early 1960s, and having some practitioners whose ideas might be termed superstitious or feudal, it was not above criticism.

In addition those traditional medical doctors who had reverted to private practice after the collapse of united clinics in the 1960s also provided competition for the emerging barefoot doctors who were financed by co-operative medical services. Their methods were attacked:

> Prior to the establishment of co-operative medical service the witchdoctors and witches of the commune always took advantage of the misfortune of others to practice blackmail and extortion.(106)

> The witchdoctors and witches of Taoerh Commune bitterly hated the establishment of a co-operative medical service, and they jumped forward to undermine it. On the one hand they hypocritically gave 'free medical treatment' to win over the masses. On the other hand they threatened the poor and lower middle peasants saying 'Once you join the co-operative medical service I'll have nothing to do with your medical treatment'.(107

While some local traditional practitioners (as opposed to college-trained traditional doctors in xian hospitals) were described as 'witches and witchdoctors', the methods of traditional medicine were being popularised and used both by the mobile teams of doctors and by the barefoot doctors. Acupuncture, moxibustion and plant drugs were all cheap methods of treatment.

## BAREFOOT DOCTORS AND TRADITIONAL MEDICINE

In the late 1960s, towards the end of the Cultural Revolution, the barefoot doctors were lauded for their skills and political standpoint, and the medicine they practised which had elements of both traditional and Western was a subject of praise. Western medical physicians were in political retreat at this time, their skills denigrated; the mobile medical teams on which they were sent highlighted the inadequacy of their training in confronting the major health problems of rural areas. In contrast, barefoot doctors were a new and more devoted type of doctor, who practised acupuncture on themselves before using it on their patients. The publication of these efforts was not only aimed at bolstering the prestige of barefoot doctors, but reassuring patients. For the acupuncture that was being practised was a 'new' acupuncture opening up previously forbidden points, with deeper placement of needles.

By the early 1970s it was estimated that 70 to 80 per cent of cases of illness were treated with acupuncture and herbs by barefoot doctors.(108)

The barefoot doctor's manuals produced by health departments used Western daignostic lables maintaining traditional sub-classifications, which contrasted with traditional medicine textbooks produced in 1959.(109) These later books expected a prior acquaintance with Western medicine.

## TRADITIONAL MEDICINE AND THE CO-OPERATIVE MEDICAL SERVICE (CMS)

Of great importance was the centrality of traditional medical drugs to the new system of health care financing - the co-operative medical service. By relying on traditional plant drugs, Dexing county in Jiangxi was able to reduce its importation of Western medicines by 52 per cent during 1969-70, thus contributing to a decrease in state expenditure of 11 per cent. In the county's production brigades, 24 per cent were able to provide free medical service by using plant drugs and 68 per cent to reduce CMS costs.(110) Another brigade was not so fortunate: 'Because the Shuishean brigade of the Paiyangiu commune set great store by foreign medicine but slighted native medicine the practice of co-operative medicine failed in the second year.'(111)

It is clear that the changes in health care during the Cultural Revolution, which popularised all that was simple, easily access-

ible and non-expert, played a vital part in the maintenance of
traditional medicine, albeit in the new combination practised by
revolutionary barefoot doctors. Had not this popularisation taken
place, it is unlikely that traditional medicine today would be
anything other than an isolated classical system.


## TRADITIONAL MEDICINE, 1970-6

*Research*
The pragmatic and empirical approach to science that character-
ised Party attitudes towards medicine at the end of the Cultural
Revolution meant a playing down of theory and research.
Traditional Chinese medical theory was regarded as having
elements of feudal superstition.

> We have to still make greater efforts to reorganise and study
> Chinese traditional medicine, discarding what is not needed
> and selecting the essential, eliminating the false and retaining
> the true in the light of modern scientific knowledge.(112)

The type of research suggested, however, was 'repeated
clinical practice' rather than laboratory research. Such practices
would be then followed by experimental research: 'and the
essence of the theory of traditional Chinese medicine and its
therapeutic theory should be explained and raised to the plane
of modern science'.(113) Such a research programme posed some
problems.

> Traditional doctors advocated supporting the upright and
> driving off evil, but in the case of physically weak patients
> dared not prescribe the heavy doses of bitter and cooling
> herbs to kill germs. The curing effect was slow to show.(114)

Since much of traditional medicine depended upon maintaining
a balance in the body, thereby preventing disease or fortifying
and supporting the body's own defences, it was difficult to
convince sceptics when the normal cause and effect process
which characterises tests for the efficacy of Western medicine
was absent.
By the early 1970s suggestions that Western doctors should
attend formal courses in Chinese medicine appear to have
been dropped. It was merely suggested that they should 'learn
from traditional doctors' by observing them at work in the
hospital. The withdrawal from pressures towards formal training is probably partly explained by the closure of both traditional and Western medical schools during the Cultural
Revolution.
The integration of Western and traditional medicine was being
demonstrated in a number of well-publicised cases of serious
illness such as polio, burns and deafmutism,(115) and was

promoted not only at primary levels but at secondary level in the hospitals, too. The development of acupuncture analgesia was seen as a triumph for a modern version of a traditional therapy and a prime example of integration. It was claimed that by 1970 more than 100,000 operations had used acupuncture analgesia.(116) Much stress was laid upon the combination of the two systems. Some of these claims of efficacy have been subsequently shown to be fraudulent, and at the time Western professionals displayed a muted scepticism towards the use of traditional medicine in those cases which required hospital treatment. From traditionalists, too, there were fears for the dilution of their subject, for they did not want it to be regarded as 'an easy-to-learn' system of rudimentary medicine. Significantly, despite extravagant claims, there was a lack of confidence in the 'new acupuncture'. 'The Peking conference on acupuncture anaesthesia agreed that all difficulties had not yet been overcome . . . severe pain occurred in some cases and not all operations or patients were suitable.'(117) 'The laws of acupuncture have not been mastered - theoretical research on the subject must continue.'(118)

The suggestion that research was necessary led to the setting up of small hospital-based programmes to study the mechanism of acupuncture analgesia in 1975. However, most public pronouncements tended to stress success and many claims were made for the new 'combined' medicine. The nature of the combination was usually to use Chinese medicinal herbs combined with standard Western procedures, traditional splinting with fractures, or acupuncture analgesia in Western-style surgery. An example of this approach is the treatment of bronchitis, diagnosed by the methods of Chinese medicine, treated by traditional medical preparations, but also utilising X-rays, pathology, microbiology and biochemistry.(119) The word 'combination' therefore covered a variety of different practices.

*Traditional medicine in the health care system*
During the ideological tussles of right and left during 1974-6 (which in the medical sphere took the form of discussion about the status and usefulness of barefoot doctors) the question of traditional medicine was not central. Clearly, it remained the basis of much primary care, either on its own or in combination with Western medicine, it was dispensed by barefoot doctors and had assumed both a popular and practical character which was politically respectable.

Many traditional medicine practitioners were not so fortunate as the discipline itself. Those who were not part of the barefoot doctor scheme, nor at the 'upper end' of traditional practice, i.e. working in the traditional medicine departments to be found in most hospitals at all levels from commune to provincial, left those rural health schemes where their incorporation had been attempted and reverted to private practice, or were deprived of their livings on the grounds of their political unreliability.

## TRADITIONAL MEDICINE 1976 ONWARDS

The fall of the 'Gang of Four' brought no sudden change in the position of traditional medicine, but by the following year TCM was swept along in the 'modernising' current which sought to regenerate economic growth and modernise the scientific and technical means of achieving it.

*Current research in TCM*
Fundamental research is stressed, and it is felt particularly necessary to evaluate those previously reported examples of successful combined drug therapy.(120) The responsiveness of China's medical practitioners to the interest in traditional medicine shown by Western countries and by the World Health Organisation, has led to a number of careful studies of the treatment of disorders by combined therapy.

Pharmacologists' research in scientific centres such as the Institute of Materia Medica, Beijing are analysing traditional medicines and searching for active ingredients. Similarly complex neurophysiological research into the mechanism of acupuncture analgesia is being undertaken as well as scientific research into mechanisms of combined treatments such as herbal medicines used in acute abdominal conditions.

All these developments point to a much more serious and wide-ranging approach to traditional medicine than has been observed over the past thirty years, and it is clear that as far as therapies are concerned, the official stance of the Chinese leadership is to support the continued development of traditional medicine. Prior to the major world conference on acupuncture analgesia, held in Shanghai in 1979, the Minister of Health, speaking of the two million patients who had undergone acupuncture analgesia during surgery, said:

> It is effective. It has stood the test of time and is still playing an important role in protecting the health of our people. It has a theoretical basis. Since the publication almost two thousand years ago of the Yellow Emperor's Classic, traditional Chinese medicine has formed a systematic theory of anatomy, physiology and pathology as well as the diagnosis and treatment of disease. This theoretical system has continued to be substantiated and built on by modern science.(121)

A less complimentary, but slightly more realistic, view of the status of traditional medicine is to be found in the 'Chinese Medical Journal':

> It should be pointed out that Chinese medicine, like other things, is not at all perfect, consisting naturally of both pearls and rubbish. . . . Ever since Western medicine was introduced to our country, sharp differences in opinion have arisen. . . . Some, casting a sceptical eye on traditional

Chinese medicine, had to regard it as unscientific, and others, devoted blindly to the classical teachings, refuse to make the slightest deviation from the old dogma. Either of the two attitudes is of course, incorrect. A real valid and valuable theory cannot stand unchallenged forever without necessary modification.(122)

Vice-Premier

Chen Muhua speaking at the traditional Chinese Medicine Conference reminded her audience that support for Chinese medicine: 'Is a consistent policy of the Party too. Any disarmamentation against or underestimation of the medical legacy of the Motherland is wrong.'(123)

Traditional medical opinion seems to be divided on the issues. To some purists who regard Chinese traditional medicine as a complete science the attempts to modernise it undermine its whole basis.

Chinese scholars, instead of demonstrating and illustrating this mature science to the rest of the world, are in fact constantly whittling away at its basis. If they were to persevere in this attitude, they are bound to annihilate the very essence of two millenniums of scientific endeavours.(124)

To others probably the majority of old traditional medical practitioners, survival, even if it involves a degree of compromise, is probably more important. Interestingly, those doctors who are undertaking laboratory and clinical research in traditional medicine are more likely to be Western trained. The research input of old traditional doctors and into the Academy of Traditional Medicine has up to the present been very limited. In 1980 a new journal of traditional medicine, devoted to research and clinical studies, was proposed. In the same year 200 traditional doctors in Shanghai were selected to teach or do research work at some medical research institutions.(125) While doctors chosen to do research work have to be under fifty years old, 'veteran' doctors are being encouraged to write down everything they know, thus systematising traditional knowledge and abolishing its private individual practitioner nature.(126) The scepticism of many Western-trained doctors in China towards traditional medicine is still a barrier. While there is widespread acceptance of traditional medicine 'because people are used to it' and 'it's good for chronic conditions', the attitude of many Western doctors is 'wait and see'. Although many Western doctors will admit of traditional medicine 'there is something in it. It is especially useful in building up the patient',(127) there are few who are committed to pioneering integration, feeling the necessity to build up their own Western-style specialties. Even the most advanced specialists, however, will admit to using TCM for some of their own illnesses (e.g. the common cold).

*Employment status of traditional practitioners*

The problem of organising and integrating traditional practitioners into the health service defeated the Republican
Government. The Communist Party has been more successful
in incorporating traditional medicine and those who practise it
into a national system of health care. In essence, the problem
has always been the same. There has always been a demand
from the indigenous population for traditional medicine. In order
that the demand could be satisfied, and that practitioners would
provide an adequate level of care, traditional doctors had to be
guaranteed an adequate livelihood within the new system.

In 1949 the expanding health care system needed the traditional doctors; their number far exceeded that of those who
were trained in Western medicine. Yet despite the need for
their services, and demand for their skills, they suffered from
lower status and inadequate salaries. As the numbers of
paramedical and Western-trained doctors increased, traditional
practitioners who offered fee-for-service treatments in the
rural villages came under pressure from the competing co-
operative medical service. These grass-roots traditional doctors,
who formed the majority of traditional practitioners, and should
be distinguished from the relatively small numbers of doctors
trained in traditional colleges, sought survival in a number of
ways. Some found new opportunities for work when co-operative
services collapsed due to economic hardship. Others retrained as
barefoot doctors, although this was not an easy option when
participation in farm work was also required. Some worked part
or full-time as independent pharmacists or undertook other
trades in order to survive. Over all of them was the constant
threat of accusations of political unreliability on the basis of
their 'superstitious practices'. It is suggested that many local
practitioners may have suffered in this way.

The result has been a decline in the number of traditional
practitioners; in 1949, according to some reports, there were
781,930, and in 1980 251,088.(128) In many cases this has been
due to death, but the impossibility of practice has also been
important. This decline has caused concern not only to the
traditional medicine 'establishment' but also to the government.

From 1978 onwards many traditional doctors benefited from the
general rehabilitation given to those disgraced under the 'Gang
of Four'. Veteran practitioners were praised in the press as
victims of persecution. The All China Association of Traditional
Chinese Medicine, which had been dissolved along with other
professional bodies during the Cultural Revolution, was
revived.(129) A survey of medical practice in Hebei province in
the same year 'discovered' many traditional practitioners who
were not working.(130) Attempts were made by medical cadres
to 'inform them of the Party's traditional medicine policy' and
opportunities to work were offered them; old doctors 'volunteered
to delay retirement so they could continue to serve socialism a
few more years'.(131) The outcome of the Hebei survey was to

identify more clearly the problems faced by traditional practitioners, who had been 'subjected to discrimination and
ostracism'.

> For those traditional medical practitioners whose status has
> been questioned since the advent of the Cultural Revolution,
> a proper resolution should be sought. . . . All improper and
> falsification cases should be overthrown and slates wiped
> clean. For those already dealt with *before* the Cultural
> Revolution [our emphasis] a petition for rehearing is
> suggested.(132)

These statements represent an attempt to come to terms with
the current shortage of traditional practitioners. Despite the
massive growth in China's health services and health personnel
since 1949, the need to balance the development of rural health
care against the expansion of urban hospital-based medicine
since 1976 explains the revival of interest in traditional practitioners. The barefoot doctors, who might in the early 1970s
have superseded them, are still insufficient in number and
quality to provide a service for rural dwellers, comparable to
that enjoyed by people living and working in cities, towns or
suburban communes. The latest moves to incorporate traditional
doctors into the rural health care system and give them 'new
and appropriate work' represent an advance on the incorporation
moves of the late 1950s, where traditional doctors were used
often as 'pairs of hands'. The growing public legitimacy of
traditional medicine and the traditional pharmaceutical industry
means that traditional doctors are now more likely to be encouraged to practise their craft.

*New training schemes*
The training of traditional practitioners is being systematised
and the aim is to

> create conditions that will promote courses for training
> teachers of traditional Chinese medicine, and for continuing
> education of practitioners . . . for the few who are especially
> knowledgeable and capable they can be transferred to focal-
> point hospitals.(133)

The Tianjin College of Traditional Medicine, closed in 1969, has
been reopened, offering a five-year course, with clinical training in an attached Chinese traditional medicine hospital.
  Twenty-four practitioners' training institutes have opened(134)
with a total enrolment of 20,000.(135) It was proposed in 1980
that in most advanced institutes the college course would be five
years long with two and a half years' basic training in traditional
and modern medicine and the remainder 'under the guidance of
veteran doctors'.(136) There is still widespread use of and
interest in the apprentice system of education which is the

'traditional way'. Even doctors trained in traditional colleges
will still spend a few years working closely with a 'teacher'.
Some traditional doctors with teaching responsibilities for
students still seek the 'one to one' relationship to pass on their
special experiences and prescriptions.

Early results of the revised college training have been dis-
appointing, at least to senior members of the TCM establishment.
Ren Yinqui, a professor at the Beijing College of TCM, recently
remarked:

> The number of traditional practitioners is decreasing and
> their professional standards are rapidly dropping. Only one
> thousand practitioners are qualified to serve as a link between
> past and future. Last year an examination was held in Peking
> to screen more than six hundred middle-aged or older prac-
> titioners. . . . However only one third . . . passed the
> examination. The results of some of the practitioners . . .
> were shocking.(137)

Proposed changes in the organisation of TCM made by Ren
Yinqui were that a special bureau should be set up to supervise
practitioners of TCM, that laws should be drafted to control
and regulate practice, and that strict foreign-language requirements for TCM practitioners should be moderated. 'A practitioner
of Chinese medicine studies Chinese medicine, not foreign
medicine. . . . It would be better to stress the study of the
ancient Chinese language with competence in one foreign
language only.'(138)

*Traditional doctors in the health care system*
The policy problem has always been to maximise the resources of
traditional medicine while removing the uncontrolled nature or
potential charlatanry of the traditional practitioner. This objective appears to have been modified by a Party decision to allow
the development of a degree of private practice, which is an
indication of the desire of both Party and Ministry officials to
provide a large volume of trained and acceptable health care
personnel as an overriding policy objective. Indeed the provision of a large, stable skilled force of traditional practitioners
can fill the gap for rural areas where co-operative medical
services have cut back on funding, or where peasants prefer
their surpluses to be re-invested in economic expansion rather
than in the local health care system. It is of interest to note that
the province which has been most forward in its promotion of
traditional practitioners is also the one where a 'fall-off' of
barefoot doctors was reported. In Hebei 'In the past three years,
five thousand doctors were dispensed with. As a result the
percentage of brigades which used the co-operative medical
service was reduced from 98.6 in 1977 to 89.9 per cent.'(139)
How far regulations of employment for traditional practitioners
will contain controls on the nature and extent of practice, as

well as geographical mobility, remains to be seen.

*Witchcraft*
Along with moves towards the restoration of traditional medicine
there are definite attempts to rid rural traditional medicine of its
superstitious elements and by training, to exclude 'witches and
witch doctors' whose activities have been increasingly reported
in the Chinese press. While doubtless an increase of such superstitious practices accompanies an augmented use of traditional
medicine, since the line between traditional medicine and superstitious practices may be difficult to draw in the case of
individual practitioners,(140) the attempt to exclude more
doubtful elements reflects a desire to integrate and consolidate
trained traditional practitioners into the health care system. In
1979, in Hunan, reports of fake medicine being sold at village
fairs, and fortune telling, appeared in the Press,(141) and in
Anhui, a circular was issued by the provincial government which
stated: 'Acts of feudal superstition performed by witches and
fortune tellers are strictly prohibited, and so is swindling by
witchcraft and witch doctoring.'(142)
A more horrifying incident from Hainan island reported a
witch's attempt to treat a bedridden girl by driving out a water-
monkey spirit, using paraffin which she set alight. The girl
was crippled for life.(143)
In all these incidents a strict line is drawn between acts of
feudal superstition, and traditional medicine and its practitioners,
but in reality the demarcation could prove difficult. It seems
likely that pressures for regulating and licensing are therefore
likely to increase, and will result in a legal framework for the
control and supervision of practitioners.

*Pharmaceuticals*
Traditional medicine pharmaceuticals have also been subject to
new regulations. There were some doubts expressed about
quality, and new administrative measures were set up to deal
with the problems. Pharmaceuticals were to be manufactured only
under licence from the state or municipality and

> the public security, industrial, commercial, administration,
> health and medical administrative agencies must work in close
> co-ordination and punish . . . illegal acts like using inferior
> or unauthorised ingredients, substituting bogus for genuine
> ingredients, mixing bogus with genuine ingredients, manu-
> facturing and selling bogus and inferior drugs and marketing
> outdated, ineffective and deteriorating drugs. Quacks and
> drug pedlars, who swindle people out of money and put their
> lives in jeopardy, must be eliminated resolutely.(144)

Traditional and modern pharmaceuticals are among the top
fifty of China's exports. One market is the large 'overseas'
Chinese population. Another is Third World countries like Algeria

and Ethiopia where Chinese health care teams have worked. The manufacture of traditional products requires less capital investment than Western medicine, even if modern technology is used, and it has been estimated that the initial outlay could be recouped in three to five years. This aspect of traditional medicine must therefore be seen as a growth point in the modernising Chinese economy.

CONCLUSION

A distinction should always be maintained between the official policy of the integration of traditional and Western medicine, and the survival of traditional medicine in day-to-day health care in China. Official policy, which is an overarching attempt to negotiate the conflicting interests of various powerful groups, occurs at a level far above the daily experience of ordinary people who, in their demands for medical assistance, use both Western and traditional medicines eclectically, to satisfy whatever they define as their health care needs. The two levels are not entirely distinct, however, for official policy does finally affect what is available for ordinary people.

The official policy to pursue recognition of traditional medicine has undoubtedly contributed to the general raising of standards of traditional practice. However, the evidence for the existence of a New Chinese Medicine which combines the best of both schools is certainly questionable and, as our chapter suggests, the word 'integration' has covered a variety of practices, theoretical, organisational and practical.

Whatever form such integration might have taken, it remains an unattained goal, whose existence was more important as a means to ensure the adequate survival of traditional medicine, than as an end to be achieved. Other factors besides official policy have contributed to the relatively healthy state of traditional medicine in China today. Among these are the manpower demands of the expanding health care system over the past thirty years, and the demands of the indigenous population and overseas Chinese for traditional medicine dispensed by practitioners whose skills include the ability to diagnose disease in the 'whole person', a style of practice uncharacteristic of Western medicine.

Both scientific and organisational policies to achieve integration have succeeded in ensuring the survival of traditional medicines. Legal measures to regulate practitioners may well, in the process of regulating and licensing doctors, deal a death-blow to integration, while promoting the existence of respectable, officially recognised and registered traditional practitioners. As far as traditional medicine is concerned, therefore, the key to official survival now lies not in integration, but in separation, and better training. The two disciplines now maintain a modest degree of respect for each other and traditional doctors can bolster their legitimacy by demonstrating the validity of their practice within the paradigm of Western medicine.

In December 1981 it was announced that an institute for combining traditional Chinese and Western medicine has been established. Yet it is to be completely separate both from the Chinese Medical Association and the All China Association of Traditional Medicine. This seems to indicate the older organisations' reluctance to wholeheartedly promote the long-established policy of integration to form a new Chinese medicine.(145)

These large-scale policy issues are unlikely to affect the continuing popularity and acceptability of traditional medicine. What they do illustrate, in Croizier's terms is the continued conflict between two main themes characteristic of modern developing China - 'that of the drive for national strength through modern science, and the concern that this process should not betray national identity'.(146)

NOTES

1 Croizier, R.C., 'Traditional Medicine in Modern China - Science, Nationalism and Tension of Cultural Change', Cambridge, Harvard University Press, 1968, p. 3.
2 J. Needham, 'Clerks and Craftsmen in China and the West', Cambridge University Press, 1970, p. 268.
3 Croizier, op. cit., p. 15.
4 Needham, op. cit., p. 268.
5 Ibid.
6 P. Huard and M. Wong, 'Chinese Medicine', World University Library, London, Weidenfeld & Nicolson, 1968, p. 47.
7 Croizier, op. cit., p. 28.
8 Needham, op. cit., p. 391.
9 Ibid., p. 265.
10 Croizier, op. cit., p. 30.
11 Ibid., p. 31.
12 Ibid.
13 E.H. Hume, 'The Chinese Way in Medicine', Baltimore, Johns Hopkins University Press, 1940, p. 59.
14 J. Needham and Lu Gwei-djen, 'Celestial Lancets', Cambridge University Press, 1980, p. 157.
15 Huard and Wong, op. cit., p. 62.
16 Ibid., p. 60.
17 M. Porkert, The dilemma of present-day interpretations of Chinese medicine, in A. Kleinman, et al. (eds), 'Medicine in Chinese Cultures: Comparative Studies of Health care in Chinese and Other Societies'. Washington Fogarty International Center, 1974, p. 64.
18 J. Spence, Commentary on historical perspectives and Ch'ing medical systems, in ibid., p. 81.
19 Jennerian smallpox vaccination was an advance on the long-standing practice of variolation common in China.

20    Jerome Chen, 'China and the West - Society and Culture 1851-1937', London, Hutchinson, 1979, p. 129.
21    Needham, 'Clerks and Craftsmen', op. cit., p. 407.
22    Wu Lien-teh, 'Early Western Medicine in China - Memorial Volume 1912-1932', Shanghai, National Quarantine Service, 1934, p. 278.
23    E.V. Gulick, 'Peter Parker and the Opening of China', Cambridge, Mass., Harvard University Press, 1973, p. 24.
24    Croizier, op. cit., p. 36.
25    Ibid., p. 38.
26    Ibid., p. 28.
27    Ibid., p. 46.
28    Ibid., p. 71.
29    Wu Lien-teh, 'Plague Fighter - The Autobiography of a Modern Chinese Physician', Cambridge, Heffer, 1959, p. 565.
30    Ibid.
31    R. Croizier, Medicine and modernization in China: an historical overview, in 'Medicine in Chinese Cultures', op. cit., p. 37.
32    Lu Xun, 'Selected Works' vol. 1, transl. Yang Xianyi and Gladys Yang, Foreign Languages Press, Beijing, 1980, pp. 58-68.
33    Ibid., p. 399.
34    Mao Tse-tung Talk to Music Workers, 24 August 1956, 'Peking Review', 37, 14 September 1979, p. 13.
35    Croizier, 'Traditional Medicine in Modern China', p. 129.
36    Ibid., p. 66.
37    Chen, op. cit., p. 131
38    Croizier, 'Traditional Medicine', p. 132.
39    Ibid., p. 134.
40    Ibid., p. 133.
41    Ibid., p. 137.
42    Ibid.
43    Ibid., p. 138.
44    Ibid.
45    This refers to the massacres that resulted when the Guomingdang forces under Jiang Jieshi turned on the trade unionists and Communists who had allied themselves with his forces for the Northern Expeditional Force. This was a serious setback for the left and was important in the later policy of making the revolutionary bases in the rural areas.
46    H. Agren, Patterns of tradition and modernisation in contemporary Chinese medicine, in 'Medicine in Chinese Cultures', op. cit., p. 41.
47    Croizier, 'Traditional Medicine', p. 153.
48    Ibid.
49    Ibid., p. 154.
50    Ibid., p. 155.
51    Ibid.

52  Ibid., p. 192.
53  Ibid., p. 160.
54  Mao Tse-tung, The united front in cultural work,
    'Selected Works' vol. III, Peking, Foreign Languages Press,
    1975, pp. 185-6.
55  Crozier, 'Traditional Medicine', p. 164.
56  Association News, 'CMJ', vol. 67, 1949, p. 403.
57  D. Lampton, 'The Politics of Medicine in China: the Policy
    Process 1949-1977', Folkestone, Dawson, 1979, p. 30.
58  Ibid., p. 36.
59  Directive on work in traditional Chinese medicine, 30 July
    1954, from Miscellany of Mao Tse-tung thought (1949-1968)
    Part I, 'JPRS', Arlington, Virginia, 1974.
60  Lampton, op. cit., p. 47.
61  Croizier, 'Traditional Medicine', p. 180.
62  'Chien K'ang Pao (CKP) (Health News)', 8 March 1957,
    'JPRS', 583 1 July 1958.
63  'CKP', 8 March 1957, 'JPRS', 225, 11 February 1958, p. 21.
64  'Chung-chi I k'an', nos. 4-8, 1957, 'JPRS', 583.
65  'CKP', 8 March 1957, 'CCIK', op. cit., p. 4, in 'JPRS', ibid.
66  'CKP', 12 March 1957, in 'JPRS', 225, 11 February 1958,
    p. 27.
67  'People's Daily', 8 January 1957, 'JPRS', 583, 1 July 1958.
68  'Chung-hua I'hsueh Tsa-chih', 'CMJ', no. 5, 1957, in
    'JPRS' 583, op. cit.
69  'CKP', 5 March 1957 in 'JPRS', 225, op. cit.
70  Crozier, 'Traditional Medicine', p. 177.
71  Ibid.
72  Lampton, op. cit., p. 49.
73  'People's Handbook', 1957, in Croizier, 'Traditional Medicine',
    p. 157.
74  'Kuangchow Jih-pao (Canton Daily)', 6 December 1956, in
    Lampton, op. cit., p. 50.
75  'CKP', 22 March 1957, in 'JPRS', 225, op. cit.
76  'CKP', 8 March 1957, in 'JPRS', ibid.
77  'CKP', 5 February 1957, in 'JPRS', ibid.
78  R. MacFarquhar, 'The Hundred Flowers', New York, Praeger
    1960, p. 124-9.
79  'CKP', 18 January 1958.
80  'CKP', 15 February 1957.
81  'CKP', 18 January 1957.
82  'CKP', ibid.
83  'CKP', 5 February 1957.
84  'Kuangming Jih-pao (Bright Daily),' 24 May 1957, in
    MacFarquhar, op. cit., pp. 126-7.
85  Ibid.
86  'CKP', 2 March 1957.
87  Speech by Li Teh-chuan, 'Kuangming Jih-pao, SCMP' 1457
    and 'NCNA', 9 October, 1959, 'SWB'/PE/W27/B/45.
88  Lampton, op. cit., p. 107.
89  'NCNA', 27 December 1958.

90  Li Teh-chuan, speech at 2nd Session of 2nd National People's Congress, April, 1960, 'SCMP', 2237, pp. 17-23.
91  Ibid.
92  'Peking Provincial Service', 'SWB'/FE/W158/B/16, 25 April 1962.
93  Doctors of modern western school persist in the study of Traditional Medicine in Shanghai, 'Wen Hui Bao', 9 February 1963, 'Sup. SCMP', 115.
94  Yeh Ch'u-ch'uan, at 2nd session of 2nd National People's Congress, 'JPRS', 6493, 3 January 1961, pp. 1-11.
95  Chin Wo Pen, Do more medical research work, speech at 2nd session of 2nd National People's Congress, in 'JPRS' ibid.
96  Ibid.
97  Ibid.
98  'NCNA', 17 August 1967.
99  'Hung-i chan pao, Pu I chan Pao (Red Medical Combat Bulletin), Suppl. SCMP', 198, p. 32.
100 'SWB'/FE/W232/B/22, 2 October 1963.
101 Ibid., B/19, 2 October 1963.
102 FE/W232/B/12, 2 October 1963, 'SWB'/FE/W222/B/27, 24 July 1963, W309/B/22, 7 April 1965.
103 'Lanchow Provincial Service', 15 October 1964, 'SWB'/FE/W/ 309/B/22.
104 'NCNA', 29 January 1966, 'SWB'/FE/W352/A/46.
105 Ibid.
106 We have taken the correct road, experience of the Taoerh Commune, Miao Nationality, 'Current Background', 872, pp. 39-41.
107 Ibid.
108 'SWB'/FE/W633/A/11, 22 July 1971.
109 H. Agren, op. cit., pp. 44-5.
110 'SWB'/FE/638/A/12, 8 September 1971.
111 'Peoples Daily', Exercise the dictatorship of the proletariat on the health front, 27 June 1975.
112 'SWB'/FE/3697/B/II/18.
113 Mao Tse-Tung thought lights up the way for Chinese science, 'Hung ch'i (Red Flag)', 2 February 1970, 'Sup. SCMM', January-April 1970, p. 62.
114 Canton 'Nanfang Jih-pao', 23 February 1970, 'Sup. SCMP', no. 275, July-August 1970.
115 PLA Hospitals combined use of Chinese and Western medicine 'NCNA', 17 January 1971, 'SWB'/FE/3588/B11/7, FE/W990/A/ 15 November 1972.
116 'SWB'/FE/W641/A/4, 17 September 1971.
117 'SWB'/FE/W664/A/1, 1 March 1972.
118 'Canton Provincial Service', 14 January 1972, 'SWB'/FE/ W656/A.
119 'NCNA', 1 October 1977, 'SWB'/FE/W952/A/1 26 October 1977 FE/W923/A/1, 6 April 1977.
120 'SWB'/FE/W977/A/1, 26 April 1978.

121 National conference on acupuncture anaesthesia, 'NCNA', 15 January 1981.
122 Chang Hsiang-tung, Acupuncture analgesia today, 'CMJ', 92, 1, January 1979, pp. 7-16.
123 Chen Mu-hua addresses a traditional medicine conference, 'Peking Home Service', 15 March 1980.
124 M. Porkert, A close look at Chinese medicine in today's People's Republic, 'Eastern Horizon', December 1979, p. 31.
125 'Shanghai City Service', 10 January 1980.
126 'SWB'/FE/6451/B11/14, 21 June 1980.
127 S.M. Hillier, interview file no. 11, July 1980.
128 WHO, 'Number of Health Personnel, All China', 1978. Personal communication 8 April 1980.
129 'NCNA', 12 June 1978, 'SWB'/FE/5841/B11/2.
130 'Kuangming Jih-pao (Bright Daily)' in Chinese, 12 December 1978, 'China Report', 073119 5292 CSO 4008, p. 23.
131 Ibid., p. 24.
132 Ibid., p. 23.
133 Ibid., p. 30.
134 Ibid.
135 'NCNA', 11 June 1980.
136 'NCNA', 14 August 1980.
137 'SWB'/FE/6901/C1/3, 9 December 1981.
138 Ibid., C1/4.
139 'Wuhan Provincial Service', 14 March 1980, 'China Report', no. 32, 'JPRS', 075518 p. 41.
140 I am grateful to Stafan Feuchtwang for this point.
141 'Hunan Daily', 22 July 1979, 'Changsha City Service', 22 October 1978.
142 'SWB'/FE/6335/BII/11, 2 February 1980.
143 'Guardian', 28 February 1980.
144 'SWB'/FE/6744/B11/6, 9 June 1981.
145 'Beijing Review', 7 December 1981, p. 29.
146 Croizier, op. cit., p. 229.

# Part Four

# SPECIAL TOPICS
# IN CHINESE HEALTH CARE

# 11 THE PROVISION AND TRAINING OF MEDICAL AND PARAMEDICAL PERSONNEL

## S.M. Hillier

The staffing of a health care system the size of China's is an immense task. The sheer size of China, and volume of work to be done, requires an enormous input of personnel if even the simplest tasks are to be attempted. Although, especially in preventive work, the Chinese have often tended to rely on the mass participation of the lay population, there still remains a need for trained people. Who these people are, their background, number and type of training, have been the focus of political conflict over the years in China since 1949.

The training of medical personnel has not been insulated from wider conflicts in Chinese politics over the role of education. Indeed at times it has been treated as the exemplary case, from which generalisations about all forms of education dealing with expert knowledge could be made. In addition to these wider issues, there has been a difficulty within the field of health care itself: the training requirements of medicine set against the service needs of the population.

The tradition of medical education in China is far older than anything in the West. Formal and what we might call 'modern' medical education antedated the Communist regime by some fifty years.

China's ancient system of traditional medicine had in the past contained a variety of practitioners each with different types of training. Some learned their craft from relatives; some had a more or less formal apprenticeship, some were pupils at medical colleges. Needham(1) notes that 'Regius professorships and lectureships in medicine implying examination date from +493. The Imperial Medical College and provincial medical colleges were then established (+620-+630) and medical degrees awarded from then onwards.' By +739 every provincial city with more than 100,000 families was legally enjoined to have twenty medical students. A typical curriculum of thirteenth-century China contained divisions of internal and general medicine, convulsive and paralytic diseases, paediatrics, ophthalmology, external medicine, gynaecology and obstetrics, stomatology, dentistry, acupuncture and the treatment of war wounds.

## MODERN MEDICAL TRAINING

By the beginning of the twentieth century several medical missionary colleges, initiatives for which began in Europe and

America, were established in China. The most famous was
Peking Union Medical College.

The style of teaching at PUMC, and at many other US-
inspired medical colleges, was very much along the American
model of medical education. There was a strong emphasis on
research, and on the expensive training of a small number of
scientific doctors who would be a vanguard in raising China's
science to new levels and, as some writers would argue, by
becoming medicine's elite, ensuring the dominance of Western
science in China. By 1937 the PUMC had graduated only 166
doctors, a tiny number when set against the health care needs
of the society.

By 1934 there were twenty-four medical colleges in China. Of
these twenty-two were founded by foreigners. Beijing had two
medical colleges, Shanghai seven, Guangzhou three, and the
remainder were distributed among the provincial capitals of the
coastal provinces, with the exception of the West China University in Chengdu, Sichuan province.(2) The schools offered a
five- to six- year course, plus a one-year internship, and
produced about 500 graduates per annum. On the whole their
curricula strongly resembled those taught in the universities of
the West, with some modifications. There was little emphasis on
public health, for in many colleges no courses were offered.
Two exceptions were Xiangya Medical College, Hunan, where
the course gave 'an introduction to the social sciences especially
psychology'(3) with 'practical work in the hospital and public
health centres', and the West China Union Medical College,
Chengdu, where the dean, W.R. Morse, questioned 'the suit-
ability of the curriculum of PUMC to our own similar institutions'
and remarked that 'China as a whole may eventually need State
education in medicine. Civic centres, rural health projects and
the development of a suitable system of provincial medicine are
all in the air.'(4)

*Medical training under the Nationalist government*
Morse's reading of the situation was correct. The Republican
Government was hoping to set up a State Medical Service and to
incorporate within that a regularised form of medical training.
It sought to improve on the meagre number of doctors of
whom(5) 65 per cent practised in the coastal provinces. Shortly
after the foundation of the National Government in 1928 a
commission on medical education had been set up to work out
curricula for medical, nursing and midwifery education.(6) In
1935 the commission finally validated the six-year course for
medical colleges and a four-year course for medical technical
schools. An outside report, originating from the League of
Nations (the Faber commission), had recommended in 1931 that
to best meet the health needs of the population, a two-tier
system of medical training was required.(7)

The report had recommended that after bringing existing
National Medical Schools up to standard, the government should

develop special medical schools in each province which would provide a basic medical training. Little attention was paid by Faber, or by the Chinese commission, to the use of auxiliary health personnel and the training of health officers, although such a course already existed in Nanking(8) and paramedical staff had already been used in a public health programme in Dingxian (Tinghsien). (9)

However, the lack of any organised system of medicine and health care meant that the recommendations for secondary medical schools went largely unimplemented, although more money was allotted to bring the university schools up to standard. Fears in the profession of providing a 'double standard' of medicine, and of competition from the greater number of lesser trained practitioners who nevertheless possessed a medical qualification, were paramount. The American representative of the China Medical Board in China, writing on the new proposals for dual education, and a state system of medical service, public health administration and health education, remarked

> The policy . . . is only workable under conditions of rigorous control at the centre. The theory that doctors who are less fully trained than university graduates will gravitate to rural areas and offer medical service at low rates to the poor has been shown by the experience of other countries to be undependable. A few, perhaps under the urge of humanitarian or patriotic service, will do so, but the majority will crowd into city centres and there compete relentlessly with other physicians.(10)

By this time, however, the weak Guomindang government was engaged in a war against the Japanese and the civil war which followed put paid to any major developments in medical education.

In 1943 an estimate of the number of doctors in the population made by Sze, Secretary General of the Chinese Medical Association, put the number at 12,000. (Later data suggest this was an underestimate.) Of these he states:

> Only 60 per cent of the total were duly qualified doctors, the balance being apprentice-trained practitioners who were permitted to register up to 1937. Seventy-five per cent are concentrated in the main ports of the six coastal provinces; 92 per cent are under the age of fifty, and 67 per cent under the age of forty; showing the relatively recent development of medical schools.(11)

With the current population of China, this meant that there was one doctor for about every 20,000 to 50,000 persons. The contribution of traditional doctors, who in fact provided the bulk of medical assistance, is omitted from these calculations. The Faber commission had noted that there were about 1,200,000 practitioners of Chinese medicine, and 7 million 'druggists'.(12) The Nationalist response to traditional medicine had been first ambivalent, and then hostile (see chapter 10), and it was clear that the traditional doctors were going to play very little part in the health service envisaged by the Western-dominated Republican Ministry of Health (see Chapter 2).

*Red base-area training*
Some doctors were members of the Communist Party and lived and worked with their fellows in the Red-base areas in Jiangxi and Yenan. The practical health needs of the red bases required a less grandiose approach than that adopted by the Nationalists to the problems of medical manpower. Elementary courses in hygiene and health were started at Chingkangshan in 1928 by Dr Nelson Fu, and by the end of the year sixteen army cadres were trained as 'doctors'.(13) The doctors looked after the army and saw to the health needs of the local population as well, when the amount of medicine permitted. A small hospital was established at Jinggangshan and later, in 1934, ten more and a public health school that graduated about fifty students per year(14) were set up. By the end of the war the guerilla Red armies had over fifty hospitals.(15) During the bitter fighting of the late 1930s and early 1940s, however, the lack of medicines rather than the lack of suitably trained manpower was a major obstacle. The Communist Party's attitude towards traditional medicine was forged during this time. Whatever their views on 'witch doctors', and 'feudal superstitions', traditional medicines, and traditionally trained healers, were a valuable adjunct to the tiny number of Western-trained doctors and auxiliaries. This was a policy which would lead to much conflict with Western-trained doctors in the years after liberation. Other sources of conflict would be the role of college-trained doctors, their length of training, the status due to them, the role of para-medical personnel. The relative importance of demands for personnel from urban and rural areas would also become a major policy issue.


MEDICAL TRAINING IN THE EARLY YEARS OF THE COMMUNIST GOVERNMENT, 1949-54

He Cheng, Deputy Minister of Public Health, speaking at a luncheon in Beijing ten months after the Communists assumed power, said that in the whole of China there were some 20,000 qualified Western-style doctors, 2,500 pharmacists, and about 20,000 nurses and midwives. New objectives would be to increase the total number of health workers to 3 million, which would include 600,000 doctors, dentists, pharmacists and technicians.(16) In addition, middle-grade assistant doctors with a two-year course were to be trained at county-level schools. The aim was to establish medical institutions in every county and district.

University-trained doctors would staff the big city hospitals,
research institutes and the county hospitals, whereas other
district health centres would be staffed by middle-grade
assistant doctors, who would also work at county level.

*Higher level doctors*
The new government was committed to the production of about
3,000 new graduates a year, and the twenty-two university
medical schools were enrolling huge classes of 500 to 600
students. Medical schools at first ran newly reduced four-year
courses(17) as well as five-year courses admitting only senior
middle-school graduates. The exception was the elite Peking
Union, which still required a three-year premedical course
before its clinical course. There was a strong tendency to
preserve the level of expertise. Party officials went to great
lengths initially to reassure the Western- or Soviet-trained
professionals of the Chinese Medical Association that expansion
of numbers would not imply a lowering of standards, for both
these groups valued expertise.(18)

On the one side the Ministry of Health was faced with having
to negotiate conflicts of 'quality vs. quantity' with these professional interest groups. On the other it was confronted by the
enormous health needs of China, which had to be dealt with,
and for which resources of money and manpower were small.
Analysis of manpower targets in the First Five-Year Plan
suggests that these were set rather low, at roughly one doctor
per 10,000 population, although this was recognised as far from
ideal.(19) But numbers graduating increased - from 2,948 in
1954 to 4,527 in 1955 and 6,840 by 1956.(20)

*Middle level doctors*
Statistics suggest that in 1950 there were about 53,000 middle-
level doctors.(21) These middle-level doctors resemble those
recommended by the Faber report of the 1930s, and the 'feldsher'
of the Soviet medical system. Their two-year training was
shorter both than the Faber suggestions or the Soviet 'feldsher',
and was to be financed by the county administration. By 1956,
176 secondary medical schools were listed: this figure, however,
covers schools of nursing, midwifery and pharmacy, as well as
'medical schools'.(22)

*Nursing*
When schools of nursing were set up, they followed the pattern
of medical schools, with an elite school in Beijing and other less
grand institutions in other cities. The Western influence at the
top was clear - nurses in Beijing celebrated Florence Nightingale's
birthday - and the movement in nursing training was essentially
to raise its status: 'Many nurses do not like nursing as a
profession and use it as a stepping stone until better work comes
along.'(23)

The training was to be two and a half years. Salaries were

raised, and better crèche facilities organised. Nursing aides
were also trained 'for non-technical work, thus allowing nurses
to concentrate more on the actual nursing care of patients'.(24)
   The style of training for all levels of staff stressed expertise,
high quality, a clear division of labour specialisation, and a
degree of elitism. Indeed, the pattern of medical education was
not dramatically different from that proposed twenty years
earlier. When questions were raised about the medical education
policy, they were done in a way that reflected the professional
dominance of medicine. It was the values of the professionals
who ran the Ministry of Health and the Chinese Medical Association which set the standards for the style of medical education,
and the numbers to be educated. By 1954 top physicians were
calling for a doubling of university-trained doctors and in 1955
courses were extended from four years to five.(25) The course
had been shortened originally because of military needs during
the Korean war. General health policies also supported these
views, by emphasising hospitals, especially in the cities.

*Lower-level medical personnel*
Although the training of paramedical staff is not much publicised
during this period, it seems that training of public health
activists was undertaken. In 1954 the Party committee had
called for expansion in the number of intermediate medical
personnel. Due to a shortage of money at local levels, and the
emphasis on curative medical care, which required a certain
level of skill,(26) this expansion did not occur immediately. By
1957, however, it was claimed that several million public health
activists had been trained by Red Cross organisations. The job
of these activists was to be: 'a nuclear force of rural sanitation,
bringing about a drop in the number of diseases and
epidemics'.(27)

*Summary*
The early 1950s therefore witnessed a generally conservative
approach to medical education, and professional doctors were
in a position to lay the ground rules in a situation where they
controlled important resources. The slow growth of the 'middle-
level' doctors relative to university-trained doctors is some
indication of this. Conflict was coming between the Ministry,
senior doctors and the Communist Party and the debate first
surfaced openly during the 'Hundred Flowers' movement.


POLICIES 1957-9: THE 'HUNDRED FLOWERS' AND THE
GROWTH OF SPECIALISATION

*Higher-level medical education*
By the late 1950s problems in university medical education were
beginning to be voiced, both by those doctors who worked in
the Ministry of Health and leaders of the Chinese Medical

Association. An article in 'Health News' in February 1957 claimed
a 37 per cent increase in the number of college medical students
since 1954. There were now twenty-nine medical colleges with
an enrolment of 44,000, but

> many problems face these medical institutions of higher learn-
> ing, the most serious of which is the lack of qualified teachers.
> Often there are between five and six hundred first-year
> students in a class and only one to three instructors are
> available.(28)

There was a shortage of clinical facilities for training, and
the course itself was too crammed:

> Too many subjects are covered in the five-year course as
> compared to the six-year course in the USSR. The five-year
> course also includes the study of Chinese traditional medicine
> and the principles of Marxism-Leninism, leaving very little
> time for practical training in medicine . . . many students are
> being taught by subprofessional personnel in the actual work.
> Clinical medicine has been sadly neglected and too much
> emphasis has been placed on basic medical sciences.(29)

In order to shorten the course of training, students had been
required to specialise in a subject before graduation, and 'major'
in a particular branch of medicine,(30) but it was now felt,
within the Ministry at least, that the problems of training and
the health requirements of the population required a less
specialised approach:

> General practitioners are most needed in the mines, factories,
> rural areas, frontier communities and among the minority
> tribes. . . . Cases have occurred where doctors trained only
> in internal medicine have had to face emergency cases in
> obstetrics, gynaecology, paediatrics and some other special-
> isation, and were unable to cope with the emergency. This is
> because students who specialise in one branch or department
> have not paid too much attention to other medical courses
> while still at medical school.(31)

It was suggested that courses become more practical:
'theoretical training should be shortened to four years and
practical training extended from half a year to one year'.(32)
This modest increase suggested by the Ministry could hardly
be called a revolutionary change. But leaders in medical education
were divided, with many pressing for a further raising of
theoretical standards. During the Hundred Flowers movement,
forums were held at Peking Union Medical College to discuss the
problem, and many discontents were aired:

> The professors thought that at present the *central* problem of

medical education was the contradiction between quality and
quantity . . . the students, due to the low education standards
in the middle schools, had a very poor foundation in foreign
languages, their knowledge of biology, chemistry and physics
is also extremely deficient.(33)

The specialists had much to say about the Ministry of
Health – they were extremely dissatisfied with the way the
Ministry had for the last few years only laid emphasis on the
development of medical establishments whilst ignoring the work
of medical education.(34)

The principal of the Medical College complained that 'Since
Liberation the students of Peking Medical College have increased
from 400 to 3,000, but there are only 700 beds in the attached
hospital',(35) and irritation was voiced by professors at the
college at the role of the Communist Party: 'Whilst the Party
committee members cannot cope with technical work, they refuse
to learn or rely on specialist advice.'(36)
Medical colleges still possessed a good deal of influence over
their own curricula. At Hunan medical college both English and
Russian were introduced into the course.(37) There were
suggestions that dental education should have five-year instead
of four-year courses.(38) Doctors who were deputies at the
National People's Congress that summer proposed six-year
medical courses instead of the current five-year ones.(39)
Unfortunately, the graduates who were being produced 'prefer
to work in large hospitals and express no interest in working
in remote regions or small clinics'.(40)
In August 1957 the Ministry of Health placed the elite Peking
Union Medical College under its 'leadership', and increased the
college's research grants and equipment. The following year a
new elite medical course opened in Peking, at Union Medical
College, which was renamed the New China Medical College. Its
eight-year course with three years of basic sciences, two years
to basic medical knowledge, two years of clinical medicine and
one year of field work with compulsory language courses in
English and Russian(41) seemed designed to satisfy all professional complaints. The problem was that such a course would
take a long time to train only a few students. From 1950 to 1958
the increase of medical graduates was 223 per cent compared
with an increase of 438 per cent in other scientific fields. Yet
in 1958, with an enrolment of 49,100, of whom 40 per cent were
women, the number of medical schools increased fourfold to
159 with courses in many higher medical schools of six years or
longer.(42) It seemed clear that in matters of higher education
the emphasis remained on a longer training even if the theoretical
content had been reduced, but an attempt was also being made
to meet demands for expansion while retaining high quality.
Expansion in this sector of medical education showed the
greatest number of students being admitted since Liberation.

Those in charge of higher medical education and research were 'left to their own devices', and some top schools increased the length of their courses. By 1959 the prestigious New China Medical College was removed from the Ministry 'leadership' it had enjoyed two years previously and placed under the direct control of the Chinese Academy of Medical Sciences. Some concessions to the ideological principles of the Great Leap Forward were made by the higher medical educational institutions. More students of peasant or worker background were admitted, students and staff worked in mobile medical teams and manual labour was introduced into the curriculum. One graduate of Wuhan Medical College described this:

Each student had to work for two months as a manual labourer. One month was spent in collective labour - a whole class was sent somewhere to work together - and the second month was made up of separate weekly assignments until a full month's working hours had been put in.(43)

*Middle and lower-level medical education*
Were developments at the higher level balanced by expansion at the intermediate and lower levels? Secondary-level institutions were by no means immune from the criticisms about quality that had bedevilled the medical colleges. There are clear signs of attempts to rectify the position by the provincial administrations in China, since these secondary medical schools were their responsibility. Numbers of teachers were increased(44) and some were sent for further training to attend spare-time courses at higher medical schools.(45)

The Great Leap Forward of 1958 led to an increase in the number of students graduating from intermediate schools. At the end of 1959 it was claimed there were over 800 medical schools with an enrolment of 240,000 students (cf. the 49,600 in higher medical schools). There were also approximately 130,000 intermediate-level doctors, more than double the number in 1950, and the number of colleges had increased sevenfold.(46)

This great expansion was an essential part of the Great Leap Forward, and the attempts at rapid industrialisation launched by Mao. Whilst higher-level medical education appeared to be moving away from the service needs of the health care system, towards the creation of a highly trained specialist group, the overall medical education policy was described as 'walking on two legs',

that is, using at the same time both traditional Chinese medicine and modern medical methods, promoting at the same time medical education at institutions of higher learning, secondary and vocational levels, encouraging both regular and spare-time training as well as full-time and part-time training.(47)

*People's Communes and mobile teams*
The major development in health care organisation during the
Great Leap Forward was the formation of People's Communes,
which were self-supporting units based on the collective
ownership of land. The communes operated their own self-
financed basic medical units, supported by the county hospitals.

A curious historical development which began during the
Great Leap Forward linked together the most prestigious medical
schools with the organisational innovations in health care on
the communes. While medical colleges were left to pursue their
courses and carry out research, a contrary movement involved
students and teachers in visiting the countryside and training
paramedical workers. Workers thus trained were the forerunners
of the world-famous 'barefoot doctors', just as the doctors and
students foreshadowed the mobile medical teams of the Cultural
Revolution.

In 1958, 10,000 doctors, nurses and other medical personnel
from Shanghai went down to the countryside to train health
workers from production brigades.(48) From Hunan medical
college 17,000 students and other personnel arrived in the
People's Communes. In one month they trained 13,000 child-care
workers and health workers.

> Some 2,500 teachers and students of the Hunan Medical College
> were organised . . . working with local medical workers, more
> than thirty medical personnel in Chenki county carried out
> a health check on commune members. . . . The medical
> students have all gained knowledge of preventing and curing
> local diseases.(49)

Throughout 1959-60 an estimated 300,000 medical workers
went to the countryside.(50) Their job was not simply to train
paramedical workers but to provide medical care where little had
existed before. The 'sector' style of health care organisation in
the cities (where a particular hospital took responsibility for
a particular area of the city) was transposed to the rural areas:
'In 1957 each college adopted a particular area as its base for
all activities, including teaching and scientific research closely
combined with production.'(51)

*Summary*
The years 1956-9 were dramatic ones for China, and medical
education was greatly affected. Policies which stressed the
'quality' approach to higher education were continued, but the
medical professional interests, which had been outspoken at
the beginning, no longer dominated the scene; those in charge
of universities maintained their position but their views no
longer shaped the entire field of medical education. Expansion
of other areas of medical training, blocked in previous years,
was able to occur because of a brief economic upturn. In fact
the greatest expansion was at intermediate levels. Thus for a

short period all styles of medical education - walking on two legs - were maintained. Intermediate levels were locally financed, while the university sector was the responsibility of central government. When economic disasters hit locally-based health care systems, intermediate and lower levels suffered while the university medical schools remained insulated.

## 1960-4 PROLOGUE TO THE CULTURAL REVOLUTION

*Higher level medical education*
Mao's prestige suffered somewhat after what were perceived as the economic disasters of the Great Leap Forward. It seems that he was no longer in a strong enough position to push for more attention to be paid to rural health care when the communes themselves were on the brink of disaster. In higher-level medical education the intake of schools fell back from the 'high' of the Great Leap Forward, suggesting that more stringent entrance requirements were being applied. The political content of the curriculum was reduced. Levels of academic work were also intensified. In one revealing account of a 'model' party secretary from Shanxi Medical College, the role of the Party in attempting to influence the style of the curriculum - usually in the direction of reducing hours spent on basic medical sciences - is delicately portrayed:

> Some students told him [the Party Secretary] 'Several lessons are taught in one session, so how can we digest what we are taught unless we read during the midday break?' He learned that the principal aspect of the contradiction had to do with faculty members . . . some faculty members said: 'Anatomy and chemistry are big subjects. How can the students learn them properly unless we teach more about them, assign more home work and conduct more tests?' Others said 'Parasitology and physiology, which are small subjects, are given so little attention that any further reduction will cause them to be completely displaced.' Immediately Li Kuei-jung's mind was lit up. He said to himself 'So this is the trouble.'(52)

Despite Party attempts at course modification, the length of medical courses was actually *extended*, with the objective of producing a six-year course in all medical schools. According to one account, all except one of the higher medical schools was running a six-year course.(53) Applications to medical schools far exceeded the number of places available with about one in thirty applicants being accepted. There are varying accounts of the class background of entrants. According to one report, the majority of university medical students were the sons and daughters of well-educated parents.(54) Another observer suggested that 'students from "worker background" number about 80 per cent of the total medical students. This however does not give too clear a picture because many children of intellectuals are also included in the "worker" class category.'(55)

All the conventional subjects were taught in the curriculum, but factory and public health work received no mention, and it has been suggested that public health work was the destination of those college graduates who failed their final examination.(56)

Compulsory manual labour was still part of the course, although in some cases (e.g. Shanghai No. 1 Medical College) it was slightly reduced from two to one and a half months,(57) and the focus in subsequent placements after graduation was towards hospitals of medium to large urban centres. This emphasis coincided with the combined objectives of both profession and Ministry bureaucracy to improve and consolidate the work of urban hospitals, a move which was supported by non-Maoist elements in the Party leadership.

Generally the political stance of doctors, students and medical educators appeared of less importance than their abilities. The 'redness versus expertness' equation was definitely weighted on the side of the expert in the majority of cases.

Between 1960 and 1964 about 84,000 students graduated from higher medical colleges, compared with 31,093 between 1956 and 1960. The increase was due to the expansion of higher medical education during the Great Leap Forward. The numbers of college-trained graduates were still considerably less than those of intermediate doctors, but the proportions changed, due to a decline in the numbers of intermediate-level doctors (see below). Overall the number of university medical colleges was reduced from the 142 that had existed at the height of the Great Leap Forward to 98 by 1963.(58) This suggests that admissions to medical schools were reduced (even though classes may have been slightly bigger) despite the increased number of graduates coming 'on stream' as a result of expansion in the late 1950s. In higher medical education, therefore, there was a tendency to contract, and emphasise lengthy specialist training and research, especially that which matched the highest levels of Western science and technology. This was combined with an urban bias in the distribution of university-trained graduates.

The growth of provincial university medical colleges meant that graduates of the most elite medical colleges in Beijing and Shanghai were most likely to remain in their own cities, and not be transferred: 'In Taiguan, for example, one doctor reported that only one girl from Peking, and two from Shanghai, have been assigned to that area in three years, the rest being graduates of Shansi province.'(59) Roughly 30 per cent of graduates from the higher-level colleges went to jobs in the countryside:(60) in real terms this meant an input into the rural areas during the early 1960s of some 28,000 Western-trained doctors for a rural population of some 600 million.

County and commune hospitals in remote areas may be staffed by a graduate of a regular medical course assisted by one or two 'middle doctors' and a few untrained nurses whom he is responsible for teaching. More often they have no medical graduate at all. On the other hand the majority of staff in urban hospitals are regular medical graduates, with experienced Western-trained doctors in charge and 80 per cent of the nurses are fully trained.(61)

*Middle-level medical education*
If the years 1960-4 witnessed a contraction in higher-level medical education, the training of intermediate level doctors presents a more complicated picture. Subsequent Red Guard publications claimed a 50 per cent drop in the total number of graduates produced over the period from 280,000 in 1961 to 40,000 by 1964.(62) The drop was probably not so great, however, since the first figure was an estimate of the total number of intermediate-level doctors produced between 1949 and 1960 (and an overestimate of 30,000 at that) compared with the numbers produced between 1961 and 1964.(63) It is difficult to judge whether the contraction in the intermediate level was as great as suggested. A recomputation of figures which Cheng has derived from official publications suggests that the real drop did not take place until about 1963-4; and that 1962 witnessed a level of production of middle-level graduates at least as great as that of the years since 1959.(64)

At first there were attempts at 'raising standards' which continued the efforts of the Great Leap Forward in the intermediate schools but these suffered the same setbacks as beset rural health care programmes. The fall-off in training may have been partly due also, as Lampton suggests, to a reduction in demand for the services of intermediate doctors,(65) either because of a total reduction in facilities, or because better qualified doctors were likely to be the first choice when funds were restricted.

The picture at one county health school in Shaanxi illustrates some of these points:

In 1960, in attempting to make the school an instrument of bourgeois dictatorship, some of the leading members of the Administrative Region Party Committee . . . condemned the school as 'irregular' and 'black' and forced it to change its period of schooling to five years and its curriculum according to bourgeois models. In 1962 they flagrantly closed the school down altogether.(66)

Cutbacks in intermediate-level education were probably not as great as has been supposed. According to one source the number of middle-level medical colleges seems to have increased from 100 in 1964 to 230 in 1965.(67) However, the proportion of intermediate-level graduates relative to higher-level graduates continued to fall through 1960-4. Whereas the ratio in 1960 was roughly three to one, by 1964 it was about two to one.(68)

Despite this, Cheng suggests that the gap between the demand and supply for intermediate level manpower was closing and that the deficiency was declining.(69) It is possible to argue on the basis of this that the cutbacks in training programmes were a rational response, given financial constraints, to the fairly satisfactory growth in this area, resulting from the expansion of the late 1950s.

*Lower-level medical personnel*
Lower-level medical personnel - paramedical workers - had first reached prominence during the Great Leap Foward, and their inception was linked with the development of the communes, and the system of health care financing which to a large extent committed the communes to their employment, and the counties to their short practical training. The idea was to ensure that there were adequate numbers of health personnel for the rural areas, but by 1961 it seemed that this attempt was to be super-seded by the creation of mobile teams of doctors from urban centres and medical schools who visited the countryside to provide medical assistance, and to teach lower and intermediate-level medical personnel.

> The Second Hospital of the Kiangsu Medical College organised two medical teams to serve commune members in rural areas. During the past two months, those teams performed more than seventy surgical operations.(70)

> A group of professors, lecturers, doctors and senior-grade students of the Changshan Medical Institute were recently organised into two groups for medical work in the country-side.(71)

With increasing numbers of higher- and intermediate-level personnel becoming available, the overall demand for lower-level personnel may have declined. The collapse of co-operatively financed health care in the communes meant that they were now an expensive and inferior source of medical manpower. As one later report put it:

> In August 1961 the agents of China's Kruschev made a sinister report, viciously smearing the health workers in production brigades and ordering them to stop work. This new public health force, created during the Great Leap Forward, was then destroyed. In Shen Mu County the number of health workers declined from 3,900 in 2,500 production brigades in 1958 to 300 by 1961.(72)

At the time it seemed that, since communes might not be able to support them, their expansion should not be encouraged.
In the rural areas, what health care remained available tended to be at county level, and it was here that State resources were

concentrated. Consequently the demand for lower-level, partly skilled personnel was less, and decisions about resources tended in the direction of improving the fabric and equipment of county hospitals and providing better services to patients rather than training individuals, especially at the lower levels. Hospital conditions were bad:

> only a dilapidated shed used as a horse-treating station and with three huts that could collapse at any time. The weed around the huts was knee-deep, and the place was infested with mosquitoes and flies. It became a marsh in the rainy season.(73)

As one disgruntled patient remarked: 'Even the lavatory of the army hospital I once stayed in was better than your hospital.'(74)

*Summary*
The policies of medical education during the period 1960-4 represent a change from those pursued during the Great Leap Forward. Later commentaries during the Cultural Revolution would suggest that reactionary groups in the leadership had taken advantage of the country's economic difficulties in 1961-2 to pursue their own particular direction, but it would appear that their actions were not so much full-scale deliberate policies as a response to a situation which had already been created over the previous few years. Medical graduates at the highest level continued to be encouraged, those at the intermediate level appeared plentiful also, but their number was not increasing; basic-level health personnel declined in numbers because of the concentration of facilities at county hospitals.

Contrasted with the Great Leap Forward, the period is one of contraction and retrenchment. Economic difficulties were bound to produce some cuts, but their direction and impact might have been greater if a previous situation of expansion had not prevailed. The problems of providing an adequate system of health care to the rural areas had not been solved during the Great Leap Forward, nor were they, despite the creation of a hospital in every county and a clinic in every commune by 1965, ended during this period. By 1965 the whole question of rural health care became a cause célèbre, and this fundamentally altered the nature of events.


THE CULTURAL REVOLUTION, 1965-70

Why was medical education one of the first areas to be subjected to radical attacks by Mao in his bid to bend the system and style of government to what he thought to be appropriate for China? Mao's prestige and power were still far greater than those of any other person in the Chinese leadership, and in retrospect it seems that the key to understanding the situation lies not so much in the triumph of one set of policies over another (for indeed although differences existed between Mao and the Ministry of Health on many issues, divisions were fewer), but in *who* should determine policy. In other words, a political struggle was emerging, transforming and deepening policy splits and, in Mao's actions at least, asserting the differences which existed between himself and certain elements of the Party and state bureaucracy, in this case the Ministry of Health.

During the period preceding the Cultural Revolution modest expansion in health care had taken place despite serious financi strictures. However, the problem was, as acknowledged by bot Mao and everyone else, a problem of maldistribution of health care resources between urban and rural sectors which was only slowly being resolved.

What was a rural area and what was an urban area? Was a county town an urban centre in the way that a provincial capita might be? Clearly the current policy of the Ministry which had sought to place the level of resources at county level need not necessarily be interpreted as an 'urban-based' policy. The most important thing about it was that it was a policy which ensured control by the Ministry of facilities and training. Any devolution below that level would certainly shift the balance of power away from central to local control, thus disturbing Ministry plans to consolidate a national standard of health care. Mao's interest lay almost solely in rural health services, and his belief was tha medical education policies were insufficient to meet rural health needs. In his view problems of maldistribution of medical personnel could be solved if courses were shortened and new graduates sent to the countryside. Research and the development of highly trained doctors was less important than the pressing health needs of the rural areas. He outlined a plan for solving the problems of rural health care in broad terms. After castigating the Ministry of Health as a 'Ministry of Urban Gentle men's health' he went on:

> In medical education there is no need to accept only higher middle school graduates, or lower middle school graduates. It will be enough to give three years to graduates from primary schools. They would then study and raise their standards mainly through practice. If this kind of doctor is sent down to the countryside, even if they haven't much talent they would be better than quacks and witchdoctors and the villages would be better able to afford to keep them. The more a person studies, the more foolish he becomes. (75)

Mao criticised the direction of medical work which was using scarce resources

in the study of rare, profound and difficult diseases, while

there was 'little effort to study how to prevent and improve
the treatment of commonly seen, frequently occurring and
widespread diseases' . . . I am not saying we should ignore
the pinnacles, but only a small quantity of manpower and
material should be expended on them . . . we should leave
behind in the city a few of the less able doctors who graduated
one or two years ago, the rest should all go to the countryside. . . . In medicine and health work, put the stress on
the rural areas.(76)

Such a major speech had an effect. The Ministry of Health
immediately held an important meeting to discuss it with top
Ministry cadres. The conclusion (unavoidable in the circumstances) was that they had made serious errors in neglecting
the needs of the countryside but mistakes, they maintained,
were sins of omission rather than commission. Following Mao's
speech the transfer of medical personnel was stepped up
rapidly, so that by September 1965 in Guangdong province
alone 6-7,000 doctors from hospitals at and above the 'xian'
(county) level were sent to the countryside.(77) The President
of the Chinese Academy of Medical Science who had led a team
to the countryside earlier in the year remarked 'we have begun
to open our eyes to the countryside and to understand our
peasants. Living and working among them we feel their great
worth and an urge to serve them well.'(78)

*Higher-level medical education*

*Curriculum changes and 'instant graduation'*   The January
conference of the Ministry of Health (held before Mao's June
declaration) was already responding to the political changes in
the air.
   Criticisms were growing of the abstract nature of medical
education, and these focused upon its inefficiency, in an attempt
to alter it in the direction of something more appropriate. In
Beijing 'the fundamental course was comparatively theoretical
in nature. The teachers formally explained lessons abstractly
in a manner difficult to understand.'(79)
   By March radical changes in examination methods were being
announced. Take-home papers were allowed, for 'there are no
ready-made answers in books'.(80) The most important immediate
change was that many students who were in medical college were
graduated and sent to the countryside, others who had enrolled
in 1964 or 1965 spent two years in their college, for they were
still in training in 1966. One informant said that he did not
complete the full five-year course at his medical college but
was graduated in 1967 after three years of study.(81) 'Two
thirds of the students who have graduated from Szechwan
medical college in recent years have gone to work in the rural
areas.'(82)
   At this stage, it was still possible to promise: 'Those who have

worked for two to three years in rural hospitals can apply for periods of advanced study, or post-graduate courses in big city hospitals.'(83)

The actual content of curricula was difficult to define, but what does seem clear is that the elite institutions, the major medical colleges, were going to hold out against these changes as long as possible. At a conference in September called by the Ministry of Health it was concluded that: colleges and universities 'should produce medical workers who take a firm political stand and are technically expert. *Long and short courses must be established*. The experiments of some medical schools [in sending students to the countryside and shortening courses] deserve to be imitated.'(84)

Speaking of Beijing Medical College, a top party cadre announced that 'The 8-year system of the Medical University shall go on . . . from now on it is not permitted to discuss the question as to whether it should go on or not,'(85) and the President of the Chinese Academy of Medical Sciences said 'since most of the things in the original curriculum should still be maintained, how can the number of academic years be reduced?'(86)

In 1966 attempts were still being made to retain and improve the five- and six-year courses at medical schools,(87) and it was argued: 'a political instructor can teach Marxism Leninism, but cannot remove a tumour from a patient's body'.(88)

*The closure of higher-level schools*   In the summer of 1966 the majority of medical schools were closed. One informant tells what happened:

> When the Red Guards first came to our medical school in 1966 we did not want to pay them much attention. We just wanted to get on with our studies. They were from Canton, I think. *They were not even medical students* [my emphasis]. They wanted us to make some criticism, make big posters and so forth and criticise our professors. We did not want to do this because we loved our teachers. But later in the year we did do this. One or two of the older professors were criticised. Some of our students did support all this. I didn't. I was in the middle, but I didn't want to say anything. Then the college was closed. No one was killed, but some people, some teachers, were beaten. . . .(89)

Power had effectively moved from the state and Party bureaucracy to Mao and his supporters. The situation in the medical schools, some of which were controlled by Red Guards, others by revolutionary 'work teams', others by curious coalitions of the former and sympathetic teachers and cadres,(90) was such that courses could not be held; students stayed for political discussion and 'struggle' meetings. The Ministry of Health was itself invaded by Red Guard students, who demanded that con-

fidential files be made available to them. Unsuccessful attempts
were made by senior cadres to moderate the behaviour of the
students at a forum held before an audience of medical students
at the leadership compound Zhongnanhai, Beijing.

Tao Ju, member of the reception centre of the Party Central
Committee delegated to deal with Red Guards arriving in Peking,
said:

> I went to talk with several students and a dispute ensued
> over the question of allowing Ch'ien Hsin Chung to hand over
> the data [i.e. secret Ministry of Health files]. I said: 'Your
> demand for data is revolutionary, and it is quite right that
> we support you, but the data are not returned to the Ministry
> of Health.' At that point in the meeting Vice-Premier Chen I
> interrupted angrily: 'snatching is wrong and things must not
> be snatched'.(91)

Students criticised the nature of their medical course. Writing
on the course at Beijing Medical University they said:

> The three-year pre med course was vaunted as 'an outstanding
> feature'. The 8-year course provided excellent conditions for
> the careful and painstaking grooming of the bourgeois of
> their own successors. Students were made to study the same
> courses in biology and chemistry as those taught in the depart-
> ments of biology and chemistry. In practice it is not necessary
> for doctors to learn so much about maths, physics and
> chemistry. Moreover they are forgotten as soon as the students
> leave the pre med stage. Students read many books and
> attend many lectures but have few opportunities of dealing
> with patients . . . having studied so long behind closed
> doors their minds are full of foreign rules and dead dogma.
> Practice is carried out according to specialties . . . the pro-
> longed seven--year course greatly impairs the health of
> students. The students study nothing relevant to medicine
> the first year, go nowhere near the hospital the second year,
> do nothing in connection with a patient in the third and
> fourth years and merely view him in the fifth year. In the
> eighth year students are placed on a 24 hour responsibility
> system. They are shut up in hospital wards day and night
> tirelessly practising the so-called 'basic skills'.(92)

*Medical students in the rural areas*
Nevertheless, sufficient organisation existed to oversee the
transfer of medical students to the countryside. At Dazhai,
Shaanxi province:

> No building was specially erected for the school. Four caves
> dug into the loess hillside served as classrooms, dormitory
> and kitchen. Since there was no blackboard, the students and
> teachers made makeshift ones with wooden boards from their

beds. Cardboard boxes are used as desks. In this way the
school was opened without spending a cent.(93)

In Hebei, 1,400 teachers and students from the medical school
went to the countryside, despite hostile comments that:

In the rural areas where there are no instruments and equipment how can you carry out teaching practice . . . where
roads are difficult and you may not see a single patient for
days, how can you learn? In the rural areas you will be part
farmers, part physicians. Can you regard yourselves as
college students?(94)

A wash basin used as a steriliser. Child delivery was carried
out in a bamboo reclining chair. They did not spend a single
penny of state funds in building up a laboratory, an operating room and several wards.(95)

Obeying Chairman Mao's teaching that 'working is studying
. . . some first-year students could independently examine
patients and treat diseases commonly found in the countryside'.
Experiences were salutary: 'They soon found that seven out
of the ten prescriptions [they gave] were not taken to the
pharmacy but were pasted on the wall by peasants.'(96)
  Costly prescriptions for Western medicine were out of the
question - cheaper traditional methods were necessary, and this
required a reorientation of medical education towards a greater
consideration of traditional methods. Medical education was
described as 'essentially practical'. When presented with a badly
scalded child, the students consulted their textbooks, in which
it was stated that the patient should be put in a germ-free
room and treated with ultra-violet rays. 'The angry students
threw the book away saying "what we have learned in the past
cannot be used".'(97)
  By 1968 new plans were drafted for three-year courses in
medical education, and new admission policies decided upon.(98)
Medical colleges were to enrol 'barefoot doctors and health
workers', and those who were recommended by their work units
as suitable. There was to be no entrance examination, and direct
admission from school was to be disallowed.


POST-REVOLUTIONARY DEVELOPMENTS -
'BACK TO THE CITIES'

By 1969 the Cultural Revolution was in its downturn. Revolution
ary committees had been set up at all levels of government, and
in the factories, schools and universities. These organisational
units were backed by the Army who had been brought in to
reinforce law and order and contain what were viewed as more
extreme revolutionary elements. The consequence of such

changes for medical education was that schools and colleges
began to readmit students, and by 1970 were beginning courses
once again.

At the outset of the Cultural Revolution Mao had demanded
that half of the staff of urban hospitals and colleges should
go to the countryside. In effect, about a third finally went,(99)
but even this left the urban hospitals and medical colleges
depleted. The medical colleges, in reopening courses, began to
stress the need for urban as well as rural teaching material. At
Jilin Medical University, the college authorities declared that:

> it is also necessary to appropriately integrate the college or
> university *with the city* in accordance with the teaching and
> learning needs of students. . . . In our opinion, a teaching
> force should remain in the university headquarters for guiding
> the teaching and learning companies and carrying out research
> on doubtful and difficult cases of disease and on essential
> high level, difficult and advanced items. The university head-
> quarters is not only the command headquarters for the teach-
> ing and learning companies but also the base area for making
> improvements.(100)

The major medical colleges were among the first to begin
courses, but in addition were running courses in their rural
bases to train intermediate medical workers whose development
is discussed below.

*Intermediate and lower-level medical workers*

*Lower-level specialists* At the September 1965 conference on
medical education it was decided to set up large numbers of
secondary medical schools in the rural areas. These colleges
included the conventional middle-level colleges which have been
discussed, but also, 'spare-time' colleges, where students
studied from six to eight hours per week. Central China had
twenty-one such colleges, with small intakes of fifty students.(101)
Students in intermediate colleges and spare-time colleges were
expected to do physical labour in factories and communes, and
attend their courses in the evenings. The courses lasted three
to five years.(102)

Courses were also instituted for various technical specialists
- X-ray, dentistry, 'tumour recognition' - for the so-called
'xian doctors'. These were graduates of intermediate-level
schools, who still formed the majority of county hospital staff.
Some intermediate medical personnel including nurses were also
promoted to senior posts, and others allowed to continue to
higher education.(103)

Two model peasant health workers were described in the
national press:

> One is a 1963 graduate from a hsien medical school who had a

three-year course of medical study and farm work. He is in charge of the health of five hundred peasants. He stays a farmer. The second a middle-school graduate is in charge of her brigade's team of three. Her knowledge comes from the evening courses which the commune health centre provides for all village personnel. They are at once physical labourers and guardians of the people's health. It is true that they lack advanced theoretical knowledge, but they will make progress through practical work. The important thing is that they have the honest desire to serve the peasants.(104)

By the end of 1965 these conventional intermediate-level 'xian' courses were being reduced from four to three years, and the curriculum included an increased amount of traditional medicine.(105) Where there was a substantial amount of manual labour, as in the model Jiangxi courses, they remained four years in length.

They [the students] spent four to six months annually helping with farm work. [There is] one year of elementary medicine when students work in hospitals as assistant nurses doing various odd jobs. They do one and a half years more advanced study on endemic local diseases, and work as assistant doctors and members of medical teams. They also work one and a half years as hospital interns.(106)

The major medical colleges – Beijing and Shanghai – opened combined farming and study colleges for three-year courses and enrolled 'middle school graduates from local peasant families'.(107) At the same time 'millions of volunteers are being trained in the communes to popularise hygiene and health knowledge'.(108)

In addition over one million of these peasant health workers, forerunners of the barefoot doctors, were trained rapidly in one- to three-month courses at county hospitals. As well as the inter- mediate doctors, a new type of health worker was beginning to emerge.(109)

*Barefoot doctors – lower-level generalists*   One of the functions of the medical teams sent to the countryside was the training of rural medical workers, both intermediate doctors and bare- foot doctors. The entire strategy of mobile medical teams and part-time schools employed from 1965 onwards can be seen as a massive subsidy of manpower for training and treatment, given by the urban areas to the rural areas. Even the smallest 'xian' was required to transfer personnel to the new focus of health care – the commune, and within the commune the brigade. Since, however, the transference of personnel from urban areas was not sufficient to solve the problem of the rural areas, generating a medical health care system manned by and financed by those selfsame rural areas appears to have been an extremely imagin- ative and efficient solution to the problems of rural health care.

Thus the 'barefoot doctors' came into being.

The term 'barefoot doctor' was first used around 1968 to describe the large numbers of peasant physicians being trained.
A flexible approach towards training has usually characterised
the health care system of China. However, the concept of a
part-time health worker working in his or her own native
commune was an original one. It is not known who was actually
responsible for this policy. A report in 1966 records the first
details of barefoot doctors:

> A new type of peasant physician who is both a medical worker
> and a peasant is coming into being in every part of China.
> With the current campaign to extend the medical services . . .
> group after group of city doctors have been going into the
> countryside and large numbers of graduates of city medical
> colleges have been assigned to work in county hospitals or
> commune clinics. *But this is only part of the answer* and in
> order to ensure that adequate medical and health services
> become available to peasants everywhere part-study part-
> farming secondary medical schools are being set up to train
> secondary medical personnel amongst the peasants locally.

> The teachers are the doctors of the hospital and the students
> are all young commune members who have completed their
> courses at junior middle school.(110)

This described the barefoot doctors almost completely, failing
only to mention that potential candidates are chosen by their
communes and their wages derived from work points paid by the
brigade. Methods of training differed in length, and were
carried out in three-month sessions which accumulated a total
training of between eighteen to thirty months. By 1968 it
looked as if the training period might become shorter and that
'barefoot doctors' was a term increasingly used to describe
many types of basic local worker. From this time onward the
role of the mobile team diminished while that of the barefoot
doctor was augmented. It is not known how rapidly the number
of barefoot doctors increased after the first reports of June
1966, but by 1968 the suburban communes around Shanghai
had about 6,000 barefoot doctors, an average of 1.8 per
production brigade. The Shanghai barefoot doctors were themselves in charge of training an 'underforce' of 25,000 volunteer
health workers.(111)

*The new rural health infrastructure*   The expansion of rural
health services which had taken place included a hospital in
every one of China's 2,500 rural counties, and a hospital or
clinic in each commune. The former were financed by the state,
but the latter by production brigades in the communes who
contributed to a welfare fund. The brigades themselves sometimes
had small clinics as well, depending upon how wealthy they were.

County hospitals employed a few high-level graduates or
rusticated veteran doctors who had been sent to the countryside
The majority of their staff were intermediate-level graduates.
In rare cases commune hospitals also had graduate medical
staff, but more usually intermediate-level doctors, and traditiona
doctors. These were supplemented by a force of barefoot
doctors, some of whom would be based in the commune hospital,
others at brigade clinics, and occasionally at production team
level. In addition, volunteer health workers, who would work
occasionally in sanitation campaigns, also existed. The patient/
barefoot doctor ratio varied considerably from commune to
commune. In some a barefoot doctor was in charge of several
brigades – that is up to 3,000 people. In others he or she had
general responsibility for the twenty or so families of a production team.

This expansion of services required staffing, which accounts
for a departure, by the late 1960s, from the original barefoot
doctor model to include many kinds of workers, and also a change
in the type of responsibility. Originally the barefoot doctor was
seen as the basic general health worker, and as a link in the
referral chain, but by 1969-70 the feats of barefoot doctors in
'performing difficult and advanced surgery' were lauded, and
their efforts seen as equal, even superior, to that of college-
trained doctors. At first their popularity was based on their
willingness to serve the peasants, and their accessibility as
'little red doctors', but later it was held that their strength lay
in the reliability of their political outlook and their practical
close contact with their patients. The original commune clinic
training of 1965-6 had, it was stated, led to 'bourgeois ideas'
among barefoot doctors.

> Some purchased a thick volume that cost nine yuan a copy
> and showed off by carrying it round with them in villages.
> Some of the barefoot doctors were unwilling to be barefoot
> any longer but were keen to become city doctors in white
> smocks.(112)

When training was reduced in some areas to a two-month
'training class' which included much political study, including
that of the 'three constantly read articles',(113) together with
'the teaching of medical skills closely related to the problems
of the area,' the resultant barefoot doctors were, it was
suggested, far superior either to previous models, or to the
college graduates:

> There was one doctor who claimed to have studied for some
> twenty years in school, but he once mistook appendicitis for
> ordinary gastroenteritis. The disease became worse and
> peritonitis resulted because treatment was delayed. A bare-
> foot doctor was then fetched who immediately made the correct
> diagnosis and saved the patient's life.(114)

Modifications also took place in the recruitment of barefoot doctors. Although the original idea was 'from the commune back to the commune', there is evidence that barefoot doctors did not always come from communes. Indeed, some were educated youths from the cities, sent to the countryside.(115) Yet others from the cities volunteered to become barefoot doctors, as a means of ensuring themselves a place at medical school later.(116)

By 1970 the barefoot doctors were a well-established fact of rural health care. Supported and financed by production brigades, they were undertaking a large proportion of basic health work, so that about only 10 per cent of cases were referred upwards. Their training and skills were variable, but in general they provided a cheap, effective and efficient means of closing the rural-urban gap.

*Higher medical education policies 1970-6*

*Changes in curricula*  By 1970 courses at university medical schools were beginning to start again. They were short, only three years in length. A specimen curriculum employed at the Beijing Medical College has been provided by Dimond(117) and the content stressed the requirements of rural health care - how to treat common diseases without the aid of sophisticated equipment; how to analyse stool specimens for parasitic ova; how to obtain clean drinking water, treat trachoma, and carry out surgery in primitive conditions. Dimond notes that nine months of the students' three years were to be spent in the countryside, twelve months in the city doing basic medical sciences, studying preventive and traditional medicine, six months in clinical training, and seven months in manual labour.

No entry examinations were held and barefoot doctors were favoured entrants,(118) although they should have reached junior middle-school level. Students had to be of worker, peasant or soldier origin, and be recommended by the unit or commune. Sixty per cent of the entrants in Beijing in 1970 were women, and 80 per cent were barefoot doctors.(119) Although the details of curricula varied in various medical schools - time in the countryside ranging from nine to twelve months, basic medical sciences ranging from four months in Beijing to twelve months in Tianjin - the emphasis on rural health matters and manual labour was about the same. The major medical colleges were the ones where political struggles had been the greatest, and their abolition as centres of elite medicine and professional power by the new entry requirements was a definite political move, which reflected the attitude of the Maoists towards the allocation of university places.

Students who had spent a long time in the countryside and who 'counted on their fingers the whole day long to figure out when they could go home',(120) were now able to make up membership of the large entry classes - 470 at Shenyang, 360 at Beijing, 500 at Tianjin, 350 at Zhongshan.(121)

*Open-door schooling*   Provincial health authorities now exerted
a degree of control over provincial medical colleges, but policies
varied depending on the degree of radical commitment of the
provincial government. In Lioaning province one third of the
provincial medical college was moved 'permanently' to the
countryside,(122) whereas in Guangdong, Zhongshan Medical
School's rural teaching base was tiny compared to the city
complex of five affiliated hospitals, one of a hundred beds.(123)
Nevertheless Zhongshan was described as being run 'with the
door open' with its rural teaching base providing opportunities
for students to work in the rural areas.(124) In Anhui the
medical college established 'five permanent bases and over thirty
temporary centres for training in the countryside'.(125)

*Mood of the medical colleges*   Apathy and fear characterised the
teachers in medical schools. Some had been severely criticised,
or sent to the countryside as a punishment. Many had been
made to undertake heavy manual labour for the first time in their
lives. Most had been forced to practise in conditions they would
ideally not have chosen. Although not everyone regarded this
as a bad experience, the Cultural Revolution had left some of
the older doctors with physical and psychological scars. As one
professor said: 'I'd rather sell bean curd than engage in
scientific research',(126) and another: 'When you commit a
blunder in teaching someone will grab you by the hair and shoot
you.'(127) Others said:

> since we are not clear how the revolution in medical education
> should be carried out and how universities should be run,
> it is better for us to wait and see. Let other fraternal colleges
> blaze the trail and it is not too late for us to act 'when the
> meal is prepared'.(128)

> In Chungshan Medical College, to encourage action, a student
> put up a dazibao [wall poster] bearing the title 'clinical
> teachers should get up!' Following this, a clinical doctor put
> up a dazibao saying 'It is not that we do not get up, but that
> the Party Committee of the hospital has not sounded the bell!'
> Seeing the poster, a deputy secretary of the Party Committee
> shook his head and said 'It is not that we do not sound the
> bell, but that the Party Committee of the college has not
> provided us with a bell.'(129)

Clearly, if the medical schools were to function successfully
this mood among the medical establishment would have to be
overcome!
    The people who now controlled the Ministry of Health had
achieved their positions during the Cultural Revolution. Since
they were directly under the control of the Politburo, and Mao
himself, any policy changes which implied a deviation from the
correct revolutionary line would render them politically suspect.

All the same, they were faced with the task of administering health services and overseeing training on a scale which was vast, even though much power and responsibility had now devolved to communes and brigades running their own medical services. Paradoxically, therefore, over-centralised control, as Lampton(130) points out, meant incomplete attention to many areas like research, or urban health care, and decisions on these were difficult to make. It follows, therefore, that medical schools, although in most senses far weaker than they were in 1960-4, still retained a measure of institutional strength and insulation. This, together with the necessary abilities of their staffs in clinical work and teaching, placed them in a relatively strong position to determine staffing and curricula.

*Political changes of the 1970s* In 1972 changes began to be felt in higher medical education. These coincided with a softening of anti-intellectual attitudes. One of the most important events was the return to his post of Qian Xinzhong, the Minister of Health who had been criticised and dismissed in 1967. He was a man known to be sympathetic to professional standards and research.

By the end of the same year over 80 per cent of senior professors, doctors and cadres of medical schools who had been sent for political re-education were rehabilitated.(131) At Zhongshan Medical College 'although the traditional influence of the bourgeoisie is strong, because the young teachers have no experience, it still needs the service of old teachers and has assigned seventy old teachers to leadership posts'.(132)

In the medical curriculum, there was talk of 'strengthening basic theoretical studies . . . work must proceed on a long-term basis, by a painstaking and careful manner'.(133)

Problems in the educational standard of those admitted to medical school was evidenced by the fact that schools began to introduce six-month 'preparatory' courses before the official one began. This had to be done cautiously:

> Acting on Chairman Mao's teaching . . . Sun Yat-sen Medical College (Chungshan) has changed from a six-year system to a three-year system. *With the addition of a six-month fundamental course* the total length of schooling now adds up to three and a half years.(134)

There were also 250 graduate students there in 1974.(135)

By 1975, however, political developments had reached the stage where the Maoist elements launched another attack on those in the Politburo, particularly Deng Xiaoping who had been rehabilitated. With the illness of Zhou En-lai (the protector of many an ageing cadre and the behind-the-scenes encourager of scientific research) and Mao as well, factions headed by the 'Gang of Four' tried to re-establish their interpretation of the Cultural Revolution line, in a bid to direct the future policies of

China. Protection and praise of the new medical graduates was part of this and a forceful defence of the 'new' short-course medical graduates was marshalled.

Second-year students are generally able to perform surgery on piles, fistula, appendix and hernia as well as diagnosing and treating common diseases.(136)

Their attitude to their work was devoted, their diagnostic skills superior, they were tireless in their work for patients, showed initiative in teaching, undertook dangerous procedures and intervened in serious cases to good effect.(137)

Despite these remarks, however, the curriculum continued to be modified in favour of greater amounts of study. Wen and Hayes (1975),(138) Dimond (1971)(139) and Roser (1977),(140) who collected data on the course at No. 2 Medical College Shanghai, all described courses of about three years. The writers, comparing 1971 and 1973 curricula, noticed a general decline in the amount of curriculum time devoted to manual labour and to political study. In the early 1970s the majority of graduates were expected to go to the countryside for permanent settlement, but by 1976 only half were assigned there.(141)
The undoubted benefit of the shortened course was that it produced graduates who were simply trained, more quickly. Although by no means ideal, the course found favour amongst the more pragmatic since these new graduates made good the shortfall of doctors which occurred when medical schools were closed - probably some 120,000.(142)

*Post-Mao developments in higher medical education*  In 1976, shortly after the death of Mao Zedong, the so-called Gang of Four were deposed from their positions of power, to be replaced by Hua Guofeng, and a reinstated Deng Xiaoping, a man committed to policies of modernisation. A nationwide movement to examine priorities in science and technology, industry, agriculture and national defence began. It was clear that medical curricula would once again be scrutinised to consider how far they were fulfilling national objectives. In a comment on the publication of volume V of Mao's works attention was drawn to his remarks that:

politics and professions form a unity of opposites in which politics is predominant and primary . . . but it won't do to confine oneself to politics and have no technical or professional knowledge. Our cadres in all trades and professions should strive to be proficient in their work and be both red and expert.(143)

Medical colleges began to enrol research graduates and Qian Xinzhong, speaking on his draft plan for medicine and health

at the 1978 National Science conference, emphasised that
research and new technology equipment would be provided to
raise China's medicine to advanced world levels.(144) The 'Chinese
Medical Journal' remarked 'study of basic medical sciences and
research on the fundamental problems of life and diseases cannot
be further delayed'.(145)

A visit to medical schools in 1978 evinced the knowledge that
courses at medical schools were being lengthened to five years
'because students lack basic theoretical knowledge'. Students
who expected to graduate in 1978 were being told to stay on for
another year's study, and there are reports of students being
withdrawn from long field assignments.(146) The courses as
from 1978 consisted of three(147) years' preclinical teaching
and two years' clinical training with four months' study of
traditional medicine. The elite medical course of the Chinese
Academy of Medical Sciences which also retained four months'
traditional medicine was once again eight years. At Guangzhou
No. 2 Medical School, students spent twelve weeks in the
countryside. For half the time they performed manual labour,
and for the other half worked as members of mobile teams or
alongside barefoot doctors or in the commune clinics. At
Sichuan Medical College it was reported that students performed
about eight weeks of manual labour during their entire four-
or five-year college courses.(148) In 1981 at Zhongshan when
asked about manual labour a student smiled and said 'one week
a year'.(149)

Multiple-choice examinations were held, and if a very high
mark was obtained, students were qualified earlier. A few went
on to post-graduate research or specialist training, but the
majority worked as general hospital doctors specialising in
medicine or surgery. Doctors applied for positions and were
assigned to them by the provincial health bureaux. 'If it was
psychiatry, I would be sad', remarked one student.(150)

In 1978 when entrance examinations were held, the pass mark
was lower for students of worker-peasant-soldier origin than
for high-school graduates who formed between 20 and 30 per
cent of the college entry.(151) The policy of admitting barefoot
doctors to higher-level medical schools was, by then, in abey-
ance, their admission to intermediate schools and special barefoot doctor training schools being more likely.(152)

Now, high entrance qualifications are required for medical
school students have to take six papers covering basic sciences
and English. One informant, a professor at a provincial medical
school, said 'When the results come out, Beijing has the first
choice. After they have "creamed off" those, we take the next
three hundred on the list.'(153)

*Numbers of higher-level graduates* Latest manpower statistics
from China suggest that the number of Western-trained
physicians is 447,000 compared with the 120,000 graduates of
1964.(154) As the first group would contain a greater proportion

of those born before Liberation, this suggests that, during the
years when colleges were open, an average of almost 30,000
graduates a year were being produced. This is more than the
number of graduates before the Cultural Revolution, but the
shorter course probably accounts for the difference in amount.
If the longer five-year course obtains, there should be some
temporary fall in numbers. There has been no call as yet to
increase the number of higher-level graduates. The assignment
of graduates to particular tasks is an important indicator of
whether the current situation distributes a greater number of
higher-level medical personnel towards the rural areas than
before the Cultural Revolution. We are told that roughly 100,000
medical workers had settled in the countryside between 1970
and 1976,(155) but what proportion were higher-level graduates
is unknown. Importantly, these 100,000, taken as a proportion
of the total number of Western-trained higher level and intermediate doctors, amount to less than one seventh of the total
of 781,930.(156) In 1973 in Jilin province, of the city medical
workers sent to the countryside less than 3 per cent settled
there.(157)

*Organisational changes and medical training*   The current change
in direction emphasises research and increases the demand for
higher-level graduates, but it remains to be seen whether the
failures of graduate distribution that occurred before the
Cultural Revolution will be repeated to the ultimate detriment
of the majority of Chinese - the rural population.

Recent suggestions for the reform of medical training seem
to consolidate the distinctions between the various types of
doctor. As well as improving training for barefoot doctors (see
below), three levels of medical training are envisaged. At the
top, it is suggested, should be the 'forty medical colleges and
universities established before 1958' who train 'doctors, teachers
and researchers of a still higher medical quality . . . the length
of schooling can be extended to six or eight years as suitable'.

Next come the 'doctors for prefectural hospitals and large
and medium-sized city hospitals' who study 'a five-year course',
and whose graduates 'should be guaranteed to have quite a
high standard of medical proficiency'.

At the third level come 'doctors for county hospitals' who
would be senior middle-school graduates with a three-year
course trained at provincial, municipal, autonomous regional
or prefectural hospitals. These trainees 'will be enrolled, trained
and employed locally, and that way they will feel at ease'.(158)

These distinctions spell out clearly the attempts being made
to reorganise, improve and rationalise medical training. What is
obvious is a complete departure from the fluidity of roles,
skills and training of the past ten years and a re-emphasis upon
different classes of doctor with different levels of skill. For
this to work for the maximum benefit of all the population, an
efficient and potentially costly system of referral of patients

from lower to higher levels will be necessary. Experience in
other parts of the world, especially Western countries, suggests
that different classes of doctor produce first-, second- and
third-class medicine, which operates to the detriment of those
for whom first-class services are not available. It seems clear
that although impressive steps have been taken toward the
provision of general medical care for rural areas, the bias in
favour of the cities will remain.

*Lower-level medical personnel*
In 1978 statistics released by the State Statistical Bureau to the
World Health Organisation put the number of 'feldsher' doctors
- the first time this Russian term has been used for many
years - at 423,410. Figures are also given for auxiliary personnel, technicians, nurses and midwives. The total number of
these amounts to 1,336,059.(159) However, there was no mention
in the list of barefoot doctors.

The omission of the barefoot doctors seems a matter worthy of
note: current Chinese estimates of numbers vary from 1.8 to
1.4 million. In 1970 there were, it was claimed, 1.1 million
barefoot doctors. Their employment was intimately tied to the
economic level of the commune. As part farmers, part paramedics,
their income was calculated from work points using the time rate
system, where points are allotted based upon the number of
days' work performed during the year. The barefoot doctors
also received fees for medicines and assistance at child delivery.
In some cases they made up a partial salary from these, or this
money helped payments for the work points credited to them
during the time they spent in health work, roughly one third
of the year.(160)

As early as 1971 criticisms of and by the barefoot doctors of
their levels of skill and conditions of work were voiced. In a
highly publicised letter to 'People's Daily' three barefoot doctors
suggested that hours of farm work and medical work needed to
be appropriately arranged and that barefoot doctors should be
guaranteeed to 'make no less' than other brigade members with
comparable skills and workload. These barefoot doctors noticed
the relatively high turnover of staff in some brigades due to
conditions of employment. Illness occurs at all times, and work
could sometimes be extremely exhausting for the conscientious
barefoot doctor. As well as attending to the sick, the job
included preventive work, and the cultivation of herbs for the
traditional medicines which form a substantial part of his or her
armamentarium.

The barefoot doctors were much praised in the beginning, and
their short one-year training, of which 50 per cent was practical
health work, seemed enough. First official criticism of the
training and style of rural medical work came when Fu Yichen,
deputy secretary general of the Chinese Medical Association,
visiting Toronto, said that as many as 80 per cent of the population living in the countryside rarely see a qualified physician

and were usually seen only by barefoot doctors.(161)

From the point of view of the medical profession's establishment, bare-foot doctors were certainly not the answer to rural health care problems. The CMA's views had not really changed since the 1950s, but the idea that enough graduate doctors could be produced to ensure that all Chinese had a qualified doctor available was unrealistic.

The Party leadership did not agree with the professionals. One section, the most radical faction, would definitely have supported barefoot doctors under any circumstances, mainly for ideological reasons. Another section, most closely allied with the Ministry of Health, supported the retention of the barefoot doctors for practical reasons. What worried them, therefore, was how to make the scheme work. They were concerned at levels of responsibility undertaken by barefoot doctors and the relationship between them and qualified physicians. 'Some people erroneously held that it was sufficient just to have the barefoot doctor and at one stage they neglected to give play to the role of professional staff.'(162)

This inevitably led to mistakes which were criticised. One barefoot doctor reported:

Once a young woman of No. 3 production brigade complained of an acute bellyache. Knowing that she had painful menstruation before, I mistakenly thought she was suffering from that ailment and gave her pills to kill the pain. Some three hours later her bellyache sharpened, I had no choice but to take her to the county hospital. A diagnosis revealed that she was suffering from peritonitis due to rupture of the appendix. A handful of class enemies declared provokingly. 'If a girl could cure a patient, a yellow cat would laugh 'til it's blind. . . . Doctors must be old. It isn't safe to let a young girl treat you.'(163)

The suggestion made by Deng in 1973 that barefoot doctors should 'go from barefoot to straw sandals, and from cloth shoes to leather shoes' and improve their training skills was, despite strong opposition from radicals, taken seriously, for worries existed about the viability of the barefoot doctor scheme, if they were unable to convince peasants that they were capable of adequate treatment.

Improving and lengthening training costs money, however. The model two-year course in Shenmu county, Shanxi province, consisted of one year's study and one year's agricultural work, which paid for the costs of administration, laboratory tests, tuition and the cook's wages.(164) The one million barefoot doctors, and three million 'sanitarians' existing by 1975 had generally emerged by this method which still seemed to make more economic sense. The tendency before Mao's death was still to stress the importance of practical training and criticise those barefoot doctors who 'always hope that they will put on white uniforms and mouth masks'.(165)

Of Qinghai province it was later said that 'the public health departments dared not devote energy to improving barefoot doctors' cultural and medical knowledge. The result was a sharp decline of this new thing, the barefoot doctors, and the closing down of most co-operative medical stations.'(166)

*New training schemes*   It seems that in response to criticisms barefoot doctor colleges began to be set up and the impression is that training was consolidated and made more systematic. Students received study work points from their brigades, and returned to them to do relatively small amounts of manual labour, and small amounts of health work during their two-year course.(167) By 1976 it was claimed that 'there are more than 1,100 barefoot doctor universities . . . some places have begun a system under which city doctors rotate their duties with barefoot doctors'. A cautionary note was sounded by radicals - 'these are good methods, but if we let them plunge headlong into vocational affairs in alienation from the actual class and like struggles, we will lead them astray'.(168)

After the fall of the Gang of Four in 1976, training and re-training proceeded apace without any such stricture. New text-books for barefoot doctors were brought out and in Qinghai ambitious plans 'to train barefoot doctors up to the level of secondary medical graduates in three years' were decided. In Guangdong it was planned to give all barefoot doctors advanced training by 1980(169) which again instituted the two levels of barefoot-doctor training which were originally envisaged at the outset of the Cultural Revolution. Barefoot doctors would be trained first at the commune hospital or county hospital. A selected proportion would later receive advanced training at medical school. It was also decided that at least one-third of barefoot doctors should be women with one female barefoot doctor in each production brigade.(170) Barefoot doctors were now clearly described as 'a *supplementary* force in rural medical service'.(171)

At the National People's Congress held in 1980 one of the resolutions passed was that the name 'barefoot doctor' should be changed, and since then the term has been replaced by the Western description 'paramedic'.(172)

The new training schemes for barefoot doctors have coincided with an injection of resources into county hospitals from 1978 onwards. Ideally, the barefoot doctor scheme and the county hospitals should be complementary aspects of the health care system, but the barefoot doctors' survival depends upon the success of the co-operative medical system in the brigades, which in its turn will only function if the barefoot doctors are efficient. If the brigade system collapses, patients then move to the county hospitals, where queues lengthen, standards of treatment fall and demand for state finance to improve county hospitals increases.

The number of barefoot doctors seems to have declined from
1.8 million(173) to about 1.4 million(174) between 1976 and 1979.

Most recent evidence suggests no special effort to increase
their numbers, although pressures for improved training continue. Among some sections of the medical profession it seems to
be hoped that their role will diminish *vis-à-vis* the assistant
doctors, which would produce a personnel structure similar to
that of the 1950s.

How viable such a new direction would be is open to question,
given limited financial resources. A premature departure from
the flexibility of practice, training and levels of expertise which
have been a feature of China's health care system for a considerable period of time may be an unwise jettisoning of its
greatest strength.


NOTES

1   J. Needham and Lu Gwei-djen, China and the origin of
    qualifying examinations in medicine, in 'Clerks and Crafts-
    men in China and the West', Cambridge University Press,
    1970, p. 379.
2   Prospectus of medical schools and colleges, 'Chinese Medical
    Directory', 1934, 'CMJ', 49, 1935, 999-1031.
3   Ibid.
4   W.R. Morse, Medical education in a mission school, 'CMJ',
    49, 1935, pp. 868-86.
5   Ibid.
6   C.K. Chu, The revised medical curricula, 'CMJ' 49, 1935,
    pp. 837-46.
7   Knud Faber, 'Report on Medical Schools in China', Health
    Organisation, League of Nations Report 1931, Appendix 1,
    'CMJ' 49, 1935, pp. 1063-5.
8   J.B. Grant, The Faber Report on medical schools in China
    and after, 'CMJ', 49, 1935, pp. 934-7.
9   S.D. Gamble, 'Ting Hsien', Stanford University Press, 1968.
10  Henry S. Houghton, Trends in medical education, 'CMJ',
    49, 1935, pp. 938-41.
11  V.W. Sidel, Medical personnel and their training, in J. Quin
    (ed.), 1972, 'Medicine and Public Health in the People's
    Republic of China', G.B. Risse, Thomas Springfield, Illinois
    p. 132.
12  Ibid.
13  Han Suyin, 'The Morning Deluge', London, Panther Books,
    1976, p. 241.
14  Cheng Chu-yuan, Health manpower: growth and distribution
    in M. Wegman et al. (eds), 'Public Health in the People's
    Republic of China', New York, Josiah Macy Jr Foundation,
    1973, pp. 139-57.
15  'NCNA', 24 June 1949.
16  Ho Cheng on the medical situation, 'NCNA', 2 August 1950.

17   Cheng Chu-yuan, op. cit., p. 146.
18   Association News, 'CMJ', 67, 1949, pp. 399–403.
19   Cheng Chu-yuan, op. cit., p. 141.
20   Ibid. p. 147.
21   People's Republic of China, State Statistical Bureau, 'Ten Great Years', Peking, Foreign Languages Press, 1960, p. 222.
22   Cheng Chu-yuan, op. cit., p. 149.
23   'CKP', March 1957, in 'JPRS', no. 583, CSO NY/33/3, pp. 43/5.
24   'CKP', 22 February 1957, in ibid.
25   Cheng Chu-yuan, op. cit. p. 146.
26   D. Lampton, 'The Politics of Medicine in China', Folkestone, Dawson, 1979, p. 54.
27   'People's Daily', 21 August 1957.
28   'CKP', 19 February 1957, in 'JPRS', 583.
29   Ibid.
30   Kung Nai-chuan, New China's achievements in health work, 'CMJ', 71, 2, March-April 1953, pp. 87–92.
31   'CKP', February 1957, in 'JPRS', 583.
32   Ibid.
33   'Peking Kuang-ming Jih-pao (Bright Daily)', 7 May 1957, in R. MacFarquhar, 'The Hundred Flowers', London, Stevens, 1960, p. 124.
34   Ibid., p. 128.
35   'Bright Daily', 20 May 1957, in ibid.
36   Ibid.
37   'CKP', 19 March 1957, in 'JPRS', 583.
38   'CKP', 1 February 1957, in 'JPRS', 583.
39   'NCNA', 8 July 1957.
40   'NCNA', 1 June 1959.
41   'NCNA', 19 August 1957.
42   L. Orleans, 'Professional Manpower and Education in Communist China', Washington, National Science Foundation, 1960, pp. 136–40.
43   'Current Scene', vol. I, no. 26, March 1962, p. 5.
44   'CKP', 22 March 1957.
45   'CKP', 26 March 1957.
46   Li Teh-chuan speech at 2nd National People's Congress, 'NCNA', 4 April 1969, 'SCMP', 2237, pp. 17–23.
47   Ibid.
48   F.P. Lisowski, The emergence and training of the barefoot doctor in China, 'J. Jap. Soc. Med. Hist.,' 25, 1979, pp. 339–92.
49   'NCNA', 13 March 1959.
50   'NCNA', 13 March 1959, 6 December 1958, 16 May 1959, 14 November 1960, 'SWB/FE/W66/B6.
51   'NCNA', 27 January 1961, 'SWB'/FE/W96/A/4.
52   'Jen-min Jih-pao (People's Daily)', Peking 15 July 1961, 'SCMP', 2545, p. 16.
53   Marie Sieh, Medicine in China: wealth for the state, Part I,

'Current Scene', vol. III, 15 October 1964, pp. 1-12.
54    Lampton, op. cit., p. 155.
55    Sieh, ibid.
56    Ibid.
57    'SWB'/FE/W203/B/22, 19 February 1963.
58    Cheng Chu-yuan, op. cit., p. 147.
59    Sieh, op. cit.
60    'NCNA', 11 January 1961.
61    Sieh, op. cit.
62    Chairman Mao's 26 June 1967, directive, 'Sup. SCMP', 198, p. 34.
63    Cheng Chu-yuan, op. cit., p. 149.
64    'NCNA', 23 November 1964.
65    Lampton, op. cit., p. 156.
66    Deepening the revolution in medical education, 'CMJ', 2, 2, March 1976, pp. 87-92.
67    Cheng Chu-yuan, op. cit., p. 149.
68    Computation of data in Cheng Chu-yuan, ibid.
69    Ibid.
70    'SWB'/FE/W/172/B/7, 5 July 1962.
71    'SWB'/FE/195/B/11, 9 January 1963.
72    The orientation of the revolution in medical education as seen in the growth of barefoot doctors, 'Hung Ch'i (Red Flag)', no. 3, September 1968, SCMM (Survey of China Mainland Magazines), 628, September 1966, p. 3.
73    An Hsuan-hung Hospital that serves the peasants, hospital built through self reliance and thrift, Hung Ch'i, 11, 1965. 'CB' (Current Background), no. 496, p. 37.
74    'Current Background', op. cit., p. 44.
75    Mao Tse-tung, Directive on Public Health Work, in Stuart Schram(ed.), 'Chairman Mao talks to the People', New York, Pantheon, 1974, pp. 232-3.
76    Ibid.
77    Medicine for rural areas, Canton Yang-ch'eng Wan-pao, 15 September 1965, 'SCMP', 3550, p. 11.
78    China directs its medical services to the 500 million peasants 'NCNA', 28 September 1965, 'SCMP', 3550, p. 15.
79    We are confident of running part-farming part-study medical class, Peking 'Kuang-ming Jih-pao', 11 May 1965, 'SCMP', 3471, p. 5.
80    'NCNA', 21 March 1965.
81    S.M. Hillier, interview file no. 8, July 1980.
82    'SCMP', 3532, 31 August 1965.
83    Ibid.
84    'NCNA', 9 September 1965, in 'SCMP', 3637.
85    Thoroughly criticise and repudiate the 8-year course promoted by China's Kruschev, Peking 'People's Daily', 17 December 1967, 'SCMP', 4100, p. 5.
86    Lampton, op. cit., p. 191.
87    Ching Kai, Health work serving the peasants, 'CMJ', 85, 3, March 1966, p. 146.

88  Can politics cure disease, 'China News Summary no. 113',
    in Lampton, op. cit. p. 213.
89  S.M. Hillier, interview file no. 3, July 1980.
90  S.M. Hillier, interview file no. 4, July 1980.
91  They came to see Mao Tse-tung, 'Supp.' 'SCMP', January
    June 1967, 11 November 1966.
92  Thoroughly criticise and repudiate the 8-year course
    promoted by China's Kruschev, op. cit.
93  The Mao-Liu controversy over rural public health, 'Current
    Scene', vol. VII, no. 12, 15 June 1969, pp. 1-18.
94  Medical education must follow the road of thorough revolu-
    tion, Peking 'People's Daily', 24 August 1968, 'SCMP',
    4254, p. 5.
95  Shanghai medical team carries on tradition of Red Army
    Hospital, 'SCMP', 4294, p. 22.
96  'People's Daily', 24 August 1968.
97  Ibid.
98  Hupeh Provincial Revolutionary Committee, 'SWB'/FE/W46/-
    A/5, 19 March 1968.
99  The Mao-Liu controversy, op. cit.
100 Medical education must be oriented toward the countryside,
    Peking 'People's Daily', 8 July 1969, 'SCMP', 4459, p. 7.
101 'Wuhan Provincial Service', 11 November 1964, 'SWB'/FE/-
    3398.
102 'SWB'/FE/3345, 23 November 1964.
103 'NCNA', 19 March 1965, 11 May 1965, 23 May 1965.
104 Young peasant medical workers commended in China's
    national press, 'Health News', 12 August 1965.
105 New developments in Chinese medical education, 'NCNA',
    9 September 1965.
106 Simplified medical courses in rural China, 'NCNA', 12
    November 1965.
107 China directs its medical service to the 500 million peasants,
    'SCMP', 3550, p. 15.
108 Ibid.
109 'NCNA', 11 September 1965.
110 'NCNA', 19 May 1965, 'SWB'/FE/367/A/16.
111 The orientation of the revolution in medical education as
    seen in the growth of barefoot doctors, 'Hung Ch'i (Red
    Flag)', no. 3, September 1968, 'SCMP', 628, September
    1966, p. 3.
112 Ibid.
113 Ibid.
114 Ibid.
115 Ibid.
116 S.M. Hillier, interview file no. 7, July 1980.
117 E. Grey Dimond, Medical education and care in the People's
    Republic of China, 'Journal of the American Medical Assoc-
    iation', 218, no. 10, 6 December 1971.
118 The re-orientation of medical education, 'Hung Ch'i',
    op. cit.

119 V. Sidel and R. Sidel, 'Serve the people. Observations on medicine in the People's Republic of China', Boston, Beacon Press, 1973, p. 115.
120 Occupy and transform the educational battlefront with Mao Tse-tung Thought, Canton Congress of Red Guards, July 1969, 'Sup. SCMP', 258, pp. 18-25.
121 Sidel and Sidel, op. cit., pp. 111-17.
122 Forever carry forward the tradition of the Red Army Health School, 'Hung Ch'i', no. 6, 1 June 1971, 'SCMP', 708, p. 135.
123 Lampton, op. cit., p. 228.
124 'SWB'/FE/W732/A/1, 11 July 1973.
125 Medical college conducting open-door schooling, 'CMJ', 2, 2 March 1976, p. 153.
126 Thoroughly transform the original ranks of teachers, Chungshan Medical College Revolutionary Committee, Canton Red Guard Congress 17 June 1970, 'Suppl. SCMP', 276, p. 20.
127 Ibid.
128 Penetratingly carry out mass criticism in the revolution in education, 'People's Daily', 11 September 1969, 'SCMP', 4498, p. 1.
129 Strengthen the ideological revolutionisation of Party Committees, Peking, 'People's Daily', 9 December 1971, p. 42.
130 Lampton, op. cit., pp. 257-8.
131 A general review of Communist affairs in 1972, 'Asian People's Anti-Communist League', Taipei, 1973, p. 118.
132 Continue to implement the Party's policies towards intellectuals, 'Hung Ch'i', no. 10, 1 October 1972.
133 Ibid.
134 D. Lampton, Trends in health policy, 'Current Scene', vol. XII, no. 6, 1974, pp. 6-7.
135 J. Prybyla, Notes on Chinese higher education 1974, 'China Quarterly', 62 June 1975, p. 272.
136 Raise the level of medical treatment techniques in the course of practice, 'Hung Ch'i', no. 3, 3 March 1973.
137 Beat back the right deviationist wind to reverse verdicts on the health front, 'Hung Ch'i', no. 4, April 1976, 'SCM' 76-11, 867, p. 2.
138 Wen Chi-Pang and Charles Hayes, Medical education in China in the post Cultural Revolution era, 'New England Journal of Medicine', 8 May 1975, pp. 998-1005.
139 E. Dimond, Medical school curriculum in the People's Republic of China, 'JAMA' 236, 1976, p. 1489.
140 Bruce Roser, Medical education in China in 1977, in 'New Doctor', no. 6, September 1977, p. 20.
141 'NCNA', Peking, 25 June 1975.
142 Estimate based on the annual production of graduates, prior to 1966, and the fact that no new graduates appeared until 1973-4.

143 Mao Tse-tung, 'On the question of correctly resolving contradictions among the people', speech delivered on 27 February 1957.
144 SWB/FE/W997/A/1, April 1978.
145 'CMJ', vol. 4, no. 1, January 1978, p. 4.
146 S.M. Hillier, travel notes, March 1978.
147 M. Lessof and J. Dale, Meeting enormous health needs – medical education, 'China Now', 1980.
148 S. Pepper, Chinese education after Mao, 'China Quarterly', 81, March 1980, pp. 1–65.
149 S.M. Hillier, travel notes, March 1981.
150 Lessof and Dale, op. cit.
151 S.M. Hillier, travel notes, March 1978.
152 S.M. Hillier, travel notes, March 1981.
153 J.A. Jewell, personal communication, January 1982.
154 State Statistical Bureau, 'Number of health personnel' All China, 1978, private communication, Division of Health Statistics World Health Organization, Geneva 8 April 1980.
155 'NCNA', Peking 25 June 1976.
156 State Statistical Bureau, 'Number of health personnel', All China, op. cit.
157 'NCNA', 28 February 1973.
158 Zhu Xianyi, Call for reform in medical training, 'NCNA', 'SWB'/FE/6901/C1/3, 9 December 1981.
159 State Statistical Bureau, 'Number of health personnel', All China, op. cit.
160 'Liaoning Provincial Service', 18 March 1972.
161 'CBC', Montreal, 'SWB'/FE/W699/A/1, 7 November 1972.
162 'SWB'/FE/W701/A/1 29 November 1972.
163 Raise the level of medical treatment techniques in the course of practice, 'Hung Ch'i (Red Flag)', no. 3, 3 March 1973.
164 G.B. Riss, 'Modern China and Traditional Chinese Medicine', Illinois, Thomas Springfield, 1973.
165 'NCNA', 14 May 1975, 'SWB'/FE/W827/A/1.
166 'SWB'/FE/5841/B11/4, 17 June 1978.
167 A barefoot doctor college set up in Kiangsu, 'CMJ', 2, 2, March 1976, p. 151.
168 'Hung Ch'i', no. 7, 1 July 1976.
169 'SWB'/FE/W1014/A/1, 17 January 1979.
170 Barefoot doctors making progress, 'Ta kung Pao (Impartial Daily)', 20 July 1978.
171 For further details of all aspects of barefoot doctor training see F.P. Lisowski, op. cit.
172 'SWB'/FE/6537/BII/3, 1 October 1980.
173 'NCNA', 5 June 1978.
174 'NCNA', 27 June 1979.

# 12 PSYCHIATRY AND THE TREATMENT OF MENTAL ILLNESS IN CHINA

S.M. Hillier

## MENTAL ILLNESS IN CHINA AND THE WEST - COMPARATIVE CONCEPTS

The organisation of psychiatric facilities in China on any scale had to await the arrival of the Communist government in 1949. What is available now is an enormous advance on what was available at that time, but growth in this sector of the health services has been somewhat slower than that in other areas. This probably reflects the relatively low priority allotted to mental illness in a country which has successfully attempted to wipe out an enormous burden of infectious and parasitic disease. Mental illness also appears to carry a stigma, as it does in the West, although those engaged in treatment go to considerable lengths to re-educate patients' relatives and work-mates, and ensure that jobs are kept open. There may also be a real difference in the incidence and prevalence of disease between China and the West, thus requiring fewer facilities. Writers who have discussed the subject appear to conclude that the incidence and prevalence of mental illness is much lower in China than in the West.

Two arguments are put forward to support the idea. The first concerns the large-scale and impressive removal by the Communist government of various forms of social pathology. Examples are the removal of venereal disease and related abolition of prostitution; and the dramatic change in the status of women. The abolition of the damaging trade in narcotics, removal of narcotic addiction and humane treatment and cure of addicts are achievements which Western governments have shown themselves unable or unwilling to match, and the long-term effects of these measures cannot be underestimated. The poverty, starvation, ignorance and social breakdowns which characterised China in the first half of the twentieth century are no longer prevailing features of that society. There is greater security of employment, greater prosperity, and a well-developed system of welfare and health care.

Half the population, however, do not remember pre-revolutionary days. Their lives have been lived within a socialist society which has experienced some degree of social upheaval. The Great Leap Forward of 1958-9 and, more importantly, the Cultural Revolution of 1966-70, were periods equally of political growth and anarchy, of social regeneration and social breakdown. The mental health consequences of these developments are not known about at all.

378

In the absence of comparative figures for pre- and post-revolutionary periods it is therefore difficult to draw conclusions: nevertheless observers who knew China before 1949 and since are convinced that post-revolutionary society has benefited not only the material condition of the Chinese, but their psychological condition as well. The tackling of the social problems described above has undoubtedly removed from China many of those problems like alcoholism and drug addiction – which are regarded in the West either as mental health problems in themselves, or as factors which contribute to mental illness. It may be, however, that there are other sources of social stress in Chinese society which, whether similar in form or different to that experienced in the West, are implicated in the development of mental illness. All these arguments assume, of course, that social factors do play an important part in the etiology of mental disease. Not all psychiatrists, either in the West or in China, would agree with this. There are many who would support an organicist or hereditary theory of disease. And mental illness itself covers a very wide range of behaviour from 'problems of living' to the bizarre hallucinations of schizophrenia.

The second argument which is used to support the suggestion that the incidence and prevalence of mental disorders are less in China than in the West is usually based on numbers of beds in mental hospitals as an indication of rates of mental disease. These are unreliable for several reasons. The number of beds available is an indication of supply rather than demand or need for treatment; and the supply of a certain type of treatment, i.e. hospitalisation. Therefore the figures do not relate to those sufferers who may be dealt with by alternative methods – for example by community care programmes. Bed numbers may also be an indication of the priority given to the hospital treatment of one disease rather than another, or a function of the number of staff available to care for psychiatric patients in hospital. What figures there are for China suggest shortages in the provision of psychiatric beds, and plans to increase their number.(1) There seems to have been no attempt such as has been made in the UK to decrease the number of psychiatric beds. It would be just as fallacious to argue from an increase in the number of psychiatrists or psychiatric beds available in China that rates of mental illness are increasing. Such figures may merely indicate that more attention is being paid to the problem of the psychiatrically ill, as indeed seems to be the case.

A further complication, of a conceptual nature, must also be considered. Psychiatry, perhaps more than other medical specialties, is culture bound, particularly with regard to 'functional' mental disorders, those disorders of unknown etiology. These symptoms, which are manifested through behaviour, are defined, ultimately, by the degree to which such behaviour is culturally unacceptable. Wide variations in diagnosis have been shown to exist among Western psychiatrists(2) and the problem is compounded when observers attempt to compare

Western and Chinese diagnostic categories. Chin and Chin
writing in the 1960s suggested that there were four major mental
illnesses in China - schizophrenia, manic depressive psychosis,
paralytic mental stupor and neurasthenia.(3) These are rather
broader than Western categories. Psychiatry in China now uses
the standard International Classification of Disease for both
organic and functional psychoses. However, the definitions of
neuroses of various types and phobic states are more likely to
go under the general term of 'neurasthenia'. The use of this
term is still not clear, even in 1980. Some ICD syndromes like
alcoholism and drug addiction are absent for reasons described
above. It is unlikely that their treatment would, in any case,
be recognised as the province of the psychiatrists. Other types
of illness with which psychiatrists deal in the West - anorexia
nervosa, or hyperactivity in children, seem extremely rare.

Sexual problems, which according to Freudian psychiatrists
in the West are implicated in neurotic disorders are less likely
to be seen as mental problems in China. When such problems
exist, they are more likely to be regarded as physical ones
which can be cured by drugs prescribed by a physician. Popular
culture still emphasises the link between potency and the consumption of certain types of 'medicine' and such medicines in the
form of pills, powders or tonics can be readily bought at
pharmacies for consumption by men and women. Homosexuality,
which Western questioners have been repeatedly told does not
exist, is now admitted to occur. Again, unlike in the West, its
presence does not seem to call for the assistance of a psychiatrist
Impressions suggest, however, that life for a homosexual person
can be extremely difficult in China, and the ensuing state of
mind, rather than the condition itself, may well bring some
homosexuals into treatment. It should be remembered that
psychiatric attitudes in the West towards sexuality in general
and homosexuality in particular show quite a large degree of
variation, with some psychiatrists regarding homosexuality as
an illness which requires treatment while others regard the social
prejudice against homosexuals as rendering such persons
vulnerable to psychiatric illness.

Seeking psychiatric treatment, either in the UK or in China,
depends in the first instance on the recognition either by the
patient or his family that something 'is wrong'. We in the West
are only just beginning to understand the processes by which
people define and label themselves or others as in need of
psychiatric assistance. We know almost nothing about this process in China; we do not know the extent of, or tolerance
towards, bizarre behaviour, anxiety, depression or phobias,
or of the existence of syndromes which do not occur in the West.
Evidence from Chinese communities outside the People's Republic
describe the treatment by shamans ('Tank-ki') of a host of acute
relatively minor psychiatric problems which include examination
worries, family squabbles, infidelity, agoraphobia and hysteria.
Indeed the role of the Tang-ki can be seen as that of a counsellor

as much as a healer. Major psychotic problems, especially chronic ones, are outside the scope of the traditional healer, but the evidence from Chinese communities abroad suggests a tendency to use agencies like fortune tellers or shamans for help with personal problems. Writers have also noted the Chinese tendency to complain first of somatic symptoms, and only later to talk about psychological problems. Evidence also suggests that Chinese patients' psychological difficulties are much more likely to be related to pressures for educational achievement, intrafamily conflict and pressures to conform. Western patients are more likely to suffer from problems relating to sexual competitiveness, loneliness, crises of independence.(4)

These data on Chinese psychiatric problems are drawn from Taiwan. In the People's Republic the existence of fortune tellers and shamans, although not unknown, is relatively rare, and they certainly do not appear to be a major source of consolation or assistance. As to those psychiatric problems described in the Taiwanese data, it is likely that even if similar problems exist in the rest of China, there is a strong countervailing social ethic of collective responsibility and service to society which might reduce their prevalence.

In looking at incidence and prevalence of mental illness, therefore, conclusions are difficult to reach; the problem arises partly from the disease entities themselves: Western psychiatrists still puzzle as to what can justifiably be called mental illness, and how true prevalence can be measured if we only have data on those receiving treatment. The problems in understanding the position in China could be partially overcome if more data were available from that source.

## EPIDEMIOLOGY OF MENTAL DISORDER

*Pre-revolutionary epidemiological data*
Pre-revolutionary epidemiological evidence on the prevalence of mental disease is small. Lamson, writing in 1935, estimated the incidence of mental disease to range from one in one thousand to three in one thousand.(5) Venereal disease, an important cause of mental illness, was prevalent, and in 1949 was estimated to affect 5 per cent of the population in cities and 10 per cent in the national minority areas.(6) Drug addiction, which the Nationalist government had attempted to suppress in 1935 with a six-year programme, was a widespread problem. In the 1930s there were 300,000 addicts in Beijing alone and 40 million opium users in China as a whole.(7) The eradication of both venereal disease and opium addiction in the early years following the establishment of the Communist government removed these causes of mental illness. Whereas in 1949 sufferers from general paresis (late stage syphilis) formed 10 per cent of hospital population, in 1965 they represented 2 per cent of patients.(8)

## POST-REVOLUTIONARY EPIDEMIOLOGICAL DATA

Between February 1958 and February 1959 the Hunan Provincial Health Department sponsored a survey of psychosis in Hunan Province.(9) The survey covered 1,424,751 people in People's Communes, small towns, and the cities of Changsha and Hengyang. In the communes 587 cases, or 1.27 per cent of the population, were found. The rate for schizophrenia was 0.77 per thousand and these comprised 60 per cent of patients. The second highest prevalence was in puerperal psychosis - 0.15 per thousand. Among the study population, over half of whom were aged forty or more, the rate for senile psychosis was 0.09 per thousand, and for manic depressive psychosis 0.06 per thousand. In the cities of Changsha and Hengyang the prevalence rate for all psychoses was higher than in the country-side - 1.46 per cent. As in the countryside, the largest number of patients were diagnosed as schizophrenic, and similarly the second highest prevalence was of puerperal psychoses. Lower rates were recorded for senile psychoses and for manic depressive psychoses. The researchers also noted that the number of female cases far outnumbered males, although a comparison with hospital data in a study by the same authors showed males were twice as likely to be hospitalised. Some but not all of the sex differences could be explained by differential access to treatment. They noted that female patients were over-represented in three major diagnostic categories - first-stage psychosis and senile psychosis, paranoid psychosis and manic depressive psychosis, whereas male patients were over-represented among syphilitic psychotic patients.

The survey showed that over half the psychotic patients were over forty years old. This contrasts with the in-patient data collected by the authors where 70 per cent of hospitalised patients were between twenty and thirty-nine years old. Many of the survey group were chronic patients with a lifetime history of illness, who had been kept in their families before any modern treatment was available. In fact somewhere between one-quarter and one-third of psychotic conditions had remained untreated, which reminds us again of the difficulty of obtaining accurate rates of psychiatric morbidity when only users of psychiatric facilities are counted.

This epidemiological study, which surveyed rural and urban prevalences of mental illness and compared the findings with an urban hospitalised population, produced a picture whose broad outlines would be confirmed by subsequent investigators. However, the diagnostic categories used by the psychiatrists in this study were different from those now employed by Chinese epidemiologists using the ICD. The effect of these differences in classification may be to assign lower prevalence to schizophrenia, while retaining as a separate category 'paranoid psychosis'. The field survey did not include mentally retarded persons or epileptics, although epileptic and syphilitic psychoses were included in the in-patient survey. The authors themselves also admitted that they did not include in the study patients whose illness had been gradually resolved, nor those suffering from neuropathy or sick personality. The authors also noted that the numbers of patients suffering from depressive psychoses might be underestimated because the symptoms are less likely to draw public attention.

Equally important, the total population was relatively youthful, which would explain the low prevalence and incidence of mental diseases related to ageing.

Liu(10) has carried out one of the first modern epidemiological studies of mental illness in his home province of Sichuan. This huge western province, the largest in China, has a population of 98 million people. His survey, carried out between 1973 and 1975, covered 426,789 persons. The prevalence of mental disorders averaged 6.74 per thousand with many cases of schizophrenia and mental subnormality. The prevalence of schizophrenia was higher in women, and in urban areas. The prevalence of mental handicap was higher in men, and in rural areas. Depressive psychoses were relatively uncommon.

In an analysis of the incidence of mental illness between 1964 and 1973, Liu provides data which shows that two peak years of incidence of schizophrenia were 1967 and 1971. Whilst it is most unwise to draw conclusions from incidence figures, these peaks correspond to two turning-points in the Cultural Revolution. The first follows the occurrence of widespread violence, the second the involvement of the army to restore order. However, these figures are specific to Sichuan only.

Xia and colleagues at the much-visited Shanghai Psychiatric Hospital made a general survey of the prevalence of mental disease in Shanghai and its environs in 1972-3. The average prevalence rate of mental disorder was 7.8 per thousand. Prevalence was slightly higher in the urban areas (7.86 per thousand) than in the rural areas (6.67 per thousand). As in Liu's study morbidity due to mental retardation was higher in rural than urban areas. The incidence, from incomplete data, was 20.2 per thousand in the rural areas and 10.8 per thousand in the urban areas.

Schizophrenia ranked first among the various mental disorders with a prevalence of 4.2 per thousand and a higher rate in urban than in rural areas.(11)

Liu Jieqiu, in her investigation of Xuhui district, Shanghai, found a prevalence rate of disease of 6.7 per thousand, with schizophrenia as the primary manifestation, followed by mental retardation. She noted that the standardised rate of incidence of mental disorders differed according to differences in educational status and income, and was higher after 1970 than before,(12) but did not say where the difference lay.

Shen and her colleagues looked at the incidence and prevalence of severe mental disorders in Haidan district of Beijing, consisting of four suburban communes. Overall prevalence was 7.09

per thousand. The prevalence of schizophrenia was 1.82 per
thousand, reactive psychosis 0.26 per thousand and manic
depressive psychosis 0.07 per thousand.(13)

Comparison with data from other countries is always slightly
misleading because of difference in diagnosis, in sample populations and in methods of case-finding. However, UK data
suggest higher rates of depressive psychosis, but far lower
rates of schizophrenia and mental subnormality than in China.
The difference in the disease profile could partly be due to
differences in the ages of the sample population, the UK's
containing a greater proportion of persons aged sixty-five
and over.(14) Sex differences in morbidity are less pronounced
in China than in most Western data, where, from the age of
fifteen onwards, the female excess over males becomes
increasingly pronounced.(15) However, the Chinese data do
suggest that prevalence rates for women over forty are more
than double those of men.

Overall prevalence derived from British studies shows higher
morbidity in the British population. For example, compared with
Shanghai and Beijing figures, one year prevalence in Camberwell
London, and Nottingham stands at 20 per 1,000 and 19 per
1,000 respectively; but these data include both minor and major
psychiatric illness, whereas the Chinese data concentrates on
severe psychosis only. When figures for severe psychoses are
compared, the differences still obtain with overall prevalence of
severe psychosis almost seven times greater than in China.(16)
However, the Beijing and Shanghai data were derived from an
initial list of suspected mental patients produced by barefoot
doctors who had received one week's training in psychiatric
screening. Subsequently diagnosis was verified by trained
psychiatrists.

## CLINICAL EVIDENCE OF MENTAL DISEASE

### Clinical studies of mental illness

*Classical times*  The earliest clinical records of neurological and
mental illness go back to the fourteenth century BC, when treatment was sought for headaches, dizziness and painful joints.
All these symptoms were thought to be caused by the ill effects
of 'wind'. Epilepsy was also considered as a 'wind' disease. In
'Kuo Yu', published in 500 BC, a case of loss of speech is
recorded, and Lu's 'Book of Spring and Autumn' gives an
account of cures for paralysis. The Chinese medical classic,
the 'Nei-Jing', carries detailed descriptions of loss of speech
and describes cases of paralysis and cases of insanity due to
excessive fear. The first full-blown description of instantly
recognisable syndromes of mental illness appears in the writings
of the Ming dynasty physician Wang Kentang. In his 'Standards
for Diagnosis and Treatment' he divides nervous and mental dis-

orders into three kinds. In the first kind, which he calls 'insanity' the patient is

> sometimes violent, sometimes stupid, singing and laughing or sad and weeping. He gets no better even after months and years. The common name for this disorder is 'wind in the mind'. Those with frustrated ambition are liable to be so affected.
>   The second kind is mania:
> The patient is garrulous and boisterous, raving, stubborn and violent. He abuses everyone indiscriminantly, friends, relatives and strangers. He may even climb to any eminence at hand, take off his clothes and run away climbing over the wall or onto the roof in a way that no normal person would be able to do. He may tell of things that were never seen.
>   The third kind Wang calls 'fits':
> The person subject to fits becomes dizzy and cannot recognise people. He falls to the ground, having convulsions and suffering from jerks over which he has no control.(17)

*Modern times*

Data for the modern period are derived mainly from hospital records. These give a remarkably consistent picture of the types of patient being treated for mental illness. Xia reports on studies carried out between 1935 and 1956 at one of the mental hospitals in Shanghai. Of the 4,506 mental patients treated over this period 74 per cent were schizophrenic, the great majority under forty. There were no sex differences. The majority of cases were of the paranoid schizophrenic type, and the major etiological factor was thought to be neurological - due to 'a weak type of higher nervous activity', with environmental and genetic factors accorded lesser importance.(18)

In 1966 Chin and Chin suggested that schizophrenics constituted 30 to 35 per cent of all mental hospital patients. Manic-depressive psychoses ranged from 7 to 14 per cent of all mental patients, and neurasthenics (the major diagnostic category of the neuroses employed in China), accounted for 60 per cent of all out-patient work in the mental health department at the Beijing College of Medicine.(19)

Sidel,(20) writing in 1971, reports that in the Shanghai Mental Hospital about 50 per cent of the patients were schizophrenic, the majority being young adults. Most were of the paranoid type. The psychiatrist told her that depression and post-partum depression were relatively rare.

Kagan(21) in Tianjin in 1972 found that conventional diagnostic categories appeared to have been abolished, and patients were graded only as to whether their illness was 'light', 'moderate' or 'severe'. In Shanghai in 1973 the Science for People delegation was told that the majority of patients in the out-patient department were 'neurotic' or 'psychoneurotic', but that the majority of in-patients were schizophrenics.(22) This was confirmed by D. Ratnavale (1973), who added that the in-patients were mostly

aged between twenty and thirty-five, and just over half were
suffering from schizophrenia.(23) Low incidence of depressive
syndromes, post-partum psychosis and suicide were also
reported. Walls,(24) who visited the same hospital in the autumn
of 1973, reported that 60 per cent of the patients there, and 50
per cent of the patients in a similar hospital in Nanjing, were
schizophrenic. However, he and his colleagues report that the
out-patient department was mainly concerned with the treatment
of discharged rather than new patients, although 'in some cases
the out-patients suffer from neurasthenia or epilepsy'.

Several writers - Walls, Ratnavale, and the Science for People
delegation quoted the fact that the proportion of child patients
has declined steadily over the years. The ten-bedded psychiatric
unit included in the new psychiatric hospital in Shanghai has
been converted to other use. Lowinger,(25) in 1980, described
China's leading (and only) child psychiatrist as treating children
and adolescents suffering from disciplinary problems, autism,
and hyperactivity caused by brain damage. Liu(26) says that
the two major problems as far as children are concerned are
epilepsy and mental subnormality, but that hyperactivity and
bedwetting are also occasionally diagnosed. Anorexia nervosa is
rare.

In Leung's(27) report from Shanghai in 1975 83.7 per cent of
patients were classified as schizophrenic. She also mentioned
a very small number of patients, 0.4 per cent, who were admitted
for alcohol and drug intoxication. In the same year, during his
visit to a mental hospital in Changsha, Loshak(28) reported 'for
the first time also', Chinese doctors admitted that crimes such
as compulsive stealing, sexual assault and psychopathic murder,
occur in China, although such cases are extremely rare'.
Recent reports of such crimes in Chinese newspapers support
this statement. Such events do happen, but are regarded as
sensational and shocking, and seem to be used to add weight
to the establishment view in China, that law and order has
suffered a severe breakdown during the period of the 'Gang of
Four'.

John and Emily Visher,(29) visiting Shanghai in 1977, were
told that 'the number of young schizophrenic patients is steadily
increasing - the doctors are baffled as to the reason'. Manic
depressive patients formed a very small proportion of the total
- 1.4 per cent. Some epileptics were treated as in-patients but
the majority were given out-patient treatment, together with
the neurasthenic patients. 'Neurasthenia' appears to cover
psychosomatic complaints and feelings of depression or anxiety.
As to organic brain syndromes, there seems to be some confusion
as to whether these were seen as types of schizophrenia, or as
separate diagnostic entities.

The large proportion of schizophrenics among in-patients seems
to be confirmed by reports from other parts of China. Jules
Masserman, visiting the Guangzhou Mental Hospital in 1978, said
that 80 per cent of patients admitted are schizophrenic,(30) and

a similar figure is given for schizophrenia in Sichuan by Liu
in 1980. Liu said

> About 80 per cent of all in-patients are schizophrenics, the
> simple or catatonic types being less common. Less than 5 per
> cent of patients have affective psychoses, including hypo-
> mania, chronic mania and manic depressive psychoses.
> Involutional melancholia is less frequently seen than in the
> 1950s. Confusional states and organic psychoses associated
> with physical conditions can also be found and a case of
> alcoholism or drug dependence upon hypnotics might be seen
> once in a few years.(31)

Neurosyphilis has disappeared since the 1950s. Ninety per
cent of the out-patients were neurotics, many of whom presented
with symptoms of headache or insomnia. They could be
depressed, or anxious. Hysteria was fairly rare and the total
number of hysterics had decreased. Obsessive compulsive states
were uncommon, and agoraphobia was rare.

It has also been noted that the numbers of parasuicide cases
which afflict UK casualty departments do not appear in anything
like the same amount.


## FACILITIES, RESOURCES AND PSYCHIATRIC TRAINING

The earliest record of the existence of mental hospitals is in the
Guan Ci which was compiled in -300, from the writings of Kuan
Zhong (-700). It is not known whether care was custodial, or
whether active treatment was attempted.(32) By the time of the
Ming dynasty there were regulations governing the insane, but
mostly people were cared for by their families. Those thus
cared for fared only a little better than those who were confined
in institutions. As late as 1926 Macartney was writing:

> Mental patients constitute a very helpless class in China. If
> caught upon the streets doing anything wrong they are
> arrested, thrown into prison and treated as criminals. If they
> are harmless and wander in the streets, they are mocked and
> laughed at and often stoned. Their families usually treat them
> as strangers and confine them in a dark room . . . their
> closest relatives usually disown them, although there may be
> true affection shown by a family for a psychotic member,
> especially if he be a son.(33)

It is likely that the breakdown of law and order which accompanied the decline of the Qing empire made its effects felt in the
care of mental patients too, and that in earlier times they may
have been treated more kindly.

The medical missionary movement, which was instrumental
in introducing Western medicine to China, was increasing its

influence throughout the nineteenth century. In 1870 Dr John Kerr of the Guangzhou (Canton) Hospital urged the setting up of an asylum 'where the inability of such patients might be demonstrated and pupils instructed at the same time'.(34) In 1897 a small thirty-bedded hospital was built on a site Kerr had purchased at his own expense. The hospital, an Asylum for the Insane, was expanded to five hundred beds, but closed in 1937.

Other major cities in China also built mental hospitals. By 1906 there was a refuge for the insane for seventy-five patients built in Beijing, which by 1936 was reorganised into the Beijing City Psychopathic Hospital with 200 beds. It was used as a teaching hospital for students from Beijing Union Medical College. In Suzhou, in 1923, a psychopathic ward was opened in the Elizabeth Blake Hospital. The mentally sick of Shanghai were kept during the first quarter of this century in St Joseph's Hospice, but later a philanthropist, Le Pak-hong, provided the money to build a hospital for the care of patients with nervous and mental diseases at Minhong, a Shanghai suburb. This hospital, called the Mercy Hospital, had 500 beds, up-to-date equipment, and extensive grounds. Shanghai's no. 1 and 2 teaching hospitals opened neuropsychiatry wards in 1940. These hospitals also took cases from Nanjing, which although it possessed diagnostic facilities had no accommodation for patients. Shanghai also had a Buddhist hospital, the Therapeutic Institute for Nervous Diseases, established in 1939. After the Japanese occupation of Shanghai in 1944, the treatment of mental illness at these hospitals ceased.

Following the Sino-Japanese War, a psychiatric hospital was established in Nanjing, and the hospitals reopened, but on the eve of Liberation in 1949, there were still fewer than 6,000 psychiatric beds for 450 million people and these beds were concentrated in large mental hospitals in the four main cities of China, Beijing, Shanghai, Guangzhou and Nanjing.(35)

## POST-REVOLUTIONARY DEVELOPMENTS

During the mid fifties the task of building the psychiatric services got under way. Old facilities were enlarged and re-equipped, and sixty-two new psychiatric hospitals were built, at least one in each province. Beds increased to about 14,000, and small hostels were built for those who were chronically mentally ill and homeless. Sir Robert MacIntosh, who visited China in 1958, recalls being taken to visit a large new mental hospital in Shanghai which had 424 beds.(36)

In 1952 when the Chinese Society of Neurology and Psychiatry was established there were only one hundred neuropsychiatrists in China.(37)

Psychiatry was a post-graduate subject, but not of very high status. Trainees were usually assistant doctors with a three-year training from a middle-level medical school. There was a

large increase in enrolments and a dramatic upswing in the
number of psychiatrists who qualified in 1958-9. By 1957 there
were 436, but by 1959 the figures had more than doubled to
900 (see Table 12.1). In part this increase was due to an
overall expansion in education and the shortening of courses.
By 1960 most of the fifty medical colleges had departments of
psychiatry. In addition there were part-time study courses and
paramedics and cadres were encouraged to learn about the care
and treatment of the mentally ill. The tiny number of nurses
engaged in psychiatry had increased fourteen times by 1958.
Clinical research, especially into those illnesses with a high
incidence like schizophrenia and neurasthenia, was encouraged.(38)

Table 12.1 Psychiatric beds, hospitals and psychiatrists in
China and UK, 1949-80

|  | 1949[78] | 1957[35] | 1959[38] | 1978[a] | UK 1978[b] |
|---|---|---|---|---|---|
| Beds | 6,000 | 20,000 | 24,000 | 42,195 | 166,556[41] |
| Hospitals and institutes | 4 | 50 | 60 | 219 | 500 |
| Psychiatrists | 60 | 436 | 900 | 4,000[35] | 2,992[b] |

Sources:
(a)  WHO Statistics, 'Hospitals and Hospital Beds. All China'.
(b)  'Health and Personal Social Services', London, HMSO, 1978.

In the early 1960s the whole organisation of health care was
affected by economic disasters, but worst hit were those aspects
which relied on short-course or spare-time training to staff
them. Municipal hostels and local medical schools could not be
afforded. It has been suggested that the pattern of growth of
facilities was maintained, but no new hospitals were built and
developments were largely in the field of research. Laboratory
experiments into psychopharmacology, biochemical metabolism,
physiology of the higher nervous system and psychological
testing were all pursued.(39)

The Cultural Revolution of 1966-70 witnessed the virtual
abolition of psychiatry in the medical curriculum. The number
of hours spent studying the subject was reduced to a quarter
of the original. Since many medical colleges were closed until
1970, teaching and research almost came to a standstill. However,
some large-scale investigations and epidemiological studies were
carried out.

The expansion of paramedical training - the barefoot doctors
- meant that there was an opportunity to staff an expanding
network of prevention and treatment for mental illness. The barefoot doctors used both traditional and Western methods of treat-

ment. Today they are being trained to undertake screening and
treatment programmes.(40) When medical colleges reopened in
1970 psychiatry remained essentially a course taken after
graduation. Today doctors who work in mental hospitals, with
the exception of those from academic departments of psychiatry,
are recruited from junior middle school, and have a three-year
training as assistant doctors. Thus their academic standard is
not generally as high as other graduates of medical colleges,
even those who were 'three-year graduates' of the 'worker-
peasant-soldiers' entry in the education experiments of 1970-6.
At the time of writing psychiatry is being taught in the undergraduate curriculum of the medical college, but still with a
considerably reduced number of hours, and takes up about a
month to six weeks of a four- or five-year medical college
course.(41) At present it is estimated that there are somewhere
between 3,000 and 4,000 psychiatrists in China, a number which
was originally calculated by Walls in 1973(42) and remains
virtually unchanged.


## FACILITIES AND RESOURCES IN PRESENT-DAY CHINA

After the immediate turmoil of the Cultural Revolution had
ceased, some innovative experiments began which form the
basis of the present organisation of treatment. Three-tier networks of prevention and treatment were formed, called, in
urban areas, the 'city-district-neighbourhood' and in rural
areas the 'county-commune-brigade', and in industrial or mining
areas 'hospital-district-locality'.(43) Many mass prevention
stations were set up, and in factories and workshops nursing
groups and medical teams were created to deal with the mentally
ill for whom hospital care was unavailable or expensive. There
was a real attempt to include psychiatry in the expanding system
of health care, and to uniformly plan psychiatric care.

Evidence from Shanghai suggests that three-tier networks,
which can involve lay community activists in care and surveillance
of patients, may be more appropriate to a densely populated city
than to dispersed rural populations. The problem of the care of
the mentally ill in rural areas is far from solved, although
institutional care at one of the city hospitals or local mental
illness hostels seems the most likely form.

Visits of Westerners to facilities for the mentally ill have been
relatively rare events over the last thirty years. From 1971
onwards, however, an increasing number of Western (particularly
American and British) psychiatrists were invited to look at the
care and treatment of the mentally ill in China. These accounts,
while interesting, provide strictly limited data from which to
judge the state of psychiatry in China. They are based only on
visits to hospitals, and largely one hospital at that. A summary
of the information is provided in Table 12.2.

The picture that emerges is of large mental hospitals in provin-

cial capitals and in the largest cities of China, Guangzhou,
Beijing, Shanghai, Tianjin and Nanjing; a number of smaller
hospitals of approximately 300 beds in county towns, and hostels
which supplement them. There are an unknown number of the
latter but a rough estimate assuming a similar hostel/population
ratio for all China as that of Sichuan, given by Liu, suggests
about 500. The number of mental hospitals in China, for a
population of approximately one billion, is about 219. The UK,
with a population of 48 million, has 480 hospitals.(44) At present
in China psychiatric hospital beds form 4 per cent of the total
number of hospital beds,(45) compared with approximately 35
per cent in Britain.(46)

Table 12.2  Provision of facilities in some major mental hospitals,
1959-78

| Reporter | Year | Place | Beds | Psychia-trists | Nurses | Other staff | Total staff |
|---|---|---|---|---|---|---|---|
| McIntosh | 1959 | Shanghai | 446 | n.a. | n.a. | n.a. | n.a. |
| Sidel | 1971 | " | 916 | 61 | 169 | n.a. | n.a. |
| Ratnavale | 1973 | " | 1,000 | 61 | 218 | 227 | 556 |
| SFP | 1973 | " | 996 | 61 | 261 | 263 | 585 |
| Walls | 1973 | " | 974 | 61 | 213 | 309* | 583 |
| Leung | 1973 | " | 1,000 | n.a. | n.a. | n.a. | n.a. |
| Visher | 1977 | " | 1,000 | 86 | 295 | 373** | 754 |
| Ratner | 1978 | " | 1,000 | 83 | 295 | 376 | 754 |
| Masserman | 1978 | " | 1,000 | 83 | 296 | 376 | 754 |
| Kagan | 1972 | Tianjin | 500 | 47 | 259 | 104 | 410 |
| Masserman | 1978 | Guangzhou | 1,000 | n.a. | n.a. | n.a. | n.a. |
| Masserman | 1978 | Beijing | 100 | 24 | n.a. | n.a. | n.a. |

* my calculation
**includes 41 medical technicians

Writers who have, over the past decade, visited the same
mental hospital, have reported different bed numbers and staffing levels in the same hospital. Slight differences may be due to
differential reporting, but it is likely that larger differences
do represent actual changes in numbers. In Table 12.2 two points
appear. First, with regard to the Shanghai data, staffing levels
improved after 1976, both in staff numbers overall, and in
trained staff. Unfortunately there were no visits from 1974 to
1976, so it is not possible to identify the point of change more

precisely. Second, more favourable physician/bed ratios exist in the smaller hospitals, especially those which are specialist psychiatric units in medical colleges, for example at Tianjin, Nanjing, and Beijing. Not shown in the table are the figures given by Liu (1980) for Sichuan province where he quotes a patient/doctor ratio of twenty-five to one, which is about double that for Shanghai. A further point about Shanghai is important. Several writers have mentioned the existence of two large mental hospitals in the city, although no one had visited the second which deals mainly with chronic cases. Here the proportion of trained staff to patients is lower, as calculated from figures given by Xia.(47) This hospital has 1,000 beds and 272 Staff, both psychiatrists and nurses. Altogether Xia notes that there are about 2,000 mental hospital beds in the counties and districts of the Shanghai municipality, and about 600 doctors. These figures must include staff and beds at smaller outreach hospitals. We do not know the level of training of these health workers, or the extent of their responsibilities for care in factory and neighbourhood clinics. The role of paramedical and lay personnel in the treatment of the mentally ill appears much more relevant in the case of community care, where community activists are mobilised under the overall direction of hospital doctors (see below).

## Out-patient facilities

*Primary care*  Psychiatric care in China is characterised (as is other hospital care) by very large out-patient departments, where patients may come, with or without appointment, to be seen. In psychiatry, out-patient attendances are used, as in this country, for diagnosis and admission decisions, as well as follow-up of patients after treatment. From what has been written over the last decade about the facilities for the treatment of the mentally ill, it emerges that out-patient facilities are an important feature of the system. At the Shanghai Psychiatric Institute, for which most details are available, Ratnavale and the SFP delegation noted that in 1973 the Out-patient Department handled about 400 patients per day. It had eleven doctors and nine nurses. Masserman, in 1978, reported that the huge Guangzhou Mental Hospital had a correspondingly large out-patient department handling about 1,200 patients daily, and that the 100-bed teaching and research department in Beijing saw about 300 out-patients daily. In the United Kingdom psychiatric out-patient clinics are usually to be found in the out-patient departments of large general or teaching hospitals. The number of patients seen per day would be considerably lower. However, minor psychiatric illness, with which the out-patient department of the Chinese hospital largely deals, would be presented to the general practitioner in Britain.

*Community care*   In Beijing in order to remove the pressure on the city's 2,500 mental hospital beds, many patients are now treated at home. Between 1977 and 1980 about 1,700 patients were so treated. Since many of these cases were thought to be due to social problems, treatment at home where: 'doctors better understand their moods and mental state' is advised. Treatment is based on discussion with family, friends and work units.

Each of Beijing's ten districts has a clinic and a network of prevention and treatment centres has thus been constructed. Local patient surveys are carried out every six months. Patients either receive treatment at home or at the neighbourhood psychiatric clinics, which employ psychiatrically trained personnel. The essential aim is to keep patients out of hospital and prevent 'institutionalisation' of patients developing,(48) which would hinder their return to normal life.

## THEORIES OF MENTAL ILLNESS

*Classical times*
Traditional Chinese medical theory held that all disease including mental illness resulted from an imbalance of the two basic life forces. 'Those who contrary to the laws of the four seasons, dissipate in their duties, and if Yin is not equal to Yang, the pulse becomes weak and madness results.'

In traditional theory, mental diseases were originally classified as 'wind' diseases. The earliest record of mental disease is apoplexy or 'zhong feng', which meant 'overwhelmed by wind'.(49) The 'wind' theory was still in evidence in the eleventh century. In 1060, when the Imperial College of Medicine was founded, nervous and mental diseases were separated from internal medicine. Of the 120 students enrolled at the college, 30 were assigned to the class for 'wind' diseases. Some later Yuan dynasty physicians challenged the idea of 'wind' etiology, believing many diseases to be caused by 'fire' - excessive heat in the internal organs.(50)

The Ming dynasty physician Wang Kentang wrote in his 'Standards for Diagnosis and Treatment' (1602) that the common name for insanity is 'wind in the mind'. These classifications still hold in traditional medicine, while alternative folk theories of the etiology of mental illness caused by possession by evil spirits, which have been in existence for several thousand years, are still extant in some parts of the People's Republic of China.

*Early modern theories*
By the late nineteenth century those psychiatric hospitals which existed under Western auspices utilised neurological theories extant in Western psychiatry, for example, in 1880 Dr A.H. Woods, physician to the Guangzhou (Canton) Christian College,

was invited as neurologist to the Guangzhou Hospital. In 1919
he was appointed associate professor of neurology and psychiatry
in Beijing and started training Chinese doctors in the field.
The work begun by Woods flourished, and the psychiatry and
neurological departments became well established centres, publishing 'social and psychological studies in neuropsychiatry in
China' in 1939.(51)

*Post-revolution theories*
After the 1949 revolution, and probably influenced by the
relationship with the Soviet Union, the theories of the Russian
psychologist Pavlov gained currency. These theories eschewed
the existence of subconscious and unconscious parts of the
mind, seeing mental processes and understanding as proceeding
through a series of learned images. Impaired understanding,
which was how mental disease was conceptualised, could be
rectified through correcting the imbalance between inhibitory
and excitatory cortical reflexes. Chin and Chin write:

> mental disorders exist when the balance of the excitation and
> inhibition functions of the nervous system is disturbed, or
> when the nervous system is rendered incapable of working at
> its full capacity due to excessive pressures of the environment,
> physiological disease or impairment, or incorrect attitudes and
> thoughts.(52)

Koran draws a parallel between this theory and the descriptions of balance in traditional theories which employ the concepts
of Yin and Yang and remarks: 'One can imagine that this
similarity may have aided the acceptance of Pavlovian ideas.'(53)
There is little resort to Freudian theory, and the theories of
Adolf Meyer, which Cerny(54) writes 'were widely accepted in
Chinese psychiatry before 1949' were strongly repudiated by
the psychiatrists in Nanjing visited by Kagan(55) in 1972. At
that time etiological theories stressed that mental illness was a
contradiction between the individual's 'subjective understanding'
and 'objective reality'.

The importance of environmental factors such as social stress
as etiologic or provoking agents was virtually abandoned during
the Cultural Revolution and immediately afterwards. Social
psychiatry has never been strongly established, despite the
fact that in a recent Beijing study 51 per cent of schizophrenics
were found to have suffered 'acute psychogenic trauma or
chronic persistent stress before the onset of disease'.(56)

Community care programmes organised in Beijing stated that
home treatment was more effective because 'most cases are
caused by social problems, disappointment in courtships, unhappy
work situations and examination failures'.(57)

Latest work suggests a revival of interest in organic and
genetic theories of mental illness. Workers at the Beijing mental
hospital have noted abnormalities in the metabolism of 5 HT (a

chemical agent in the brain) in chronic schizophrenics and in some acute schizophrenics. Although they admit that 'in some instances the disease develops in subjects under severe and persistent stress', they note the importance of genetic factors and conclude: 'Whether the environmental factor *previously so stressed* influences brain biochemistry, and in what way, needs further investigation.'(58)

A follow-up study of 704 cases of affective psychosis in Shanghai showed that 294 (41.8 per cent) had a positive history of mental disorders among their relatives, and proposed a model of inheritance of affective disorders. These kinds of research can be seen as examples of a growing interest in the organic and genetic features of psychosis (an interest not pursued since the Cultural Revolution) and represent a definite change in direction in the theories of mental illness now extant in China. At present it is not possible to judge whether theories are eclectically applied, or whether there is the beginnings of a new orthodoxy in the care of the mentally ill.(59)

## METHODS OF TREATMENT

*Traditional*
Cerny in his summary of the literature from Eastern European and Russian sources, notes four aspects of traditional treatment detailed within them. These are ignipuncture, acupuncture, breathing exercises and plant- and animal-based drugs.

The first two were often combined. Insomnia, anxiety states, vertigo and headaches are treated by this method. Cerny reports that acupuncture has also been used in schizophrenia, manic hysteria and dementia paralytica.

In the medical text of the Yellow Emperor -(2698-2589) the Ling Shu section expounded on the use of acupuncture in mental illness. In -400 the renowned physician Bian Que noted in his textbook that by inserting needles in the Fengfu point, he was able to cure 'madness'. A later physician, Huangfu-mi (+282) in his textbook on acupuncture described madness. Patients 'talked a lot, ran about, were suicidal and hallucinated'. He treated suicidal and hallucinated patients by needling the Fengfu point, and those who were aggressive by the Shenzhu point.(60)

However, the use of acupuncture for mental illness was not widespread, probably, as Wong suggests, because needling at the Fengfu point, which is located near the brain stem, had had fatal results!

In 1956 the Hebei mental hospital began using acupuncture as a method of treatment for patients suffering from various forms of schizophrenia. They viewed acupuncture as being similar to ECT, and an 84 per cent success rate was claimed for its use.(61)

In the 1970s there were fifteen reported visits made to psychi-

atric hospitals by Westerners. Acupuncture was clearly still in
use, up to 1978, although sites, periods of treatment, length of
treatment sessions, and success rates varied.

Ratnavale(62) in Shanghai described how acupuncture was
used in those syndromes characterised by excitement, anxiety,
apathy, catotonic stupor and depression. Leung's(63) description
of acupuncture used during her 1975 visit in Shanghai is very
similar to that of Ratnavale, although she noted that the
Shenmen point, rather than the Neiguan point on the wrist
was used. Both these points are related to the pericardium
and the heart. In traditional theory, the heart 'houses the
mind'. It was noted that the use of acupuncture seemed to be
confined to treating the hallucinations and delusions of schizophrenia. In contrast, Walls noted that acupuncture was also
used in the treatment of neurotic patients both in hospital and
the out-patient department.(64)

By 1978, however, changes in the attitude towards acupuncture could be observed. Loshak(65) on his visit to Changsha
reported the remarks of a leading psychiatric instructor at the
Hunan Medical College, who stated that he did not believe
acupuncture worked well for mental illness. In Shanghai in
Masserman's(66) 1978 report the number of points used was
considerably less extensive than in the early 1970s. He also says

> To enquiries as to the 'gate' theory opioid release or other
> rationale for acupuncture, the reply was always 'We are
> investigating these questions . . . the confidence of the
> patient in the skill of the acupuncturist is essential.'

A much more rigorous attitude towards the use of acupuncture
and its effectiveness was also exhibited by Liu, a psychiatrist
practising in Sichuan. In his description of treatments used
in the mental hospitals of his home province he said 'acupuncture therapy is available for treatment of neuroses in every
general hospital and mental hospital' and 'some neurotic patients
respond well; conversion hysteria may show dramatic remission
. . . but the results of these treatments have still to be evaluated with control groups'.(67) Privately some psychiatrists
have also mentioned the 'placebo effect' of acupuncture which
makes it a 'cheap and effective form of therapy'.

A new emphasis on the scientific evaluation of traditional
therapies appears to be part of current thinking. The Department of Psychiatry at Beijing Medical School is studying the
mechanism of acupuncture. While the policy of combining traditional and Western treatments for syndromes on the same
patients persists, however, rigorous methods are required to
separate out the effects of particular therapies, either singly
or in combination. Visits to hospitals at the end of the 1970s do
suggest that the widespread use of acupuncture in a variety of
cases has declined, and a more conservative policy of utilisation
is being adopted.

*Traditional drugs* Drugs of plant, animal or mineral origin are basic to the pharmacopoeia of traditional Chinese therapy, and as such have always been used by traditional doctors and folk healers in the treatment of mental illness. They were used as sedatives, or to produce therapeutic convulsions, and appeared to be administered according to the theory of 'balance' or the beliefs in the need to shake the body in order to drive out evil spirits. As a 'wind' disease psychiatric and neurological ailments (which were not distinguished etiologically) would be treated as other types of wind disease.

At the National Health Conference of 1950 the importance of traditional medicine in the new organisation of medical care was stressed. Since then the emphasis upon the use of traditional drugs has waxed and waned, since psychiatrists in the late 1950s and early 1960s were more likely to stress the need to develop drugs like the major tranquillizers used in the West. In general, however, it can be said that the role of traditional drugs in psychiatry was of lesser importance than the other traditional method - that of acupuncture. They appear in Sidel's account(68) (1971) as 'a little herb medicine' whose therapeutic action is not specified. Kagan(69) (1972) also briefly refers to herb medicines, but the most complete account comes from Liu(70) (1980). He describes the testing of a folk herb 'Parasiticus on Coriaria sinica Maxim' in mental hospitals in Sichuan. He reports that in a series of 960 schizophrenic cases, 60 per cent showed some improvement in symptoms. Three effective elements, Tutin, Coriamyrtin and Coriatin were obtained from the herb. Its administration produced seizures and vomiting in patients, showing its ancient use as a form of drug-convulsive therapy. Masserman says that herbal skin plasters were employed at the hospital in Shanghai for psychotic restlessness, which is reminiscent of the hydrotherapy and mustard baths recommended at earlier times in Britain. He also mentioned a non-addictive hypnotic drug called Maotin, which is used.

*Modern psychiatric methods*
In the early 1950s the main modern methods of treatment available to psychiatrists everywhere were electroconvulsive therapy, sleep therapy, psychotherapy, psychosurgery and insulin shock therapy. Physical methods of restraining violent patients were also used. These methods were also used in China by psychiatrists, in the immediate post-revolutionary period. Western psychiatry has now largely abandoned insulin shock therapy because of the associated risks of brain damage and death, but it is still used in China. On the other hand, psychosurgery in China was declared illegal in the mid 1950s. At present it is only permitted for behaviour disorders due to brain damage.

During the mid to late 1950s sleep therapy and hypnotherapy were added to insulin, non-convulsive electrical therapy and ECT, and combined with tranquillising drugs which had revolutionised world-wide the therapeutic approaches to mental

illness. A major conference held at Nanjing in June 1958
reaffirmed the need for research into the physiology of the
higher nervous system.(71) The Pavlovian influence upon
Chinese psychiatry remained paramount during this period,
but there was also an attempt to modernise ancient psychiatric
theory and practice, in particular that which emphasised an
overall analysis of the patient and his circumstances. In therapeutic terms, this complementary approach led to a development
of psychotherapy, group therapy, and work therapy (see
below).

There is very little information about the therapies used
during the early part of the Cultural Revolution. It is likely
that here as in other health fields the types of therapy and
practice used by fully trained psychiatrists were largely jetti-
soned, especially if they were expensive, or could not be
readily and simply applied in the expanding rural health network. It appears however that in some of the larger city hospital
remnants of the methods and theories of the early 1950s still
existed.

Sidel, in 1971,(72) emphasised that ECT and insulin were no
longer used. To Kagan in Tianjin these were described as
'bourgeois methods' and the explanation given was because the
methods were of Western origin and required expensive equipment which was not available in the rural areas. Taipale at
Shanghai in 1972 reported that psychiatrists had abandoned
the organic theory of mental illness and that they believed that
the symptoms of mental illness were linked with social experiences, usually the patient's private interests set against those
of the collective. The decline in the use of insulin and ECT was,
it was claimed, related to this change in notions of etiology.(73)
In the following year Ratnavale reaffirmed that ECT and insulin
were not in operation in Shanghai, as did Walls, but the latter
added that ECT was being used in Nanjing. He was told:
'insulin shock and ECT are used in schizophrenia, insulin more
than ECT if regular measures fail in a given case. It is not used
in depression, since cases get better as a rule.'(74)

Shock therapy (ECT) was out of use in Shanghai in 1975
during Sophia Leung's visit. She was told that shock therapy
was discontinued since the Cultural Revolution 'for humanistic
reasons'.

The visit of the Vishers in 1977 took place at a turning-point
in psychiatric treatment. They reported the use of locked wards
and restraint and Loshak in Changsha in 1978 wrote:

> In one ward, several patients lying on hard wooden beds
> were being given insulin injections to induce coma . . . later
> the Chinese psychiatrists admitted they realised this treatment
> was considered outdated in the West.(75)

Masserman, visiting Guangzhou and Shanghai in 1978, noted
that the psychiatrists he met were well acquainted with genetic,

neurophysiological and pharmacologic behavioural and various integrative psychosocial approaches to human conduct. ECT was used occasionally for agitated states, and laser beams were used as a new method of point stimulation, being directed at the earlobes of patients for the treatment of hallucinations.

Liu gives the fullest description of ECT, adding that it is often used without anaesthesia due to lack of trained anaesthetists or drugs, a practice which carries the risk of producing bone injury or dislocation. He states that insulin coma therapy is practised now less and less, and that sleep therapy, used in the 1950s for neurasthenia and anxiety states, posed problems in management and has been since abandoned.

*Drug therapy* The transformation of the treatment of the mentally ill by the introduction of psychotropic drugs occurred in China as elsewhere. However, serious problems of shortage affected the ability of psychiatrists to administer these drugs. There were also problems of quality control, since drugs were not imported but manufactured in China itself. At present, problems of shortage still exist, but problems of quality seem to have been overcome. By 1956 the Chinese pharmaceutical industry was producing chlorpromazine, reserpine and meprobamate, and at the Nanjing conference in 1957 it was confidently asserted that an adequate supply of drugs was being provided, and increasing numbers of mental patients were being treated with modern pharmaceuticals. Economic problems in the early 1960s meant that drug treatment was not so readily available. During the Cultural Revolution little is known as to the extent of use of this therapy, but it is likely that it continued although in a restricted form since departments of psychiatry in many medical colleges were closed.

By 1971 'seriously ill' patients were reported as being treated with small doses of chlorpromazine, e.g. about 26 mg daily. The main thrust of therapy at this time was intensive group and labour therapy, supported by tranquillising drugs. Taipale reports relatively small doses of chlorpromazine - 200 mg daily for schizophrenic patients and the use of lithium carbonate in the treatment of mania. The Science for People delegation, visiting the main mental hospital in Shanghai in 1973, remembered:

> the patients were selfdirected, organised and reasonably quiet. No one was aggressive or calling attention to himself by exhibiting bizarre behaviour. This observation was so noteworthy that we asked if everyone in the room was medicated. They replied that most of the people were on low dosages of tranquillisers. It was clear from the attentive expressions of these patients and their level of physical activity that no one was 'doped up'. The games being played all required a high degree of concentration and motion co-ordination. No one was vegetating in front of a television set.(76)

Other writers at that time support the evidence of low dosage, between 200 and 300 mg daily, but Walls remarked that the maximum daily in-hospital dosage in Shanghai was about 600 mg of chlorpromazine in 1973. He said 'the tendency to use increasing doses of phenothiazines seems to have occurred in China as it has in the West'. Out-patient dosages were about 200 mg. Between 1975 and 1977 drug therapy was accorded less prominence, but from 1973 onwards it again occurred in the reports. Hospitals in Sichuan routinely give 600 mg of chlorpromazine to patients on admission, and use the same type of drugs as in the West for schizophrenia and affective psychoses like depression. As Liu says: 'The dosage range of psychotropic drugs in China is not different from that in Western countries.'(77)

Neurotic patients who are mainly treated as out-patients are given minor tranquillisers like benzodiazepines, but usually not the more expensive tricyclic antidepressants which together with lithium carbonate are reserved for the use of in-patients.

*Psychological and social therapies*
The use of various kinds of social and psychological therapy were part of the programme of psychiatric development in China from the mid 1950s onwards. The use of tranquillising drugs meant that physical restraints could be abolished, and social and psychological therapies became easier to use. However, these therapies have usually been regarded as important in their own right, and although they have been used in conjunction with drug therapy, they have also been used independently. By 1957 labour and sports therapies had been introduced into hospitals in the treatment of chronic mental illness and patients were required to do productive work. The Nanjing conference in 1958 affirmed an 'open door' policy for the mentally ill, and it was proposed to 'put an end to irrational restrictions imposed on them, thus granting them a better chance to share normal life with the mentally healthy'. A Russian psychiatrist noted that during his visit in 1959 mental patients went about freely in town, visiting bookshops, cinemas and parks.(78)

The work and sports therapies introduced at this time can be seen to reflect various ideas in Chinese psychiatry and Chinese political thinking. The idea that every person was part of society, with a contribution to make, was a fundamental part of the political philosophy of the Communist Party. Therefore work therapy which also produced useful items was an expression of this. Sport and exercise and collective work reflected a view of mental illness which was a mixture of political, psychiatric and traditional cultural ideas. From Confucius came the idea of the primacy of correct behaviour and attitude over emotions; from socialist and communist theory the importance of collective aims over individual desires. Pavlov, the Russian psychologist, introduced both the theories of dysfunctional nervous excitation and the behaviour therapy available to right it. From Lenin was derived the dialectical notion that correct (i.e. healthy) individual consciousness is characterised by a recognition of social goals, and that an inward-looking individualistic consciousness is *per se* unhealthy since it can only reflect the outside world in a distorted way. The theories and therapies were based on altering perception and thus altering behaviour. Unconscious ideas had no status in these formulations, for although prior to the revolution some Freudian theory, and some ideas of the psychobiologist Adolf Meyer, were accepted in Chinese psychiatry, these were rapidly abandoned in favour of Pavlovian theory. In Tianjin in 1974 in reply to a question on Freud the answer came swiftly:

We oppose him and we also oppose Soviet revisionists who stress individual biochemistry as the cause of mental illness. Sexual repression is not a cause of mental illness because sexual repression as a cause of mental illness is tied to bourgeois experts' analysis of society. Freud serves the bourgeoisie in their rule over others. He attempts to cover up class struggle by stressing only internal causes. (79)

During the Cultural Revolution psychological and social therapies became very prominent. When one declared aspect of the Cultural Revolution was to produce attitude and behaviour changes on a huge scale, it would have been unusual for mental patients to be excluded from the process. Although, as we have seen, drug therapy continued to be used, the number and variety of social therapies increased considerably and continued to enjoy prominence up to the mid 1970s.

In the early 1970s Sidel reported how psychiatric hospitals were using the army model of organisation, and dividing patients on the wards into divisions and groups called 'a collective fighting group' within which sicker patients were paired with those who were getting better, to provide mutual support. Beneath the rhetoric of the Cultural Revolution, it is possible to discern many innovations and serious attempts at sociotherapy. Because barriers and divisions of responsibility between medical, nursing and administrative personnel were broken down, more staff were available to conduct small groups, work therapy, or reading and study sessions, and to organise follow-up care. Since most hospitals were required to send one third of their medically qualified staff to the countryside, both the opportunities for, and necessity of, alternative therapies became important.

Sidel described the study sessions which involved reading the works of Mao Zedong, the aim of which was to give patients encouragement to struggle against their illness, to support and help each other, and to realise the importance of correct thinking. A number of patients described their illness to her in lucid f somewhat mechanical terms. One summed up his attitude to his illness thus:

My trouble was that I had subjective thinking which was not
objectively correct . . . my subjective thinking was divorced
from the practical conditions and my disease was caused by
my method of thinking. . . . I was self interested . . . I
haven't put revolutionary interests in the first place, but if
I can put the public interest first and my own interest
second, I can solve the contradictions and my mind will be in
the correct way. (80)

Therapeutic optimism was the keynote of the early 1970s, and
the theme of treatment was 'education plus medication', although
we know nothing about the effect these particular forms of
therapy had on discharge or relapse rates. Reports from the
early 1970s suggest that the patient's day was a fairly full
round of closely supervised physical and mental activities with
about two hours' physical labour a day, half an hour military
training, approximately four hours reading and political study
(including studying Mao Zedong's thought) and about one hour'
physical recreation. Two hours per day were spent in 'heart to
heart talks', a form of individual or group therapy, and a
prominent part of the therapeutic process. In addition patients
swept up, washed vegetables and made beds.

Later, visitors were less likely to be introduced to individual
patients, but the group therapy, games and use of Taijiuan
still continues to the present. Throughout 1977 and 1978
patients were reported as assembling matchboxes and making
paper flowers, gardening, weaving, cleaning and 'dropping
pencils in a jar to improve concentration'. Work and sport
therapy is less emphasised, but this may have more to do with
the psychiatrists' desire to demonstrate to visitors the modern
drug therapy which they use. As a therapeutic measure, the
thoughts of Mao were still being incorporated into study
sessions in 1978, but this has now been discontinued.

Both individual and group psychotherapy are increasingly
regarded as useful methods of treatment, especially in the case
of neurotic patients. Psychotherapy is more likely these days
to be regarded as a skill which psychiatrists use in treatment,
rather than a form of lay therapy, but lay involvement and
community support in the treatment of psychiatric patients is
an important aspect of the care of the mentally ill in China.
There are also signs that other forms of treatment are becoming
available. As one psychiatrist said to Lowinger: 'If I understand
a patient's behaviour better by the Freudian theory than
Pavlovian or other theory, I am free to use it.'(81) Sexual
problems, problems of disturbed family relationship and
occupational stress, are nowadays more likely to be dealt with
by drugs, psychotherapy, and close personal contacts between
the psychiatrist responsible and the patient's family and work
colleagues, than by exhortations, self-criticism or rhetoric.

*After-care of patients*   The average length of stay for acutely
ill patients in mental hospitals in China is about three months.
While undoubtedly there are long-stay chronically ill patients,
many of whom have no families and who therefore are housed in
municipal mental hostels, hospital in-patients are the subject of
an after-care programme which attempts to be thorough and
comprehensive. A patient who is mentally ill receives paid sick
leave. If insured, or a state employee, hospital costs are
covered. A job is kept open for him, and before discharge from
hospital his factory or unit is contacted. Sometimes colleagues
will visit him in hospital before he returns to work. One serious
problem, as elsewhere in the world, is patient relapse. Masserman in Beijing noted that between 10 and 25 per cent of patients
were readmissions. It seems likely that the lack of adequate
facilities and drugs contribute to this figure.

In Shanghai and Beijing there have been attempts to combat
the readmission rate. Shanghai has set up a co-ordinating
committee for mental health which has devised a community care
programme, which uses the smaller district hospitals to oversee
family care, psychiatric care units and day centres for occupational therapy. Doctors refer patients to higher level hospitals
for regular check-ups.

Specialist psychiatric care units are staffed by the patients'
neighbours, retired workers and family members who

> observe the patient's mental condition and report to the health
> personnel concerned in case of disorderly conduct or breach
> of the peace. They help to guide and educate the patient,
> solve social or psychologic problems and administer drugs as
> prescribed.(82)

In Shanghai there are 500 such units, set up in 40 per cent of
neighbourhood committees, and caring for 10,000 patients.(83)

Another important aspect of after-care is that provided by
occupational therapy groups. A patient who is discharged partially
recovered but not yet fit to take up a full-time job is assigned to
a local OT group, where he works for money and continues to
receive antipsychotic drug therapy. The number of patients in
each group varies from ten to ninety; they are mostly suffering
from schizophrenia although some groups for the mentally handicapped have also been formed. They work a six-hour day, and
also enjoy recreational facilities. The Shanghai programme has
about one hundred OT groups, with about 2,000 patients. The
patients might expect to stay in the groups for anything up to
five years. Since the experiment is relatively new its long-term
value cannot yet be predicted, but figures provided by Xia
suggest a reduction in the relapse rate to about 10 per cent.

The groups have a higher input of trained staff than the
psychiatric care units, being supervised by barefoot doctors,
neighbourhood cadres and retired workers, who keep in touch
with the hospital doctors.

These attempts to cope with the problems of after-care of
mental patients demonstrate one of the very innovative aspects
of the organisation of health care in China - the wholesale
involvement of the lay community in caring for the patient. It
is made clear that lay involvement is not a stopgap measure,
until more psychiatrists are trained, but is an actual part of the
therapeutic process which seeks to involve those closest to the
patient in surveillance of him, and encouragement to him.

## SUMMARY

Facilities for the mentally ill are somewhat undeveloped in
China, and although the prevalence of some forms of mental
illness appears less than in the West, some of the difference
can be explained by differences in the age structure of Chinese
and Western populations.

Methods of treatment in China have always been somewhat
eclectic, often more for practical reasons than any other.
Numerous therapies have existed side by side, and these have
received different emphasis at different periods. The present
system attempts to involve the community outside the hospital
more than in the past, and to develop research into appropriate
therapies. Some progress has been made in the care and treatment of the mentally ill but, as in the West, psychiatry remains
to a large extent a 'Cinderella' service.

## NOTES

1 Liu Xiehe, Mental health work in Sichuan, 'Brit. J. Psychiat.
  137, 1980, pp. 371-6.
2 M. Kramer, Cross-national study of the diagnosis of mental
  disorders: origin of the problem, 'Amer. J. Psychiat', 125,
  1969, Suppl. 1.
3 R. Chin and A.S. Chin, (Qin and Qin) 'Psychological
  Research in Communist China, 1949-66', Cambridge, Mass.,
  MIT Press, 1969.
4 Tseng Wenshing, Traditional and modern psychiatric care in
  Taiwan, in A. Kleinman et al., 'Medicine in Chinese Cultures'
  Washington, John Fogarty Center, 1975, pp. 177-95.
5 H.P. Lamson, 'Social Pathology in China', Shanghai,
  Commercial Press, 1935, p. 410. 'Medicine and Public Health
  in the People's Republic of China', Washington; John Fogarty
  Center, 1972, p. 292.
6 Ma Haide, With Mao Tse-tung's thought as the compass for
  action in the control of venereal diseases in China, 'China's
  Medicine', 1, October 1966, pp. 52-68.
7 R. Sidel, 'Mental diseases and their treatment', in J. Quinn,
  op. cit., p. 293.
8 Ma Haide, op. cit.

9 Yang Desen, Chen Yongde and Liu Hauxing, A survey report on psychosis in Hunan Province, 'Zhonghua Shenjing Jingshenke Zazhi (Chin. J. Neurol. Psychiat.)', no. 1, March 1980, pp. 15-18.

10 Liu Xiehe et al., Survey of psychosis in Sichuan, 'Zhonghua Shenjing Jingshenke Zazhi (Chin. J. Neurol. Psychiat.)', no. 1, March 1980, pp. 7-9.

11 Xia Zhenyi et al., Mental health work in Shanghai, 'CMJ', 93, 2, 1980, pp. 127-9.

12 Liu Jieqiu et al., Epidemiologic investigation of mental disorders in Xuhui district, Shanghai, 'Zhonghua Shenjing Jingshenke Zazhi (Chin. J. Neurol. Psychiat.)', 13, 1, 1980.

13 Shen Yucun et al., Investigation of mental disorders in a Beijing suburban district, 'CMJ', 94, 3, March 1981, 153-6.

14 'Psychiatric Hospitals', Office of Health Economics, London, 1979.

15 R. Cochrane and M. Stopes-Roe, Women, Employment and Mental Health, 'British J. Psychiat'., 139, 1981, pp. 383-81.

16 J.K. Wing and Anthea M. Hailey, 'Evaluating Community Psychiatric Service: The Camberwell Register 1964-71', Oxford University Press, 1972, p. 79.

17 T'ao, Cheng Chih-fan and Chang Ch'i-shan, Some early records of nervous and mental diseases in traditional Chinese medicine, 'CMJ', 81, January 1962, pp. 55-9.

18 Hsia Chenyi, Clinical Studies of Schizophrenia in Shanghai 1935-56, 'Chin. J. Neurol. Psychiat.', 4, 2, 1958, p. 89.

19 Chin and Chin, op. cit.

20 R. Sidel, op. cit., p. 229.

21 L. Kagan, 'Mental hospital visit and revisit Tientsin', 24-26 March 1972, mimeo.

22 Science for People delegation report, 'China: Science Walks on Two Legs', New York, Avon Books, 1974, p. 247.

23 D. Ratnavale, Psychiatry in China: observations in 1973, 'Am. J. Psychiatry', 130, 10, October 1973, pp. 1082-7.

24 P.D. Walls et al., Psychiatric training and practice in the People's Republic of China, 'Am. J. Psychiatry', 132, 2, February 1975, pp. 121-8.

25 P. Lowinger, Mental health in China, 'China Now', 90, May-June 1980, p. 23.

26 Liu Xiehe, op. cit.

27 S. Leung et al., Chinese approach to mental health service, 'Can. Psychiatr. Assoc. J.', vol. 23, 1978, pp. 354-9.

28 D. Loshak, China too has its mental patients, 'Daily Telegraph', 27 November 1977.

29 J.S. Visher and E.B. Visher, Impressions of psychiatric problems and their management: China 1977, 'Am. J. Psychiatry', 136, 1 January 1979, pp. 28-32.

30 Jules Masserman, A Chinese Odyssey, 'Psychiatric Journal of the University of Ottawa', vol. IV, 4, 1978, 293-6.

31 Liu Xiehe, op. cit.

32 Lee T'ao et al., op. cit., p. 55.

33 L. Macartney, Neuropsychiatry in China, 'CMJ', no. 617, 1926, p. 626, in L.M. Koran, Psychiatry in Mainland China: history and recent status, 'Amer. J. Psychiat.', 128, 8 February 1972, pp. 84-91.
34 K.C. Wong, A short history of psychiatry and mental hygiene in China, 'CMJ', 68, January-February 1956, pp. 44-8.
35 J. Cerny, Chinese psychiatry, 'International Journal of Psychiatry', 1, April 1965, pp. 229-38.
36 Sir Robert MacIntosh, 'unpublished diaries', 1957-8.
37 R. Sidel, op. cit., p. 293.
38 Wu Chen-yi, A history of psychiatry in China since 1949, 'unpublished mimeo', 33 pages, 1980.
39 Ibid.
40 Shen Yuan, op. cit., p. 154.
41 Liu Xiehe Personal communication, 1980.
42 P.D. Walls et al., op. cit., p. 122.
43 Wu Chen-yi, op. cit.
44 'Hospitals 1977', Office of Health Economics, London, 1979.
45 Wu Chen-yi, op. cit.
46 'Hospitals 1977', op. cit.
47 Xia Zhenyi et al., op. cit., p. 129.
48 'Beijing Review', 41, 13 October 1980, pp. 28-9.
49 J.C.C. Cheng, Psychiatry in traditional Chinese medicine, 'Canad. Psychiat. Ass. J.', 15, 1970, pp. 399-401.
50 Lee T'ao et al., op. cit., p. 58.
51 K.C. Wong, op. cit.
52 Chin and Chin, op. cit.
53 L. Koran, op. cit.
54 J. Cerny, op. cit.
55 L. Kagan, op. cit.
56 Shen Yucun et al., op. cit.
57 Treating mental illness in Beijing, 'Beijing Review', 41, 13 October 1980, p. 28.
58 Shen Yuan and Zhang Wenhe, 85 hydroxytryptamine metabolism in schizophrenia, 'CMJ', 92, 12, December 1979, pp. 817-2
59 Xia Zhenyi et al., Affective psychosis: a follow up, retrospective classification and heredofamilial study, 'CMJ', 93, 6, June 1980, pp. 365-8.
60 S.W. Wong, Acupuncture and psychiatry, 'Hong Kong Practitioner', December 1980, pp. 381-90.
61 Tan Han-kuang et al., A preliminary report on the acupuncture treatment of 53 cases of mental illness, 'J. New Chin. Med.', 11, 1957, pp. 923-8.
62 D. Ratnavale, op. cit., p. 1083.
63 S. Leung et al., op. cit., p. 356.
64 P.D. Walls et. al., op. cit., p. 126.
65 Loshak, op. cit.
66 Masserman, op. cit., p. 295.
67 Liu, op. cit., p. 376.
68 R. Sidel, op. cit., p. 298.
69 L. Kagan, op. cit.

70 Liu, op. cit., 375.
71 Wu Chen-yi, op. cit.
72 Sidel, op.cit., p. 295.
73 V. Taipale and I. Taipale, Chinese psychiatry, 'Arch. Gen. Psychiatry', vol. 29, September 1973, pp. 313-16.
74 P.D. Walls et al., op. cit., p. 123.
75 Loshak, op. cit.
76 SFP delegation report, op. cit., p. 251.
77 Liu Xiehe, op. cit.
78 E.A. Popov, 'Zh. Neuropat. Psikhiat.', 59, 10, 1959, p. 1179, in J. Cerny, op. cit., p. 230.
79 L. Kagan, op. cit.
80 Sidel, op. cit., p. 297.
81 P. Lowinger, op. cit., p. 23.
82 Xia Zhenyi, op. cit., p. 128.
83 Ibid., p. 129.

# 13 DIET AND NUTRITION IN THE PEOPLE'S REPUBLIC OF CHINA

Nancy Worcester

It has been stated that the health status of today's China has been achieved more by nutritional improvements than by the direct delivery of medical services,(1) so it is appropriate that an examination of the Chinese health system should look at the interaction of nutrition and health.

Horrific descriptions of the ugliness of malnutrition are a part of Joshua Horn's(2) description of Old China, and are an effective part of the 'speak bitterness' stories of pre-Liberation which the Chinese relate to visitors and to the younger generation. But the tragic cycle of poverty-malnutrition-disease-death, still prevalent in so many parts of the world, has been virtually eliminated in New China.

Most people in China seem to have a meagre though adequate diet. Visitors to China invariably comment on the overall impression of healthiness, particularly in the rosy-cheeked children, and the lack of overt nutritional problems. By making agricultural development a primary concern of the national economy, the Chinese system aims to provide an adequate diet as one of the 'five guarantees' (clothing, housing, medical care, food, burial) promised to its entire population. A decent diet is recognised as an essential basis of good health and improving the diet has been seen as an integral part of the emphasis on preventive rather than curative medicine.

## AGRICULTURAL PLANNING AND DEVELOPMENT

When the People's Republic of China was formed in 1949, she was faced with the seemingly insurmountable problem of trying to feed her hundreds of millions of people. Indeed, China was faced with the necessity of feeding a large and growing population on a relatively limited area of land. The cultivable land per person is less than 0.4 acres in China in contrast to 1.9 acres per capita in the United States.(3) With 30 per cent less cultivated land than India and similar monsoonal ecoclimate limitations, China is managing to feed 50 per cent more people than her neighbour.(4) Inspired by Mao's teaching, 'Revolution plus production can solve the problem of feeding the population', the Chinese are now supporting one quarter of the world's population on less than 8 per cent of the world's arable land.(5) This has been achieved by changing the relations of production in the countryside and making agricultural development the

408

principal concern of the national economy.

Land reform was an essential part of the Chinese revolution. Seventy to 80 per cent of the farmland was owned by landlords and rich peasants in Old China. The masses were poor peasants, farming individually on small plots, having to hand over 60 to 70 per cent of their harvests to their landlords. Immediately after the Communist Party gained power in 1949, steps were taken to abolish the traditional land tenure system. Introducing the rudiments of socialism, mutual-aid teams were established. Peasants joined manpower teams and after paying an agricultural tax to the state government, they were able to keep their farm incomes for themselves. From 1953 to 1957 co-operative farms were formed. Production teams collectively owned the land and tools, and the peasants were paid according to their contribution. Annual grain output was reported to have increased from 154 to 185 million tons during this period. (6) In 1958, as the Great Leap Forward was initiated, the PRC took the final step in reorganising co-operative farms into People's Communes. The communes, which became the basic unit of society, were based on a three-tiered structure: the production team (a collective group of 50 to 200 people), the brigade (1,500 to 3,000 people) and the commune (15,000 to 50,000). The years immediately following the establishment of the communes (1959-61) were calamity years of severe food shortage. It remains controversial where to allocate blame for this period of hardship. The communes were criticised for having failed to fulfil their economic role and state policy was criticised for favouring heavy industry at the expense of agriculture, but bad weather may have been the main culprit. However, this crisis did provoke a re-emphasis on agricultural policy and by 1961 production brigades and production teams were largely responsible for the planning and management of agricultural production. Food production was increasing again by 1964.

Reliable information on agricultural production in the 1960s to early 1970s is scarce. Reliable statistics from China are obscure for most topics, but this is particularly true for agricultural information for reasons of non-availability, continuous changes in coverage and reporting systems, occasional deliberate mis-reporting and lack of impartiality. (7)

Agricultural policy has gone through dramatic changes since the arrest of the 'Gang of Four' in 1976 which signalled the end of the Cultural Revolution period. The Minister of Agriculture reviewed(8) some of the measures and policies adopted in the late 1970s:

Decision-making power has been given to the production teams, enabling them to develop production in the light of local conditions; various systems of responsibility in production have been established with rewards allocated according to output; the purchase prices of some kinds of agricultural produce and byproducts have been raised, thus increasing the

income of the peasants; more flexible policies have been
adopted concerning the private plots, family sideline production and country fairs, activating the rural economy; and the
state has cut taxes and quotas for state-purchased grain.

Under the new responsibility system of management in production, contracts are signed between the collective and the
peasants (or a group of peasants) specialising in a certain type
of work.(9) The system is based on public ownership but puts
into practice the principle of 'more pay for more work'.(10) An
editorial in 'People's Daily'(11) states,

At present over 90 per cent of the production teams in China's
rural areas have adopted the system of responsibility in
production in various forms. Working hard to improve the
system of responsibility in production further is an important
guarantee for achieving a bumper harvest in agricultural
production this year.

China continues to be vulnerable to natural catastrophes.
Heavy floods in the south-west, north-west and north-east and
a severe drought in the north in 1981(12) meant that China had
to make her first appeal for international relief in more than
thirty years.(13)
Despite natural disasters, China's grain output for 1981 proved
to be close to that of the bumper harvest of 1979.(14) Total
grain output in 1980 was 2.8 times that of 1949.
It is easy to appreciate the remarkable achievements China has
made in her agricultural production, but it is difficult to
evaluate these in relation to the needs of the growing population.
While emphasising the need for the increased agricultural production, China has in recent years pursued a massive family planning
programme (see chapter 14). Reports indicate that this combined
effort has enabled China's increased grain output to outstrip the
rate of population growth(15) and that China's grain output has
increased at an average rate of 0.5 per cent in the past thirty
years. The annual rate of population growth has averaged about
twenty per thousand (0.2 per cent) during the same period,
and they conclude that although the standard of living is still
fairly low, great advances have been made.


FOOD DISTRIBUTION AND RATIONING

China has not only worked to produce food for her growing
population - attention has been paid to the storage, transport,
and distribution of foods to enable the food to reach the people
it is meant to feed.
A food rationing system was introduced in China in the mid-
1950s and has been operating since that time. To many, the
concept of rationing implies restriction. To the Chinese, who

can still remember widespread famine which resulted from maldistribution of food during years of poor harvests, rationing is a guarantee of at least a minimal diet.

Food is rationed according to sex, age, and physical labour. The decisions of which foods to ration, the ration quantities, and the proportion of the adult ration to be allocated to children are made at the local level.

It is recognised that the energy requirement is greater for manual than sedentary work, so manual labourers receive a higher quantity of grain rations. The average non-manual adult grain ration seems to be about fifteen kg per month (180 kg per year) in urban areas. This works out to be about one pound of rice per day per person. Westerners living in China have difficulty learning to consume this quantity of rice! (16) Etienne(17) commented in 1977 that during his visits to 'advanced and very advanced' communes, grain rations varied from 155 kg per year to 360 yer year. Rations were probably smaller in 'less advanced' communes not regularly visited. It is apparent that although everyone is guaranteed a minimum grain allocation, peasants working in rich production teams receive a higher grain ration than peasants working in poor production teams. This difference will undoubtedly become more marked as richer areas are able to modernise more quickly than poor areas.

In the countryside the entire year's grain ration is distributed soon after the harvest. The family collects its yearly ration from the grain store and will then be responsible for its storage in special storage huts or in earthenware jars. Most of the ration will be taken in rice or wheat flour but coarser grains (maize or sorghum), processed foods (noodles), or beans may also be included in the ration.(18) In urban areas grain is obtained through the use of ration books and is distributed in monthly allotments. Grain for the urban areas comes from the state granaries where grain is taken on the basis that the oldest is used first. Consequently, although the Chinese appreciate the distinct flavour of fresh rice, people in the cities seldom have fresh rice. They are more likely to comment on this lack of freshness than on the restricted quantity.(19) Since the early 1950s there have been state regulations about milling of wheat and rice which prevent overmilling, and this has helped to guard against vitamin deficiencies such as beriberi.

In addition to food grains, vegetable oils are also rationed on a national basis. Municipalities will ration other products if they are not available in sufficient quantities to be sold at an approved price. Meat, particularly pork, and sugar are often rationed. Eggs, poultry, popular types of fish, and bean products (bean curd) may be rationed in some areas or may be alternatives within the meat ration.

A 19 November 1981 circular by the Ministry of Food stressed that

the policy on supplies of grains and edible oil at specific

quantities and at fixed prices upon the presentation of coupons and tickets will be our country's principle for a relatively long period of time. We must persistently and unswervingly implement it.(20)

The coupons can be used to purchase grain, food made from grain, and cakes, or to dine at restaurants. The circular also emphasised that grain shops in cities and townships must store grain for residents, including the surplus grain left unconsumed from ration coupons.(21) This practice is meant to encourage the consumption of grain in a planned and economical way.

Everyone in China should be covered by the rationing system. Pensioners in urban areas will have a ration book. In the countryside the collective welfare fund provides 'the five guarantees', including food, for the elderly.(22) It appears that the only people who fall outside the ration system are those who have moved to cities without permission and so have not been given a ration book, and former landlords who still refuse to carry out manual labour.(23)

Food rationing has not only made it possible for China to more equally distribute the available food within the population, it has also enabled China to establish a reasonable level of agricultural exports.(24) This is also, of course, essential in providing more varied food products for New China. In cash value, every ton of rice exported is roughly equivalent to two tons of wheat imported.(25)

China is minimising on the loss of food by spoilage between production and consumption by improving on grain storage facilities. There are granaries in every county, commune, brigade and production team. Brigades and teams store their own collective grain and grain sold to the state or paid in taxes in county and commune granaries. Granaries have become 'showpieces' which the Chinese are proud to exhibit to visitors. It is reported that grain spoilage in the granaries is generally less than 0.2 per cent and some places have succeeded in keeping it at 0.1 per cent.(26)

Transporting food long distances from the fertile regions of China, through the mountains to the cities, has always been a problem. Historically, governments have found it easier to import grain from world markets than to depend on the internal transport system.(27) Since the early 1950s China has nearly doubled her railway network (from 24,000 km to 55,000 km) and roadways have been increased from 100,000 km to 750,000 km,(28) but limited transport facilities continue to restrict the variety of foods, particularly perishables, available throughout the country. Improvement of the railway, waterway, and road systems is considered a priority in the modernisation programmes ahead.(29)

The Chinese believe their cities should be as self-sufficient as possible. Much of the produce in an urban food market comes

from within the city or surrounding countryside. Hansen and
Risch(30) describe seeing vegetables being grown on vacant
lots, in small plots around factories and museums, and even
along the runway of an airport. It is claimed that Shanghai
grows 80 per cent of its food within the city and surrounding
countryside.(31) Fish, an excellent source of many nutrients,
is playing an increasingly important role in the diet and cities
have begun to raise fish on quite a large scale. Figures from
cities show that the total area of fish ponds built between 1974
and 1978 was equivalent to one third of the country's total
area of fish ponds before 1973.(32) Chicken and pig farms are
also being set up near large and medium sized cities to reduce
lengthy transport of produce. It was reported that the Beijing
area now has 121 chicken farms which in 1978 provided the
local market with 27 per cent of the poultry purchased by the
Beijing municipality.(33)


## PRIVATE PLOTS

'Private plot' refers to a small plot of land, usually near the
family living quarters, peasants have been allowed to keep for
growing their own food. Attitudes towards the private plot
closely reflect changing emphasis in domestic policy. During the
establishment of collective farms (1953-7), peasants were allowed
to keep private plots for growing fruit, vegetables, and rearing
animals for their own consumption. Any surplus had to be sold
directly to the state. During the Great Leap Forward (1978)
private plots were abolished, but they were re-established by
1961. During the late 1960s private plots came into increasing
political disfavour in the period of the Cultural Revolution and
the 'Gang of Four' banned most private plots as remnants of the
private ownership system. Since the downfall of the 'Gang of
Four' private plots have been restored. These plots had been
limited to 7 per cent of the total farmland of collectives, but a
Communist Party circular published in April 1981 allowed for
private plots to be expanded up to 15 per cent.(34) The exact
amount allocated to private plots is determined at the local level.
   In the mid 1970s it was estimated that even though private
plots made up less than 0.5 per cent of the tilled soil, they
contributed approximately 15 to 20 per cent of the proteins,
vitamins, and minerals of the diet because of the meats, fruits,
and vegetables which were usually grown on them.(35)
   Peasants are now allowed to sell the surplus from their private
plot at free markets. Certainly this trend may mean that there
will be more variety available for some people. But this tendency
also has potential for widening already existing differences in
what is available for people to eat. If the gap in food availability
is widened, it will be as important as ever to ensure that the
'basic diet' is as adequate as possible for the majority of the
population.

## THE CHINESE DIET

The Chinese diet has changed very little throughout history and
has always been based upon those foodstuffs most easily grown
in each region. Consequently the 'typical diet' varies enormously
from one part of China to another and may even vary distinctly
from one season to another. Carbohydrates are the principal
component in all Chinese diets because the high carbohydrate
plant foods are those most easily grown and stored. Rice is the
staple food in the south of China. A range of grains is consumed
in North China where farming is more difficult. Wheat is the
major grain in the diet there but is varied by millet, maize,
and gaoliang (sorghum). In contrast to the south, the north
China diet does not contain as much rice but will contain soya
beans and peanuts. Wheat and rice are used interchangeably
in central China or may be replaced with millet, maize, and
kaoliang.(36)

Influenced by the theory of the Yin and Yang, oppositeness
and complementarity, and the five tastes, the Chinese combine
different foods with one another and achieve a diversified diet.
Typically, small amounts of freshly prepared mixed vegetables,
and often a soya bean product, will be added to the grain.
Sweet potatoes, traditionally a low prestige food, provide an
important supplement to the diet. Although the Chinese diet is
largely vegetarian, particularly in the rural areas, families may
have very small amounts of meat - pork, chicken, or fish -
perhaps once a week and on special occasions. In north China
lamb and mutton may also be used. Eggs may play a role in the
diet especially for families who have their own chickens. The
intake of fruit varies greatly, depending on the season. When a
fruit is in season, everyone consumes huge quantities of the
raw fruit which is of variable quality for a week or two, then
no more will be available until the following year.(37) Throughout most parts of China milk and milk products are not a regular
part of the diet.

Seasoning, as well as actual availability of food, is greatly
influenced by the geographical region.(38) South Chinese
(Cantonese) food makes use of a wide range of seasonings based
on sea and fruit flavours. North China (Beijing) foods are
commonly flavoured with soy-based condiments, vinegar, and
pepper. Both the north and south China cuisines make use of
freshly prepared, lightly cooked vegetables. In contrast, in
isolated areas of west China (Sichuan) where the food supply
has been less dependable, preserved foods play a more important
role in the diet. The Sichuan cuisine is thus noted by the strong
flavours of the dried foods, spices, and salts.

Table 13.1 summarises estimates of average monthly individual
food availability for China (1974 FAO figures) and the UK (1973
figures).(39) These figures are very rough estimates for both
countries and are undoubtedly calculated differently. Actual
individual food consumption may be drastically different from

the calculated food availability. This comparison suggests that the average British person consumes nearly ten times as much fat and sugar and nearly seventy times as much milk as the average Chinese person. Cereal consumption is at least twice as high in China as in the UK. Obviously the way in which it is consumed will also be drastically different as the Chinese consume whole grains while most of our cereals come in a very refined, processed form. Potato, fruit, vegetable, nut and fish consumption appear remarkably similar in the two diets, but the individual types of foods in these groups make very different contributions to the diet. For example, potatoes in the English diet will be of the type which contribute to the vitamin C content of the diet. In contrast, sweet potatoes in the Chinese diet will contribute to the vitamin A content.

Table 13.1 Estimates of average monthly individual food availability for China and the UK* (kg)

|  | China | UK |
|---|---|---|
| Cereals | 12.42 | 6.06 |
| Potatoes | 8.59 | 8.18 |
| Other vegetables, fruit and nuts | 7.49 | 9.85 |
| Sugar | 0.47 | 3.94 |
| Meat (and poultry) | 1.57 | 5.71 |
| Eggs | 0.31 | 1.25 |
| Fish | 0.54 | 0.68 |
| Milk | 0.29 | 19.71 |
| Fats and oils | 0.26 | 2.11 |

*Calculated from 1974 FAO figures for China and 1973 figures from Wardle [39] for the UK

*Ecological view of the Chinese diet*
Ecologically, there is much that both the developing and over-developed world could learn from China's accomplishment of feeding a huge population on a relatively small area of arable land.

The Chinese concentrate on raising food for human consumption and not for animal consumption. The diet is largely vegetarian with plant foods providing most of the energy and nutrients. This practice of feeding low on the food chain – eating plant foods directly rather than first feeding animals the plant food and then consuming the meat – is an efficient way of obtaining the nutritional value from food. Table 13.2 compares the efficiency of cereals and animal foods in providing the essential nutrients and shows that if the Chinese diet were more dependent on meats and less dependent on grains, much more land would be required to provide the same nutritive value.

When chickens and pigs are raised for meat in China, they are

usually fed scraps which would otherwise not have been eaten,
rather than being fed food suitable for human consumption.
Animal waste and human waste are used for fertiliser and fed
back into the eco-system.

Table 13.2  Relative efficiency of foods as suppliers of nutrients
from an acre of land(40)

|  | Cereals | Animal Foods |
|---|---|---|
| Gross yield per acre (kg) | 350.0 | 20.0 |
| Calories ($\times 10^5$) | 12.0 | 0.4 |
| Protein (kg) | 35.0 | 4.0 |
| Calcium (g) | 100.0 | 50.0 |
| Iron (g) | 21.0 | 0.4 |
| Vitamin A ($\times 10^5$) | 3.5 | 0.1 |
| Riboflavin (g) | 350.0 | 60.0 |

The Chinese make use of a wide range of wild animals for meat.
Abbot(41) reports that snake meat is regularly on sale in
Cantonese markets along with more exotic items such as owl and
sea salamander. When meats and fish are consumed, use is made
of all edible parts of the animal.

It is not considered socially responsible to feed food suitable
for human consumption to an animal that is simply a pet. Thus
pets, particularly dogs, are only seen when they are serving a
useful role.(42) In rural areas, when dogs are kept, their meat
may be valued as an addition to the diet. The importance of
such a practice can be emphasised by recognising that the
average dog in the UK is estimated to consume the same amount
of 'grain equivalents' per day as the average adult in the Third
World.(43)

The soy bean appears in the Chinese diet in numerous forms.
It has been a practical crop for the Chinese to grow because it
mixes with other crops, adds nitrogen to the soil and produces
more protein per acre than any other (popular) humanly edible
crop.(44) It has been suggested(45) that the lack of interest
in dairy products in China may at least partially result from the
fact that soy provides many of the same nutrients more
economically.

The Chinese social/economic system has thus far encouraged
the use of ecologically beneficial agricultural practices including
the extensive use of intercropping, emphasis on organic
fertilisers, and widespread use of biological and cultural control
of insects. For a detailed description of these practices, see
Hansen and Risch.(46)

*Nutritional view of the Chinese diet*
Nutritional problems are prevalent throughout the world.
Starvation, protein-energy malnutrition, and vitamin A deficiency

blindness, are still commonplace tragedies in many Third World countries where adequate quantities of the right foods are not distributed to the people who need them. In contrast, much of the Western world is afflicted with the diseases of affluence (obesity, heart disease) caused by eating too much of the wrong foods. At this stage China seems to have minimised or eliminated overt nutritional problems and provides for her population a diet which in many ways is nutritionally superior to the average Western diet.

Large-scale nutritional studies have not been a priority in either Old or New China, so very little reliable nutritional data is available. However, the good health of the population indicates a nutritionally adequate diet and health statistics reflect the improved nutritional status of the population. Average life expectancy has changed from 35 years in 1949 to 68 years in 1980.(47) Nutritionists generally regard weight and height records as one of the easiest, most reliable means of assessing nutritional status of populations, and Chinese children thus reflect the improved nutritional status of the Chinese population. The most comprehensive study done in China (on children under fourteen in nine major cities) shows that children are 2 cm taller and 1 kg heavier than were children thirty years ago.(48) Numerous studies are now showing similar increased heights and weights. The most extreme report claims that seven-year-olds are 3.5 kg heavier and 10 cm taller than thirty years ago.(49)

Grain rationing and the Chinese tradition of a 'balanced' diet seem to ensure that most of the nutritional needs of the body are met. There was some agreement in the early 1970s(50) that active males were consuming 2,350 to 3,334 calories per day and females 130 to 300 calories less. (DHSS recommendations are 2,960 to 3,600 calories for active males and 2,500 calories for active females.) The quantity of protein taken in from grains, vegetables and animal products is certainly sufficient. It is much more difficult to evaluate the vitamin and mineral content of the diet. Calcium and riboflavin intakes appear to be low. Endemic goitre (indicating a lack of iodine in the water and diet) has been common in some mountainous areas of China. Its eradication (more complicated than anticipated) has now been brought about in at least 136 counties. The prevention of goitre, through iodising the salt and public health campaigns, has been heralded as an example of the role of preventative medicine in New China.(51) Vitamin D deficiency (rickets) has previously been a problem in some less sunny (sun can convert vitamin D precursors in the body to vitamin D) northern areas of China. An increased intake of fish products, eggs, or supplements have probably minimised the problem. However, a report(52) has mentioned rickets as a topic for study in special research units in children's hospitals and research centres, and another report(53) said that baby foods in Heilongjiang province (north-east China) are being supplemented with vitamin D, calcium, phosphorus, carotene, iron, and soya powder 'after

an investigation of pre-school children in the province'. Both
these studies suggest that rickets and other vitamin deficiencies
may still be a problem in some areas. Iron deficiency was a
common problem in Old China, but this problem was exacerbated
by hookworm which has now been controlled. Iron deficiency is
a common problem even amongst Western women so it would not
be surprising to see it in China. A Beijing study has found low
haemoglobin levels (iron deficiency) in pre-school children.(54)
Cereals have a low iron content which is poorly utilised.

A well-balanced vegan diet (a diet which excludes all animal
products including milk and cheese products) can be nutritionally
adequate, so, in theory, there is no reason why the Chinese
diet with small quantities of animal products should not be so.
The lack of obvious deficiency symptoms indicates that the diet
is probably adequate, but it is also apt to be quite marginal.
As long as a diet is marginal, that is fine - too much of a good
thing has no apparent advantage when it comes to nutrition and
there are obvious cases where overconsumption is a disadvantage
However, if a diet is marginal then it is important to make
certain that it does not 'slip' into being deficient. Storage and
cooking methods and factors which affect nutrient absorption
will be important. As there are large differences in individual
nutrient requirements, a diet which is sufficient but marginal
for most of the population will in fact be nutritionally inadequate
for those individuals with exceptionally high requirements.
There may be more sub-clinical cases of vitamin and mineral
deficiencies than has been recognised. For this reason it is
good to hear that nutritional studies are starting to be done.
It is important that when the Chinese do these nutritional
investigations they make it a priority to look at vulnerable
groups.

Although the Chinese diet is frugal by Western standards, it
provides an interesting model with which to compare. It is
heavily based on complex carbohydrates (starches) and contains
a minimal amount of simple carbohydrates (sugars). The replace-
ment of starch for sugar in the UK diet over the last century
has been blamed for many of the illnesses of Western society:
heart disease, diabetes, dental caries. The Chinese diet also
differs significantly in its fat content. Fats only contribute 10
to 20 per cent of the calories in the Chinese diet in contrast to
providing over 40 per cent in the average British diet. The
Chinese fats come almost exclusively from plant sources whereas
much of the fat in Western diets comes from animal sources, which
contain more saturated-type fats. There is absolutely no
nutritional advantage of this high fat content, and it is thought
to contribute to the high incidence of obesity and heart disease.
Chinese studies(55) have suggested that the low incidence of
atherosclerosis in (east) China is related to a low serum (blood)
cholesterol level in normal Chinese and propose that this is due
to the low saturated fat intake.

'Taking grain as the key link' has been the basis of both

Chinese agricultural policy and Chinese diet   and it has been a controversial issue. The average diet contains approximately 500 grams (nearly 1 lb) of grain per day. As early as 1960 researchers were recommending a reduction in the percentage of grain-derived calories from 80 to 90 per cent down to 70 per cent with an increased use of fats and proteins.(56) However, it is questionable whether China would have been able to adequately feed her growing population if she had tried to change the quality of the diet.

Is there any nutritional necessity for reducing the grain content of the diet? Grains are perfectly adequate sources of calories (energy). The body will take care of its energy requirement before taking care of its other needs. So if the diet were to contain adequate protein, but inadequate calories, the body would 'waste' the protein and use it for energy. Consequently, it is sensible to emphasise the use of inexpensive, easy-to-store foods as energy foods.

Grains also contribute to the protein content of the diet (500 grams of rice will contribute approximately 40 grams of protein to the diet: the DHSS suggests 45 grams as the minimum protein intake for a man) and it is this role which is most controversial. Protein quality as well as quantity is important in assessing a diet. Fed in isolation, animal proteins are superior to plant proteins, but a mixture of plant proteins can be equal to, or better than, the quality of animal protein. When fed on its own, the protein in rice and other grains cannot be fully utilised by the body. But when this grain protein is complimented by the protein from pulses or animal products, the body can use it very efficiently. The traditional Chinese diet quite naturally encourages the balance of bean or animal products with grains, but this could also be a topic for a future public health campaign.

The protein quantity and quality of the Chinese diet appears to be adequate. If the protein were deficient, children would be showing signs of kwashiorkor. The Chinese experience supports the idea, 'Look after the calories and the proteins look after themselves' (Sir Jack Drummond, Britain's former nutrition adviser).(57)

Taking grain as the key link in agriculture was a policy encouraged by the 'Gang of Four' and so is, of course, a topic for debate today. A controversial article by Liu Zhenbang of the Research Institute of World Economy of the Chinese Academy of Social Science appeared in the 'People's Daily' in 1979 stating that the per capita grain consumption in China was three to four times that of Western countries and so he proposed using more grassland for animal husbandry and changing the diet!(58) A range of replies was printed in the 'People's Daily'. One reader said simply, 'Fish, meat, eggs, and milk are better food than grain.' Several letters suggested new areas that could be used for grassland and related stories of former grasslands which had foolishly (by the 'Gang of Four' followers) been turned into farmland. A letter from the Wuhan Bureau of Agri-

culture and Forestry advocated a diversified agriculture with
food grains as the 'key but adapted to local conditions.(59)

Government policy of a diversified agriculture was emphasised
in a 17 December 1981 statement by Lin Hujia, the Minister of
Agriculture,(60) in which he said

> China adhered to the policy of not slackening the efforts on
> grain production while continuing to increase grain output.
> Efforts should be made during the Sixth Five-Year Period
> (1981-85) to speed up cotton, sugar cane, sugar beet and
> tobacco production, and to develop animal husbandry and
> small rural enterprises.

To carry out this readjustment, the area devoted to grain was
reduced by 6.6 million hectares between 1977 and 1980, but
grain output during this period rose at an annual rate of 2.7
per cent.

The diversified agriculture policy is already influencing the
Chinese diet according to surveys carried out in Liaoning.(61)
Urban monthly meat consumption had increased 11.1 per cent
in the first six months of 1981 compared to the fourth quarter
of 1980. Peasant families consumed 30 per cent more pork, eggs,
cooking oil, and wine in 1980 than 1978, and per capita grain
consumption was down.


## NUTRITION DURING PREGNANCY, LACTATION, AND CHILDHOOD

China's most valuable investment in the future is the diet
provided to expectant mothers and growing children. Good
nutrition during pregnancy and the first few months of life is
the best insurance that the child will be able to develop her/his
full capabilities.

Improving the nutritional status of women and children has
been a much needed area of attention for New China. The plight
of women and children was particularly bad in Old China during
times of food shortages. Any grain available was given to the
men so that they could work in the fields. Women were often
given only a thin gruel, grass, and leaves. Many little girls
were so calcium and vitamin D deficient, as a result of their
poor diet, that their bones could not grow properly and it was
common for women to die during childbirth as a result of early
pelvic deformities.(62)

The improved nutritional status of women has not been without
problems. Because the diet has improved so much over a
relatively short period of time, small women are now giving birth
to disproportionally large babies. (Average birth weights in
China are now very similar to ours.) This has meant an increased
number of 'difficult deliveries' which makes a large call on the
developing medical services and technology. There is an increas-

ing emphasis on the care of the woman during pregnancy, but it is not clear what nutritional advice is given to pregnant and lactating women. Folk tradition encourages the consumption of a number of protein-rich foods of animal origin(63) and market-places are reported to have special sections for pregnant and lactating women which sell such products as liver.(64) Despite the extra nutritional requirements of the body during periods of pregnancy and lactation, it seems women are not given extra food rations during this period but are allowed to buy higher quantities of rationed products. This is an obvious area which deserves attention because a marginal diet will become a deficient diet during pregnancy and lactation.

Doctors and health workers throughout China recognise the importance of breast feeding as a guarantee of good infant nutri-tion. As many as 90 per cent of infants may be breast fed.(65) In urban areas breast feeding sometimes continues for nine to twelve months. In rural areas it may continue for up to two years.(66) Women in China do not have to choose between the privileges of breast feeding their babies or returning to work, as workplaces with nurseries will enable women to feed babies during breaks at the workplace. In the few situations where breast feeding is not possible, fresh or powdered milk is avail-able, but this must be paid for by the family and there have been reports of shortages of powdered milk and formula feeds. Supplementary feeding begins by six months and initially con-sists of cereal-based porridges. Cow's milk and soy milk are used as weaning foods. Family planning which encourages several years between children, and the availability of weaning foods, prevents 'the sickness the older child gets when the next baby is born' (kwashiorkor) still prevalent in countries where there is not adequate food available for children when they have to be weaned.

Many children attend nurseries, day-care centres, and then kindergartens, and receive some or most of their meals in these institutions. The nursery diets are said to be supervised regularly to make certain that they are both nutritionally and economically appropriate for the season. Nurseries and kinder-gartens may receive 'special foods' not available at the market to improve their diets. Children's foods have been an area for fortification. As mentioned above, the Chinese Institute of Nutrition has started fortifying special milk powders, milk drinks, and fruit drinks in north-east China.(67) The Institute of Health and Pediatrics under the Chinese Academy of Medical Sciences now produce a range of specialist fortified children's foods at four factories in Beijing, Tianjin, Shanghai, and Shenyang.(68) These products have been designed to be appetising and are attractively packaged (they contain cut-out toys) so that children will like them.

The National Women's Federation and other National Depart-ments recently held a conference to specifically discuss the food needs of the 370 million children below the age of twelve in

China, of whome 35 million are two years of age or younger.(69)
Plans call for doubling the output of children's foods by 1985
in order to have a sufficient supply of the principal foods for
weaned infants throughout the country and 'to cope with
children's diseases due to malnutrition'.(70) In order to meet
this goal priority will be given to the production of children's
food in the allocation of types of cereals and oils in short
supply. Factories producing children's foods will have their
taxes reduced or eliminated altogether.(71)

## COMMUNAL FACILITIES FOR FOOD PROVISION

The availability of communal domestic services plays an important role in ensuring a good, varied diet to all members of the
population without individual domestic responsibility having
to be a priority. All factories, workplaces, and schools have
canteen facilities where good meals are provided at minimal
cost. Neighbourhood canteens provide a large selection of prepared foods which can be taken home.

China began in 1978 to produce various convenience foods.(72)
Instant foods based on traditional cuisine, requiring minimal
preparation, include noodles, rice, rice vermicelli, and frozen
dumplings. Fully cooked, ready to serve convenience foods
containing soy bean and peanut protein have proved useful for
children, the aged, and the sick. Increasing emphasis is being
put on automating the food industry and providing more modern
catering facilities so that energy now devoted to household
chores can be directed into 'production, work, and scientific
research'. Factories in China produced a total of two million
tons of processed foodstuffs in 1980 - 60 per cent more than
in 1979.(73)

A 'Beijing Review' article(74) describing ready-to-serve
noodles and dehydrated cooked rice concluded:

It is of great significance to enable people to eat better and
spend as little time as possible on cooking. If ten minutes is
saved every meal by every working person (suppose the
labour force is about one third of China's population) then
that will mean sixteen million workers will be added to the
country's total every day.

Many unemployed urban youths are setting up 'take-away'
foodstuffs on the city streets which are proving to be popular
but will also require careful 'food hygiene' control.

## SUMMARY

Improved nutrition has been one of the most important factors in
improving the health status of the Chinese population. By chang-

ing the relations of production, making agricultural development the principal concern of the national economy, and embarking on a massive family planning campaign, China has managed to produce, on a limited amount of arable land, enough food to feed her population. Improvements in the storage, transport, and distribution of food have enabled the state to work towards the guarantee to each person of at least a minimal diet.

The Chinese diet is meagre, but appears to be nutritionally adequate. Grain rationing should ensure everyone a minimal calorie intake. The traditional Chinese diet of grain supplemented by small amounts of mixed vegetables, bean and animal products provides an excellent example of a diet which is both ecologically efficient to grow and nutritionally adequate to consume.

Throughout history, much of life in China has been centred around managing to provide an adequate diet when the food supply was extremely limited. This has not changed, but the burden for this responsibility is no longer an individual responsibility. All of society is involved in trying to fulfil the guarantee of a decent diet for everyone.

## NOTES

1　Wen Chi-pang, Food and Nutrition in Joseph R. Quinn, (ed.) 'China's Medicine as We Saw It', in Washington, D.C. Department of Health, Education and Welfare, 1974, quoted in Virginia L. Wang, Food distribution as a guarantee for nutrition and health: China's experience, 'Milbank Memorial Fund Quarterly', vol. 54, 1976, p. 145.
2　Joshua Horn, 'Away with All Pests', London, Hamlyn, 1969, pp. 16-23.
3　Virginia Wang, op. cit., p. 147.
4　Gilbert Etienne, 'China: Men, Grain and Machines - Agricultural Growth and Prospects', Geneva, Asian Documentation and Research Centre, 1977, p. 41.
5　Wang, op. cit., p. 147.
6　Ibid., p. 151.
7　R.O. Whyte, 'Rural Nutrition in China', Oxford University Press, 1972, p. 4.
8　'Xinhua News Agency', 16 October 1981.
9　Ibid., 1 April 1981.
10　Editorial: Agricultural Policy, 'Beijing Review', 28 September 1981.
11　'SWB'/FE, 9 February 1982.
12　'Xinhua News Agency', 22 October 1981.
13　James Sterba, Chinese limit foreign aid to worst hit provinces, 'The Times', 29 April 1981.
14　'Xinhua News Agency', 22 October 1981.
15　Ibid., 6 July 1979.
16　Caroline Williamson, personal notes on her stay in Peking and the nearby countryside, 1974-6.

17    Etienne, op. cit., p. 30.
18    J.C. Abbott, Food and agricultural marketing in China, 'Food Policy', November 1977, pp. 326-7.
19    Williamson, op. cit.
20    'SWB'/FE, 5 December 1981.
21    Ibid., 1 December 1981.
22    Social relief in rural areas, 'Beijing Review', 26 October 1981.
23    Abbott, op. cit., p. 327.
24    Wang, op. cit., p. 155.
25    R.O. Whyte, China, in 'Rural Nutrition in Monsoon Asia', London, Oxford University Press, 1974, p. 188.
26    Storing grain, 'Beijing Review', 27 January 1978.
27    Abbott, op. cit., p. 324.
28    Etienne, op. cit., p. 39.
29    Strive for modernisation of waterborne and road transport, 'Beijing Review', 7 July 1978.
30    Michael Hansen and Stephen Risch, Food and Agriculture in China, Part II, 'Science for the People', July-August 1979, p. 36.
31    Ibid., p. 37.
32    Raising fish for cities, 'Beijing Review' 24 February 1978.
33    'Xinhua News Agency', 30 August 1979.
34    China's farmers may double size of private plots, 'International Herald Tribune', 8 April 1981.
35    Wang, op. cit., pp. 155, 156.
36    Peter Kung, Farm crops of China 1. Distribution and major crops, 'World Crops', March/April 1975.
37    Williamson, op. cit.
38    Kenneth Lo, Interview on LBC radio, London, 23 September 1979.
39    Chris Wardle, 'Changing food habits in the UK', London, Earth Resources Research, 1977.
40    'Food for a Future', London, Abacus, Jon Wynne-Tyson, 1976.
41    Abbott, op. cit., p. 328.
42    Ibid.
43    Robin Fears, Pet foods and human nutrition, 'New Scientist', 18 March 1976, p. 606.
44    E.N. Anderson and M. Anderson, Modern China, South in K.C.C. Chang (ed.), 'Food in Chinese Culture - Anthropological and Historical Perspectives', London, Yale University Press, 1978.
45    Ibid.
46    Hansen and Risch, op. cit., pp. 33-8, and Food and Agriculture in China, Part I, 'Science for the People', May-June 1979, pp. 39-45.
47    'Xinhua News Agency', 29 September 1981.
48    'SWB'/FE, 30 June 1980.
49    Jay M. Arena, Nutritional status of China's children. An overview, 'Nutrition Reviews', vol. 32, October 1974, p. 293.

50   Wang, op. cit., p. 156.
51   Treating and preventing goitre, 'Beijing Review', 10
     February 1978.
52   'Xinhua News Agency', 16 April 1979.
53   Ibid., 8 October 1979.
54   Wu I-chan, 'China's food and population policy', talk given
     at Europe-China Association Summer School, Oxford,
     August 1980.
55   Robert L. Freedman, Review of recently published work
     dealing with nutrition research in mainland China, 'Wld.
     Rev. Nut. Diet', vol. 30, 1978, p. 9.
56   Ibid., p. 10.
57   Wang, op. cit., p. 154.
58   'Xinhua News Agency', 31 July 1979.
59   Ibid., 2 September 1979.
60   Ibid., 17 December 1981.
61   'SWB'/FE weekly economic reports, 21 October 1981.
62   S.D. Yeh and B.F. Chow, Nutrition, in J.R. Quinn (ed.)
     'Medicine and Public Health in the People's Republic of
     China', Washington, US Department of Health, Education
     and Welfare, 1973.
63   Whyte, op. cit., p. 186.
64   Hansen and Risch, op. cit., p. 37.
65   Arena, op. cit., p. 292.
66   Ibid., p. 292.
67   'Xinhua News Agency', 8 October 1979.
68   Ibid., 2 November 1979 and 31 May 1980.
69   Ibid., 27 November 1981.
70   Ibid., 16 November 1981.
71   Ibid., 27 November 1981.
72   Ibid., 10 May 1980.
73   'SWB'/FE weekly economic reports, 27 January 1982.
74   Proposal for changing dietary habits, 'Beijing Review',
     1978.

# 14 FAMILY PLANNING IN CHINA

Penny Kane

## HISTORY

Individual attempts at fertility control have been a feature of
Chinese life for hundreds of years. Traditional methods are,
in fact, better documented there than in most countries of the
world, partly because references to contraceptives - such as
condoms or caps made of paper and even tortoiseshell - occur
in classical literature and partly because in the 1950s the
Chinese government made comprehensive efforts to collect and
evaluate traditional contraceptive recipes.(1)(2)

Some of these had been handed down from one generation to
another among herbalists in the same family: for example, the
belief that silkworm eggs could serve as an oral contraceptive
dates from the seventh century. While it is possible that among
the concoctions there were some which had at least slight contraceptive effect, many also produced severe toxic symptoms.
It seems likely that most women in the old China who found
themselves unwantedly pregnant resorted to the commonest
of traditional methods: abortion or infanticide.

Traditional Chinese law dealt with abortion in only two kinds
of circumstances.(3) Abortion as the result of assault was
considered a relatively light offence; 'only a little more serious
than breaking a limb or causing permanent blindness in one eye'.
Where an abortion resulted in the mother's death, an abortionist
was subject to penalties, but there was no law which prohibited
women from seeking an abortion or penalised her if she achieved
one successfully. 'Not only was she not prohibited from seeking
to abort; it may actually be inferred that the law extended some
marginal protection to her when she did so.' A foetus was
apparently not considered as a potential human being until it
was ninety days old, and then, because the life of the foetus
was integrated with, and derived from, the mother, she had a
far greater degree of freedom to abort than did her Western
sisters. 'There was a far more flexible and situational, and a
far less moralistic approach', although the woman was subject
to her husband and her mother-in-law and did owe an obligation
to her husband's ancestors to procreate.

In 1910, however, the tottering Empire introduced a new penal
code modelled on Western and Japanese laws. Under the Code,
any woman who attempted to procure an abortion, and any person
who helped her to abort, had committed an offence: no allowance
was made for therapeutic abortion until 1935, when the code was

revised. However, given the turbulence of China during the first part of the century, and the almost complete breakdown of national control, it is unlikely that this aspect of the new Code impinged much on the ordinary peasant.

Indeed, there is evidence that it did not. After Liberation in 1949, while abortion continued to be prohibited, many women nevertheless attempted it and some died from the dangerous methods they used. For what was perhaps the first time in Chinese history, these cases were reported in the Press in their grisly details, and a heated debate took place.

Those who could not effect an abortion, or who feared its consequences, often chose infanticide. Innumerable accounts by Western missionaries and others describe finding babies exposed to their deaths: Han Suyin's autobiography describes a not uncommon experience during the 1930s:

> There was the countrywoman who came a long way from Chinsien, eight li or more, to be delivered of her tenth child, because all the others had been daughters; and a neighbour of hers had been to the hospital and had acquired a son; this woman thought she too could obtain a son by coming to be delivered at our hospital. She rode in a rickshaw all the way and this must have cost a good deal; and as she lay on the obstetric table she told Ms Hsu what had happened to her baby daughters: the first was alive, and also the third; but the second had been strangled at birth by the husband and so had the fifth and sixth; the seventh had been born in a bad year, a year of famine when her belly skin stuck to her spine, and the husband had smashed her skull in with his axe; at the eighth female child the husband had been so angry that he had hurled it against a wall; the ninth was a year old and had been given away to a neighbour and now here was something in her belly. . . . Oh let it be a son, a male child.(4)

The practice survived amongst the Chinese community in Hong Kong until at least 1954, when British soldiers were accustomed to finding abandoned babies in baskets dead on the rifle range near Kai Tak.(5)

The expedients of individuals or couples to meet the realities of poverty, illness or simply too many children were seldom entirely in tune with official attitudes. China's population fluctuated considerably over the centuries, with periods of expansion alternating with those of comparative stability resulting from those Malthusian disasters of war and famine, as well as from migration and presumably increased use of birth control. One author of the 1930s who, incidentally, argued that control of population growth was an essential factor in the country's development, identified five population peaks in the history of China and among the earliest recorded reactions to an early 'boom' was the poem by Han Feize in about 500 BC.(6)

In ancient times,
People they were few and wealthy and without strife.
People at present think that five sons are not too many, and
    each son has five sons also,
    and before the death of the grandfather
    there are already twenty-five descendants.
Therefore, people are more and the wealth is less;
    they work hard and receive little.
The life of a nation depends upon having enough food,
    not upon the number of people.

Feize

In the 150 years following the middle of the seventeenth century the population doubled or trebled; the poet, philosopher and historian Hong Liangji (1744-1809), who has been described as the Chinese Malthus, developed a similar theory to his English contemporary about geometric population increase outstripping food production, and he too assumed the answer lay in the natural checks of war, disease and famine.(7) During the years 1840 to 1940 the rate of population growth was low and only about 130 million people were added. Notes on the 1935 legal code pointed out that the prohibition of abortion was not primarily to protect the foetus. 'The objective of the nation is to multiply into strength. But multiplying and strengthening depends on the people. Unless abortion is prohibited, it runs counter to the national objective.'(8) Despite evidence of continuing discussion of China's population growth, it is clear that throughout the centuries the overwhelming balance of agreement was that an expanding population was essential for a powerful China, and should be encouraged.

## THE PEOPLE'S REPUBLIC: THE FIRST PHASE

The first post-war census in 1953 reported a population of 582 million: considerably larger than expected. The official reaction by the 'People's Daily' to the results of the census was approval, with the slogan 'Six hundred million people - a great strength for socialist construction'. But the State Council, even before the census had been counted, had approved the Ministry of Health's revised regulations liberalising access to contraception and induced abortion, and had instructed the Ministry to help the masses to control reproduction.(9)

The primary reasons for the new government's acceptance of family planning seem to have been the benefits for maternal and child health and, perhaps, the greater opportunities it offered for women's development. Maternal and child welfare was certainly the argument used by Shao Lici in a famous speech to the National People's Congress in 1954, which is now regarded as marking the beginning of the second phase of China's family planning programme. A symposium on birth control was called by

Liu Shaoqi in December of that year, and resulted in the State
Council designating responsible officials from various government departments to study the question and recommend ways of
promoting family planning. 'Under the present historical circumstances' said the Party's Central Committee three months later
'in the interests of the nation, the family and the new generation,
our Party seconds appropriately planned births.'

During the 1950s the rate of population growth was well above
2 per cent per year. But advocates of a population policy, like
Professor Ma Yinchu, President of Beijing University and a
member of the Standing Committee of the NPC were unable to
get their arguments presented to the Congress and their views
were attacked as 'Malthusian'. (Ma eventually read his paper in
1957 and probably later wished that he had not: he was publicly
disgraced in 1960 and was only rehabilitated in 1979, at the age
of 98.)(10)

A clear distinction was being made between contraception,
as a way of avoiding troublesome frequent pregnancies, and
population control measures. Soviet Marxist theory argued that
if society were properly organised there could be no such thing
as a population problem: though the concrete circumstances of
the two countries differed considerably, the theory was held to
be absolute.

Mao Zedong is reported to have included in a speech to the
Supreme State Council in 1957 a statement that 'steps must be
taken to keep our population for a long time at a stable level,
say, of 600,000,000. A wide campaign of explanation and proper
help must be undertaken to achieve this aim' in order to effect
an improvement in the living standards of the people. The
speech was eventually published under the title 'on the correct
handling of contradictions among the people' with this section
deleted: possibly because of the ignorance of population
dynamics it revealed, but more probably because population
control was still an ideologically sensitive issue in a country
whose Marxism owed much to the Russian model and where
Russian influence was still strong.(11) Family planning, however, was steadily gaining ground. The rules on sterilisation
were relaxed so that existing family size was no longer a
criterion (previously it was limited to couples with six or more
children). An Office of Birth Control under the State Council
was created with representatives from government departments
and mass organisations. Responsibility for implementing the
programme rested largely with maternal and child workers at
all levels. The programme was limited to some extent by its
reliance on medical channels (which were only intermittently
available outside the urban areas) and on the mass media for
propaganda.(12) Given the large proportion of adults who were
illiterate, and did not yet possess radios, neither the carefully
explained health consequences of too frequent childbearing, nor
the exhortations to young people to give their time to study and
work, nor the personal endorsement of contraception by local

opinion leaders, could be wholly successful.

The setting up communes in 1958 which extended medical care, and the arrival in the countryside of some intellectuals, provided the beginning of an opportunity to spread the family planning message more widely, but the fiasco of the Great Leap Forward, the three calamitous years of freak weather and famine which followed, and the quarrel with the Soviets and subsequent fear of war, meant that it was not until 1962 that the next stage of effort got under way.(13) Birth control also suffered during the late 1950s from government propaganda designed to induce working women to return to their homes, and to fulfil themselves as housewives and mothers: this was a consequence of unemployment.(14)

PHASE TWO: THE EARLY 1960s

A further problem had been lack of contraceptives. The cap is seldom a very acceptable method in overcrowded homes without sanitation; the oral contraceptive only went on general distribution in the West in 1960 (although the Chinese soon began to develop their own) and methods of male and female sterilisation were less sophisticated than they have now become. Apart from condoms, the intra-uterine device was the one reliable method, but it did require insertion by a trained person, under hygienic conditions. In January 1962 the Chinese government removed all import duties from contraceptives. Given the limitations of conventional contraceptives, it is perhaps not surprising that reliance on abortion continued. Chinese doctors are credited with having invented the vacuum technique of abortion, which soon became available at the request of the woman alone. The incidence of side effects appears to have been fairly low, partly because of the innovatory technique and partly through the elimination of legal obstacles to very early termination.

To overcome the limitations of mass communication, a face-to-face approach was adopted. Home visits and small group discussions involved maternal and child health workers, cadres, women prisoners, Women's Federation members and many others in a concentrated campaign of individual persuasion. The Cultural Workers' Corps was also mobilised to present songs, sketches and plays about birth control as its members travelled around from village to village, combining propaganda with entertainment for the illiterate masses.

A further development, in 1963, was a Party directive recommending an optimal age of marriage of twenty-two for women and thirty for men. The legal age had already been raised to eighteen for women and twenty for men by the new Marriage Law introduced as one of the first acts of the revolutionary government. The optimal age, however, was suggested for a number of reasons: that very early marriage was detrimental to the health of couples, their children, and the population at

large; that the country needed the energy and time of the
young for furthering socialism; and that it gave girls, in
particular, a chance to work and become independent instead of
settling down immediately under the dominance of a traditional
mother-in-law.

## THE CULTURAL REVOLUTION

Just as the campaign to widen acceptance of family planning was
beginning to achieve results, however, it was overtaken by the
Cultural Revolution. Organised propaganda efforts, as well as
administrative structures designed to bring family planning to
those who wanted it, were submerged in factional disputes, in-
fighting, and in the disruption of all aspects of ordinary life
which were such a remarkable feature of the period between
1965 and 1968/9. In many areas it appears that the birth rate
actually increased during this time, perhaps as a result of the
bands of unattached and undisciplined young people roaming the
countryside, as well as of the lack of direction and organisation.(15)

The experience was not all negative. Cadres, and especially
doctors, sent to the country and often shocked at the conditions
they found there, were able to spread the knowledge of contraception which they had gained in the earlier campaigns. A vast
corps of barefoot doctors was created in the years immediately
following 1969, chosen for training by their local communities to
which they returned with their Handbooks (one of the six
chapters of which was on contraception). Their work was
amplified by the establishment of co-operative medical services
at the brigade level, financed with members' fees and from the
brigade's public welfare fund, and by the building or improving
of commune health centres. An intricate system of referral and
technical back-up thus came into operation providing reassurance
and support for both the contraceptive user and his/her non-
medical advisers.

Young country people, who in the past saw few options to
marriage and a continuation of the agricultural life which was all
they knew, found that for some at least there was a possibility
of further schooling, university or technical education, and a
more ambitious future. There was a questioning of established
attitudes and traditional values which gave the young a defence
against the pressure of their families for marriage and grand-
children; women, in particular, were able to find much in the
campaign to criticise Confucius which had relevance to their own
roles.(16)

The questioning of the past was well described in the 'three
breaking down and three establishing campaigns' described in
the 'People's Daily':(17)

First break down the outdated idea of 'attaching greater

importance to sons than daughters and having both sons and
daughters' and establish the new idea that 'times have changed
and today men and women are equal'.

Second break down the old concept that 'one will have more
support and help if one has more sons and daughters' and
establish the new idea that 'fewer children means better
upbringing, and one should rely on the socialist collective
economy'. Third, break down the old concept that 'giving
birth to and fostering sons and daughters is a private matter
of minor importance' and establish the idea that 'family planning is something of a major importance to socialist revolution
and construction'.

The Birth Planning Leading Group was re-established and in
1969 regional and local birth planning committees again set up
offices with small staffs to co-ordinate and administer work.
The growth rate in 1971 was 2.3 per cent; it was falling from
its highest point in the early 1960s, which may have been over
3 per cent but still added some 20 million people annually.(18)
By 1972 Dr Carl Djerassi was able to estimate China's pill
production as sufficient for 20 million women a year, and he
understood China to be self-sufficient in other contraceptives.(1
As the pill became more widely available, it often supplanted
the IUD in popularity, especially for child spacing, while the
IUD and sterilisation became used increasingly frequently after
family completion. As is often observed in other countries,
patterns of usage of contraceptives varied widely, not just
between areas but even at different centres within them, and
reflected the choices of the providers at least as much as those
of the consumer.

In addition to medical and pharmaceutical research, a number
of population research institutes were established from 1973
onwards. These were concerned with the study of demography,
population theory, and with the social and economic aspects of
family planning. From the start, they combined pure research
with empirical studies carried out in co-operation with their
provincial Birth Planning Offices and the local family planning
bodies, and they were also involved in providing short courses
for administrators and other cadres.

LATER, LONGER, FEWER

During most of the 1970s the theme which dominated family
planning propaganda was 'later, longer, fewer'. This referred
to delayed marriage, and a larger gap between children, as well
as to having fewer children overall. 'One is good, two is all
right, three are too many' was the parallel slogan which expande
the message of 'fewer' into more definite terms. (Minority
populations, from the founding of the PRC to the present day,
have not been subject to the propaganda for 'fewer'; their

numbers are small - totalling some 6 per cent of the population - and at Liberation were even declining, as the result of endemic diseases.(20) While family planning facilities are available to them, there has been no attempt to persuade them to use these except for health reasons.)

The message was introduced to the people by every possible combination of channels. At the provincial level, there were birth planning Leading Groups, whose members came from local government departments as well as from organisations such as trade unions, the Youth League and the Women's Federation. Some of the members have only part-time involvement, others are full-time paid staff. The Leading Groups' responsibilities are to provide principles and policy guidelines, leaving it to the Birth Planning Office to undertake the main day-to-day work. This includes research, co-ordination of local efforts, organising conferences and running courses for different audiences as well as providing information and publicity.

Below the provincial level, the basic pattern of organisation is repeated at every level of local government. There are leading groups complete with full-time staff as well as with local notables. Counties, and streets within towns, are divided into still smaller units each complete with a birth control cadre to do motivational work; at the lowest level, there will be one motivator for every ten families, whose efforts are backed by mobile teams and by publicity on TV, radio and film, as well as through newspapers, theatre and posters.

From 1981 they will be supplemented by local volunteers working as part of the newly formed China Family Planning Association. The FPA hopes to tap the enthusiasm of all sorts of people from actors to academics, as well as doctors and researchers, who have standing and trust in their own communities.

The extraordinarily comprehensive organisation of family planning activity also includes various specialist bodies. From the provincial to the commune level, there are groups studying contraceptive techniques. There are also specialist family planning departments in hospitals, and technical meetings are held each year to identify contraceptive problems and discuss improvements.(21)

The specific content of the mass media publicity which complements this organisational effort varies from time to time, but a booklet compiled by the People's Health Press in 1976 (which sold over 300,000 copies) provided some indication of the range of materials used.(22) The themes of the songs, playlets and dialogues cover all the main arguments of the family planning propaganda. They may attack the old beliefs that boys are better than girls; or that lavish marriages are necessary; they may praise late marriages and criticise the mothers or mothers-in-law who hurry their children on; they may show that a son-in-law can move in with his wife's family and be their support; or explain the advantages of small families in terms of health, or the opportunities for such things as education.

Some of them talk in terms of the state, rather than the
individual. A choral dialogue, chanting the various advantages
of family planning, goes:

> The significance of family planning is great indeed;
> There is no end to speaking of family planning's advantages.
> When the national economy has a plan
> Then all enterprises also show development;
> If population growth is not planned,
> Then the planned economy will be plunged
>     into chaos. . . .

Another even recruits the children to speak, in a dialogue set
in a kindergarten, in which Xiao Kang, who has a 'host of
older brothers and sisters' as well as a younger sister, complained:

> I am not a good talker,
>     and merely make random remarks.
> Father and mother are busy at their work.
> Our family affairs are in a complete jumble;
> Older brothers and sisters are of no avail.
> They bother mother until she is
>     truly frustrated.
> I, Xiao Kang, am like a little sheep;
> I run around as I please
>     and bump into everything . . .

Her little friend, who has only a much older sister, describes
how, in the evenings, her father explains their family history,
her mother teaches songs to the children, who are 'a pair of
good companions' and they all have time for political study. Xiao
Kang and her friend agree about the benefits of family planning
and decide to propagandise their 'uncles and aunts'.

But family planning is too important for universally serious
treatment, and so there are also comedies, often extremely
funny. In one sly cross-talk act between two men it turns out,
after long discussion, that the wife of one has gone to propagandise the wife of the other, whose husband, the first explains
unknowingly, 'has some ideological problems'. Still trying to
keep his identity dark, the second man denies it: 'No, no. Her
husband's ideological problems have been solved!'

They have begun by discussing a model leader of a women's
brigade. Tell us, says the second man, why she is a model:

> 'For that I must begin talking about the time
> she was married.'
> 'Very interesting. To speak about being considered a model,
> one has to begin talking about the time she was married.'
> 'It was five years ago they were married.'

'How old were they?'
'Over fifty years old.'
'Over fifty years old before she was married?'
'The two together were over fifty years old.'
'Oh.'

## COLLECTIVE BIRTH PLANNING

All these efforts, of organisation and propaganda, are addressed
primarily to the individual couple. Perhaps the most difficult
concept in the Chinese family planning programme for Westerners
to grasp was the parallel development during the 1970s of
collective decision-making on birth plans.(23) Work teams and
brigades had become accustomed to meeting from time to time to
discuss the allocation of collective resources, and it gradually
became apparent that such decisions were bound to be affected
by the numbers involved. Should a new schoolroom be built, or
a new barn? Such planning - based, in other countries, on
demographers' projections of population composition - here relied
on asking the team members their intentions. Where the plans of
individual couples, aggregated together, seemed likely to
threaten the community's overall development plans, or to conflict with the increasingly dominant national policy to reduce
population growth, the team as a whole began to try to inter-
vene.

If the number of births expected was too high, newly married
couples got priority, as did the childless and those whose
existing child was aged three or over. The claims of others
were decided in discussion. Through such discussion and
planning, couples learned that decisions about numbers and
timing of their children did not affect them alone, but had a
significant impact on their community. From information collected
by one American delegation to China it appeared that in 1977
about two out of every three births in China may have conformed
to the later, longer, fewer, norm, though not necessarily to
those more specific plans of the production team.(24)

## POPULATION CONCERNS

The bitter debates of the 1950s about whether concern with
China's population growth rate was 'Malthusian' had unhappy
repercussions on the Chinese approach to population - as
opposed to family planning - questions until the mid 1970s. As
far as possible many officials ignored them. If censuses were
undertaken, the results were never published. In speeches
for internal consumption as well as for outsiders, they continued
to repeat that there were 600 million Chinese and later arbitrarily
raised the total to 800 million.

When China, in 1974, attacked the World Population Plan of

Action drawn up in Bucharest at a United Nations population conference, her action baffled many observers and was misinterpreted by others.(25)

On the one hand, delegates denied that population growth was a serious obstacle to development, and claimed that if other Third World countries built themselves up through self-reliance and independence and tackled the problems of colonialism and exploitation by the rich countries 'the future of mankind is infinitely bright'.

On the other hand they explained that 'China pursues a policy of developing its national economy in a planned way, including the policy of planned population growth. We do not approve of anarchy, either in material production or in human reproduction.' China did not object to population policies, but only to the idea of a world plan of action on the grounds that it was for individual countries to make their own decisions, and that as demographic conditions varied from country to country, no uniformity could or should be imposed.

After the fall of the Gang of Four, however, the Chinese began to pay attention not only to the population total but to its age structure. The 'birth bulge generation' of the 1950s was now marrying; a second 'bulge' from the Cultural Revolution years was growing up, and it became apparent that these presented serious obstacles to the country's smooth development. Formal recognition of this was shown in the new Constitution adopted in March 1978 by the National People's Congress which for the first time stated that 'The State advocates and encourages family planning'. In his speech to the Congress Chairman Hua Guofeng also described family planning as 'a very significant matter' which was 'conducive to the planned development of the national economy and to the health of mother and child'.(26)

The target of a one per cent growth rate by 1980, originally set in 1975, was now given wide publicity. For the first time since the late 1950s the National Planning Bureau gave out a figure for the country's total population: 975,230,000 people at the end of 1978. At the same time a book was published on population theory by the Office of Population Research of the Beijing College of Economics. The Census taken on 1 July 1982 showed a population total of 1031,882,511.(27)

The Chinese explain that, although China's birth rate is low among developing countries, given the huge base figure, there are currently some 12 million added each year to the population. This means that, on the one hand, there are abundant manpower resources but, if 'the role of people as producers' is to be maximised, women, previously unable 'to shake off the unreasonable circumstances surrounding monotonous child-bearing, child rearing and tedious domestic chores', must be mobilised. This implies making it possible for them not only to work, but to gain equality through economic independence, and through participation in politics and the running of the nation.

Smaller families are, besides, healthier and enable parents to

give more energy and time to their children's development.
Because the pressure of expanding numbers would be reduced,
the state would also be able to devote more resources to the
next generation.

Planned growth would also result in the ability to control
according to plan the increase in numbers reaching working age
and help to make possible technical innovation and the achievement of the 'four modernisations'. Finally, a reduction in the
rate of growth would make it possible to save some of the consumption proportion of the national income which would otherwise have to be spent on the extra people. This can be used
instead either to expand production, or to improve the quality
of people's lives - or both.

Once the rationale for a population policy has been decided,
what kind of a policy is needed, and how can it be established?
On the first question, the authors make the remarkable statement that a population policy is the starting-point for drafting
the national economic development plan, as well as being an
important component of it. Thus,

> under our nation's socialist system, child-bearing is not only
> an individual and family matter, but also a major event that
> has a bearing on the scope and rate of increase of the
> population of the whole nation and on socialist revolution and
> on socialist development.

A population plan must be based on co-ordination between State
guidance and 'mass voluntarism'.

## THE ONE-CHILD FAMILY

The unprecedented level of discussion and official comment on
population problems in China, and potential policies for dealing
with them, is exemplified by a major article by Chen Muhua,
head of the Birth Planning Leading Group under the State
Council, in the 'People's Daily' in November 1979. (The office
was upgraded to the Family Planning Commission in March
1981.)(28) This outlines the necessary measures for preventing
most third-parity births by 1985 and for an overall reduction in
family size which would reduce the growth rate to 0.5 per cent
(from 1.2 per cent in 1979) by the same date. These include
strengthening leadership and birth planning work within the
Party; increasing propaganda and education so that it is conducted with a 'great fanfare'; legislation for economic rewards
and penalties 'but with rewards as the main emphasis'; improving medical skills and contraception; and the establishment of
powerful and energetic planned birth staff office units.

Speaking at a conference in Chendu shortly afterwards, she
emphasised that the public concern that family planning would
result in too high a proportion of the old, and too small a work-

force, was misplaced, and pledged that the state would introduce measures to guarantee the health of children and care for the elderly.(29)

Most importantly, she said that the focus of the family planning programme would be towards the one-child family. The aim is that one third of all families should eventually consist of a single child, in order to meet the ultimate goal of reducing population growth to zero by the end of the century (at which time China will have some 1,200 million people).

A law was drafted in early 1979 introducing nationwide economic and welfare measures for those couples who pledged to have only one child. It went to the provinces for discussion, but it appears that provincial birth control packages of incentives and disincentives which had already been introduced had produced so much controversy that the national scheme has been put into cold storage.

Typical of the packages which were introduced at provincial level is that offered in Sichuan. The incentives consist of money – five yuan a month for fourteen years for city of state employees, whose average salary will be around 40-60 yuan a month – or a roughly equivalent amount in work points for rural workers, who also get an extra half or full area of private plot, whose produce the family can sell. The child gets an adult rice ration.

There are, admittedly, other less directly financial benefits for the one-child family. More housing space is allotted it, and the child has priority in health care, in crèche provision and in schooling.

By the end of 1980 it was claimed that 1.5 million families in Sichuan, or 80 per cent of those couples who have only one child, have pledged themselves not to have a second.(30) Overall, it was claimed that by June 1981 10 per cent of all couples had pledged to have no more than one child.(31)

In place of the national incentives scheme, a letter went out in September 1980 from the Central Committee of the Chinese Communist Party to all Party and Communist Youth League members outlining China's recent population growth and how much investment is needed to support the extra people. 'Please think it over. What a positive role the money saved from all this would play if it was used to develop the economy, culture and education!' The letter calls on all Party and Youth League members, especially cadres, to take the lead in responding to the State Council's call with practical action. The rate of population growth is seen, in fact, as a major impediment to the achievement of the Four Modernisations.

The letter followed panel discussions on family planning and population at the Fifth National People's Congress. Although delegates stressed the crucial importance of reducing China's population growth rate, there was criticism of the simplistic solutions attempted in some parts of the country, such as the pressure to accept sterilisation after one child. So long as effective contraception was being used, said a Jiangxi deputy, that was enough. Coercion, the issuing of orders or employing force of punishment to promote family planning were opposed; delegates called for continuing intensive education campaigns and more research into safe, reliable and effective contraception.(32)

It would appear that comments like this, and the lack of enthusiasm for a state incentives scheme, are the outcome of too much state guidance and not enough 'mass voluntarism' during the late 1970s. Cadres at all levels were knowledgeable about the issues and concerned for the implementation of official policy, but evidence of mass involvement in the campaigns declined.

THE METHODS

Methods of contraception available in China today include all those generally available in other countries as well as a few in less widespread use.(33) Sterilisation - male and female - now probably accounts for some 30 per cent of all contraceptive practice in China; the proportions of vasectomies and tubal ligation vary considerably from province to province. Overall, female sterilisation is much the more common procedure, but in Sichuan for example, the ratio is about nine vasectomies for each tubal ligation.

The IUD is widely regarded as a semi-permanent method for those who have completed their families as well as for spacing, and is probably still the most popular contraceptive. Women undergoing IUD insertion, as well as men or women being sterilised, are entitled to paid leave, the extent of which varies from place to place.

Oral contraceptives of various types and containing various low-dose hormonal preparations are also widely used, as are injectables. A monthly oral contraceptive is available and so is a 'visiting husband' pill for occasional use by couples whose work keeps them separated for most of the year. Spermicides are manufactured in small quantities but are not in widespread use; condoms are easily available, but do not account for much of the total of contraceptive use, perhaps in part because of their indifferent quality.

All contraceptives are available free of charge, as is abortion which also entitles the woman to leave with pay. Abortion is not regarded as a method of contraception but the numbers carried out are still high; in Sichuan the ratio to live births was one to two, and in other places has been quoted as one to one.

No national figures for contraceptive use are available and extrapolations based on experience in particular localities can be misleading, but one fairly reliable estimate is that some 80 million of the 115 million married couples in the reproductive ages are currently using a method of family planning.(34)

## CONTRACEPTIVE RESEARCH

Like those involved in contraception elsewhere in the world the
Chinese are very aware of the limitations of all existing contraceptive methods and are anxious to improve them as well as to
discover new ones. Research is being carried out in a number of
institutions around the country, some of it undertaken in
collaboration with the World Health Organisation. Copper IUDs
are being developed; a natural plant abortifacient administered
by intra-muscular injection is being tested, and chemical non-
surgical methods of sterilisation are undergoing clinical trials.
A male contraceptive agent based on cottonseed oil (Gossypol)
has shown initially promising results but it will be some years
before it is sufficiently well tested for general use.(35) The
major problem identified so far is its effect on liver function.
  Research priorities are identified by the State Planning
Commission and the Birth Planning Leading Group but permission for clinical study is granted at the provincial level
following discussions among all those concerned.
  It appears that co-ordination between different research
centres is task-orientated rather than by field.(36) Tests on
potential agents are carried out on animals and once an active
agent is found further studies are carried out to determine its
mode of action and dosage. Toxicity studies are carried out on
rats, mice, dogs and monkeys; there are no standardised
procedures for which tests should be done, or how.
  Once developed, and when animal toxicity and dosage studies
are complete, the Provincial Bureau of Public Health is notified.
It calls a meeting of the hospital, drug plant and other personnel to decide if clinical trials are warranted and if so what
type.
  That campaign is too recent for any full assessment to be
made. But one small survey(37) carried out in Anhui province,
indicates some of the problems. The survey's respondents wanted
a national law on the one-child family rather than the current
local packages. It was, for example, beyond the power of some
units to satisfy the housing needs of all single-child families,
despite the incentives promised. But if there were a national
law, it is unlikely the state would find it any easier to meet
the demand.

  Despite the emphasis in official policy on financial incentives,
  the survey noted that it was the more comfortably off families
  who were most firm in their decision to stick to one child,
  while the poorest showed a reluctance to apply for a certificate
  or, having applied, wavered in their decision.
    It can be argued that the incentives are simply not high
  enough to compensate the poorer families for the loss of
  future benefits children bring. But there is considerable
  evidence from Eastern Europe, where governments have long
  practiced incentive schemes to increase their birth rates, that

each new 'package' has only a limited life. After four years or so, the impact has vanished.

Other aspects of government policy actually work in direct contradiction to the one-child family aim. The relaxations on private produce, for example, mean that the more family members there are to work the private plots, the more income the family will get. Yet the authorities are convinced such relaxations have been the key to increased food production.(38)

Despite the official emphasis on non-coercive measures, there have been reports of forced abortion and sterilisation, as well as of infanticide by couples desperate for a son. Such abuses, as the government is well aware, could lead to a massive backlash.

The State Council is walking a tightrope between what it sees as the threat of numbers undermining their country's overall achievements and the traditionalsim of the Chinese family. Propaganda on the one-child family has begun to stress the sacrifices involved and to explain their sheer necessity for China's future, rather than on the purely economic aspects of an incentive disincentive package. Social surveys, such as the one in Anhui, are not merely carried out but the findings published complete with detailed recommendations for improv- the campaign.

If Anhui is typical, family planning workers and many of those who have signed the one-year pledge want a consistent national policy expressed as a law. But the poorer families appear indifferent to the incentives and tenacious in their desire for a family and above all for a son. If a family law is to stand a chance, it would have to offer something different, perhaps by its recognition of the personal sacrifices that pledge-takers are making, and the possibilities of its abuse would have to be very firmly stamped upon.

The Chinese themselves recognise the difficulty of persuading peasants who have no pensions to risk their old age on one child; they recognise the problems for two single children marrying and having to try to look after two sets of parents; and they recognise the possible social consequence of producing a nation with such a high proportion of only children. But they are determined to try to make the policy work. What they have not yet recognised, in their preoccupation with demography, is that the very attempt to institute such a policy is inherently dangerous. If the people reject it, many of the previous gains could be jeopardised: if 'family planning' comes to mean an unacceptable 'one-child family' then family planning itself will be discredited.

## NOTES

1   Norman Hines, 'Medical History of Contraception', Baltimore, Williams and Wilkins, 1936.
2   H. Yuan-tien, Sterilization, oral contraception and population control in China, 'Population Studies', vol. 27, 3, 1965.
3   Bernard Hung-kay Luk, Abortion in Chinese law, 'American Journal of Comparative Law', vol. 25, 2, 1977.
4   Han Suyin, 'Birdless Summer', part 1, London, Jonathan Cape, 1968.
5   Peter Kane, The Welch Regiment, 1954, personal communication.
6   Ta Chen, Depopulation and culture, The Phi Tau Phi Lecture Series no. 11, Lingnan University, Canton, 1934.
7   Leo Silberman, Hung Liang-chi: a Chinese Malthus, 'Population Sudies', vol. 13, 2, 1960.
8   Luk, op. cit.
9   H. Yuan-tien, Birth control in mainland China: ideology and politics, 'Milbank Memorial Fund Quarterly', vol. 41, 3, 1963.
10  Ruth Weiss, Ma Yinchu and his New Population Theory, 'China Pictorial', no. 12, 1979.
11  See, for example, Wang Ya-nan, quoted in H. Yuan Tien, Birth control in mainland China.
12  Pi Chao-chen, China's birth control action programme 1956-64, 'Population Studies', vol. 24, 2, 1970.
13  Han Suyin, Family planning in China, 'Japan Quarterly', vol. 17, 4, 1970.
14  Delia Davin, 'Women, Work and the Party in Revolutionary China', Oxford University Press, 1976.
15  Margaret Wolfson, Serve the people, internal report, OECD, 1975.
16  Penny Kane, Population planning in China: the individual and the state, in T.S. Epstein and D. Jackson (eds), 'The Feasibility of Fertility Planning', Oxford, Pergamon Press, 1977.
17  Pi Chao-chen, 'Population and Health Policy in the People's Republic of China', Washington, Smithsonian Institute Occasional Monograph no. 9, 1976.
18  'People's Daily', Beijing, 30 July 1973.
19  Carl Djerassi, Fertility limitation through contraceptive steroids in the People's Republic of China, 'Studies in Family Planning', vol. 5, 1, 1974.
20  Joshua Horn, 'Away with All Pests', London, Hamlyn, 1969.
21  Penny Kane, 'World Medicine', London, New Medical Journals Ltd, March 1981, pp. 41-2.
22  Leo A. Orleans (ed.), 'Chinese Approaches to Family Planning', New York, MacMillan, 1979.
23  Graham Leonard, 'A report for IPPF on education for birth planning in China', internal report IPPF, International

Planned Parenthood Federation, 1975.
24  Pi Chao-chen, The Chinese experience, 'People', vol. 6, 2, 1979.
25  Statement of the Chinese delegation to the World Population Conference at Bucharest, August 1974.
26  Hua Guofeng, Unite and strive to build a modern powerful socialist country, 'Beijing Review', 10 March 1978.
27  H. Yuan-tien (ed.), 'Population Theory in China', London, Croom Helm, 1980.
28  Chen Muhua, Controlling population growth the planned way, 'Peking Review', 16 November 1979.
29  'Xinhua New Agency', 22 December 1979.
30  Penny Kane, China's great fanfare on birth control, 'People', vol. 7, 2, 1980, and personal communication from the Sichuan Office of Birth Planning.
31  'NCNA', 26 October 1981.
32  Ibid., 25 September 1980.
33  Contraceptive use in China, 'PLACT Product News' vol. 2, 1, 1980, and Penny Kane, personal communications.
34  Ibid.
35  Gossypol - a new antifertility agent for men, 'CMJ' 4, 6, 1978, and Penny Kane, personal communications.
36  Oral contraceptives and steroid chemistry in the People's Republic of China, Committee on scholarly communication with the PRC, Report no. 5, Washington DC, National Academy of Sciences, 1977.
37  A survey on single-child families, Anhui population, Population Research Office, Anhui University, 1981, discussed in Penny Kane, The one-child family, 'Times Health Supplement', 27 November 1981.
38  John Erik, China's policy on births, 'New York Times', 1 February 1982.

# APPENDIX

Table of Chinese dynasties

| | | |
|---|---:|---:|
| Shang | - 16th cent. - | 1066 |
| Zhou | -1066 - | 221 |
|    Warring States | -403 - | 221 |
| Qin | -221 - | 206 |
| Western (Former) Han | -206 - | +23 |
| Eastern (Later) Han | +25 - | +220 |
| Three Kingdoms | 220 - | 280 |
| Jin | 265 - | 420 |
| North and South Kingdoms | 420 - | 581 |
|    Liang | 502 - | 557 |
| Sui | 581 - | 618 |
| Tang | 618 - | 907 |
| Five Dynasties | 907 - | 960 |
| Song | 960 - | 1279 |
|    Southern Song | 1127 - | 1279 |
| Jin (Tartar) | 1115 - | 1234 |
| Yuan (Mongol) | 1279 - | 1368 |
| Ming | 1368 - | 1644 |
| Qing (Manchu) | 1644 - | 1911 |

# INDEX

# INDEX OF MATERIA MEDICA –
# COMMON AND SCIENTIFIC NAMES

# INDEX OF ACUPUNCTURE POINTS

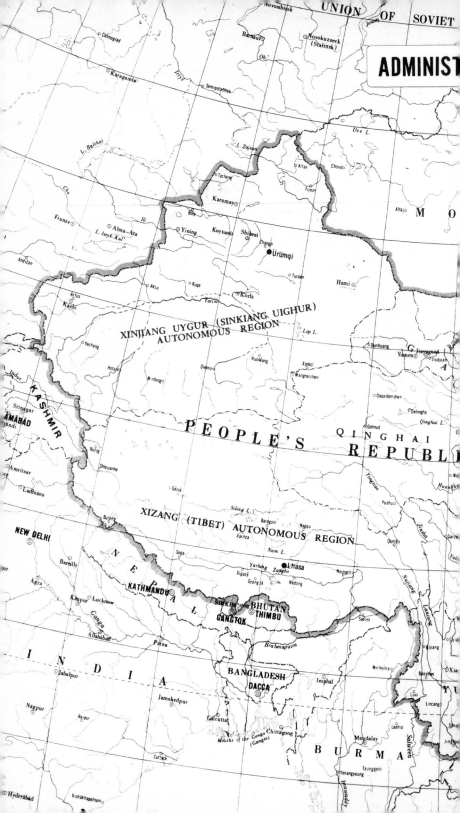